Spinal Epidural Balloon
Decompression and Adhesiolysis

Jin Woo Shin

Spinal Epidural Balloon Decompression and Adhesiolysis

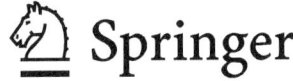

Jin Woo Shin
Department of Anesthesiology and Pain Medicine
ASAN Medical Center
Seoul
Korea (Republic of)

ISBN 978-981-15-7264-7   ISBN 978-981-15-7265-4 (eBook)
https://doi.org/10.1007/978-981-15-7265-4

© Springer Nature Singapore Pte Ltd. 2021

This work is subject to copyright. All rights are reserved by the Publisher, whether the whole or part of the material is concerned, specifically the rights of translation, reprinting, reuse of illustrations, recitation, broadcasting, reproduction on microfilms or in any other physical way, and transmission or information storage and retrieval, electronic adaptation, computer software, or by similar or dissimilar methodology now known or hereafter developed.

The use of general descriptive names, registered names, trademarks, service marks, etc. in this publication does not imply, even in the absence of a specific statement, that such names are exempt from the relevant protective laws and regulations and therefore free for general use.

The publisher, the authors and the editors are safe to assume that the advice and information in this book are believed to be true and accurate at the date of publication. Neither the publisher nor the authors or the editors give a warranty, expressed or implied, with respect to the material contained herein or for any errors or omissions that may have been made. The publisher remains neutral with regard to jurisdictional claims in published maps and institutional affiliations.

This Springer imprint is published by the registered company Springer Nature Singapore Pte Ltd.
The registered company address is: 152 Beach Road, #21-01/04 Gateway East, Singapore 189721, Singapore

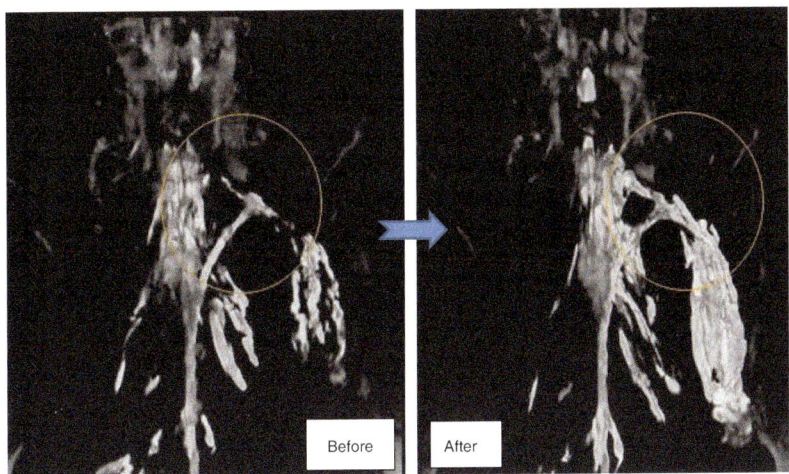

Using spinal epidural balloon decompression and adhesiolysis to overcome the limitations of existing nonsurgical treatment modalities. Mastery of this technique will yield a broader understanding of epidural procedures, including neuroplasty "Beyond the percutaneous epidural adhesiolysis"

Preface

However well imagined or planned at the outset, professional trajectories may sometimes take unexpected or unintended directions. In my case, this applies to 16 years of my life as a professor of anesthesiology and pain medicine at Asan Medical Center. While being the first in the world to develop and establish the medical basis for spinal epidural balloon decompression and adhesiolysis and genicular nerve radiofrequency ablation are achievements that I could not have fathomed when I began my career, I have derived much satisfaction from the fruition of the work and found its progression very rewarding.

As we enter into an aging society, the number of patients suffering from degenerative spinal disease will increase. However, many feel frustrated with current therapeutic modalities, including surgery, as they often fail to yield satisfactory outcomes. These unaddressed needs have fed my continued interest in novel procedural techniques, and I have often found myself explaining such frustration to those around me. Then, 1 day, my wife casually mentioned an idea about balloons: this became the advent of my conception of the balloon procedure.

Looking back, it is clear that many revolutionary inventions in one field were informed by ideas from a completely different field. I believe balloon decompression to be a similar case. The fact of the matter is that it would have been difficult for spine specialists like me to come up with an idea about a balloon. This limited imagination is rooted in an inflexibility of thought and an excessively narrow preoccupation with existing methods that make it difficult for us to conceive of the use of a balloon to attenuate hard stenosis. While I thought that the balloon was a refreshingly novel idea when I had first heard of it, I did not believe that it would be effective. However, data from initial research showed that this method achieved a startling degree of pain mitigation: an initial success that ushered the commencement of full-fledged research and development efforts. The discussion of a specialty distinct from our own tends to meet with disinterest, but the sharing of information and engagement in discussions with people from other fields can often help fuel innovation. Creating as much opportunity as possible for interdisciplinary communication and interaction has time and again demonstrated the potential for engendering progress.

When treating patients in hospital settings, people often find many areas that require improvement. However, while most people think about what is needed and how certain problems should be fixed, they do not put forth the effort required to actually fix the identified issues. While working as a professor, I often thought that while medicine in Korea has reached a world-class level of excellence, we should not be satisfied with just being able to proficiently use existing techniques or equipment; instead, we should improve such techniques or instruments and introduce novel therapeutic modalities to the world. I believe such thoughts and interests have led to the development of this procedural technique. My colleagues and students who saw the development process often told me that, when treating patients, they now think about how existing methods can change or whether they can be replaced. They have undergone a similar, desirable transformation: no longer satisfied with just learning existing medicine, they have begun the pursuit of better methods.

I did not perform many neuroplasty or adhesiolysis procedures since I did not believe that such procedures offered sufficient improvement. Rather, as I studied the balloon decompression technique, I realized why the neuroplasty or adhesiolysis operations that I had performed did not yield satisfactory results. These reasons include the appropriate selection of patients for specific procedures and the inadequate performance of procedures. In other words, I mistakenly believed myself to be an expert and blamed the technique or equipment whenever the outcome was unsatisfactory. I had lived under the false impression that I knew the subject well and did not even research the topic thoroughly.

As I became increasingly engaged in my research into balloon decompression procedure, I continued to gather and compare data on how and where to perform the procedure to increase the likelihood of improvement; all significant facts engendered by my research on balloon decompression have been included in this book. Because such information is related to neuroplasty and adhesiolysis, reading this book will help develop a better understanding of those procedures as well.

I have often felt that focusing on study or research of one specific field facilitates the understanding of other fields. I hope that readers of this book will have the same experience.

I had never thought about writing a single-volume book because I did not have anything specific to write about. Even if I was to write a book, it would simply comprise a compilation of references to foreign books or articles, which would have been too difficult a task relative to its value. However, I decided to write and publish this based on the fact that there was a need to organize the material into the form of a book since it was difficult to accurately relay all of the key concepts during lectures on balloon decompression alone. Moreover, the amount of material left precluded the retention of how exactly to apply the technique on actual patients.

This volume is the product of my attempt to include everything I know about this field. I sincerely hope that this book will be of great help to its readers.

Seoul, South Korea Jin-Woo Shin
March 1, 2020

Letter of Recommendation

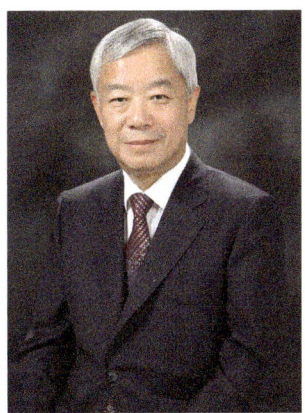

I believe it has been over 20 years since I have known Professor Jin-Woo Shin. I saw him often and became acquainted with him during his residency at Asan Medical Center, where he showed much interest in pain medicine and actively participated in society events. Since he became a professor at Asan Medical Center, we have become closer personally as well.

Professor Jin-Woo Shin is passionate about pain medicine and has demonstrated excellent performance in research, which has culminated in the publication of his work in renowned international journals and has made possible the systematization of genicular nerve radiofrequency ablation as well as the development of epidural balloon decompression, a novel therapeutic modality.

I have recently retired from the Department of Anesthesiology and Pain Medicine at Seoul National University. During my long tenure as a professor at Seoul National University, I had invested much effort into the advancement of the Korean Pain Society. I now find it personally fulfilling to see that the quality of the Korean Pain Society has been raised to a level of international recognition.

Recently, an increasing number of physicians in Korea have developed various procedural techniques and equipment that have become introduced on a global stage. Beginning in an era when we used to learn techniques from overseas, we have advanced to the point of developing excellent techniques that are being taught overseas.

Developed by Professor Jin-Woo Shin, genicular nerve radiofrequency ablation and epidural balloon decompression are outstanding techniques among those referred to above, and their academic bases have been well proven. The equipment used in epidural balloon decompression must receive certification from overseas markets, preventing overseas physicians from using the procedure at this point. However, once the necessary certification has been obtained, it will surely become a universal procedure worldwide. It is my understanding that genicular nerve radiofrequency ablation is already being received with much interest overseas since it can be performed easily with existing equipment.

This book is a compilation of two procedural methods developed by Professor Jin-Woo Shin. He has included details that will allow physicians with little experience in this type of procedure to easily and safely perform the procedure, which in and of itself demonstrates the methodical organization of his research findings to date; this book will thus prove of undoubted help to anyone interested in this procedure.

I hope that Professor Jin-Woo Shin will continue to upgrade this procedural method and develop other novel techniques.

My sincerest congratulations to Professor Jin-Woo Shin for the publication of his book, *Spinal Epidural Balloon Decompression and Adhesiolysis*.

Sang-Chul Lee
Korean Society of Integrative Medicine
Seoul, South Korea

Korean Pain Society
Seoul, South Korea

Korean Pain Research Society
Seoul, South Korea

Letter of Recommendation

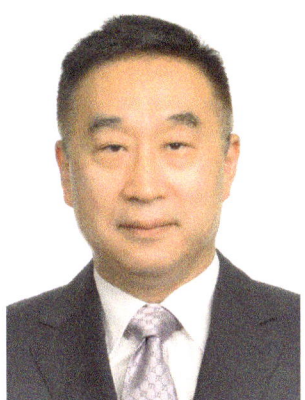

Through spinal epidural balloon decompression and adhesiolysis, the main topic of this book, we are looking at a previously unimagined horizon for percutaneous epidural adhesiolysis. Our attention is naturally drawn to spinal epidural balloon decompression and adhesiolysis since it can resolve the thirst that could not be quenched with existing percutaneous epidural adhesiolysis. From this perspective, my personal view is that the subtitle of this book—"beyond the percutaneous epidural adhesiolysis"—is not an overstatement by any means.

Spinal epidural balloon decompression and adhesiolysis can be divided into two aspects: (1) clinical trial results and (2) equipment for the procedure.

With respect to clinical trial results, I would like to express my respect to the author for having brought his extensive experience and reflections to bear and recognize the immeasurable value of this book that provides a vehicle for these experiences and reflections. This book contains the lengthy experience of the author and thus provides clinically useful information, including the appropriate selection of patients for the application of spinal epidural balloon decompression and adhesiolysis; specific details about approaches for reaching the target points; functional improvement following the procedure; and positive predictive factors. They say that the typical life cycle for the systematic review of an article is 5 years. Considering that the author is already approaching 10 years of performing spinal epidural balloon decompression and adhesiolysis, we can encounter the second renewal of the author's experience and reflections through this book.

With respect to the equipment, we must give high marks to the author for standardizing devices for the procedure. The clinical applicability of percutaneous epidural adhesiolysis, which is recommended above others to address refractory low back pain and radiating leg pain, is broadening under the generic name of epidural neuroplasty. Since the introduction of the Racz's needle ('97) and the clinical application of the Fogarty catheter by the Racz's needle ('04) in Korea through academic journals, various types of procedural equipment have been introduced for use during percutaneous epidural adhesiolysis. However, I believe that the materialization and maximization of the clinical efficacy of percutaneous epidural adhesiolysis were realized through the development of equipment for spinal epidural balloon decompression and adhesiolysis.

In pursuing a novelty development process, we can guess at the struggles the author faced when methodizing the spinal epidural balloon decompression and adhesiolysis procedures.

I believe that publishing an original work is an ultimate joy that can be felt only by the author. Once again, I would like to express my blessings and respect to the author as well as to the immeasurable value of this book.

Jae-Chol Shim
College of Medicine Hanyang University
Seoul, South Korea

Korean Pain Society
Seoul, South Korea

Letter of Recommendation

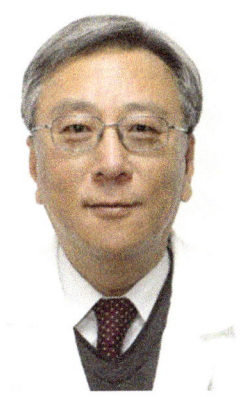

In addressing degenerative spinal diseases commonly encountered in pain clinics, especially spinal stenosis, procedures such as regular nerve block not only show limited therapeutic effect, but the improvement effect lasts only a short time, and the disease may recur in many cases. In addition, even surgical intervention often yields unsatisfactory outcomes. Accordingly, various catheters, including the Navi and Racz catheters, have been developed and used as nonsurgical therapeutic modalities. However, no procedure can improve pain and function by actually expanding the stenosed space.

As a result of using the ZiNeu catheter with its added ballooning function, areas with adhesion can be removed within a short period of time by mechanically expanding the space—although not to the extent of surgery. Using this method not only produces the excellent mitigation of pain and improvement of motor functions, such as walking, but a sustained effect of a relatively longer duration and lower recurrence rate. This method thereby offers a revolutionary therapeutic advance in addressing chronic degenerative spinal diseases.

Professor Jin-Woo Shin, the developer of the ZiNeu catheter and author of this book, is a person who possesses an enthusiastic personality, infinite love for pain medicine, and inexhaustive curiosity. I had the opportunity to work together with him and noticed his unrelenting personality, which made him incapable of overlooking even the smallest detail, so much so that he almost risked becoming a nuisance to his colleagues. Although there have been others who took an interest in the Fogarty catheter and attempted to use it, I believe it is Professor Shin's personality that played a major role in applying such an idea to an actual product.

This book represents the meticulously organized thoughts, efforts, and procedural experiences of Professor Shin to date, as well as the knowledge he accrued through extensive research. I am confident that this book will be very helpful in promoting the understanding of not only balloon decompression but also neuroplasty and adhesiolysis, as well as help to inform the actual execution of these procedures.

I believe that the level of pain medicine in Korea has already reached a world-class level. If we always think about the possibility of generating more effective treatment modalities and strive to improve areas that are lacking, such efforts will lead to the further development of outstanding novel techniques and equipment.

Lastly, I extend my endless praise to Professor Jin-Woo Shin for his efforts and passion, and I eagerly anticipate the day when the ZiNeu catheter will be used throughout the world.

Chung Lee
Pain Clinic at Korea Cancer Center Hospital
Seoul, South Korea

Asan Medical Center
Seoul, South Korea

Letter of Recommendation

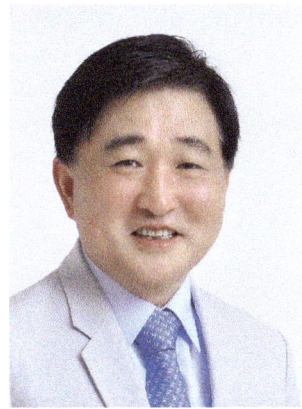

My sincerest congratulations to Professor Jin-Woo Shin for the publication of his book, *Spinal Epidural Balloon Decompression and Adhesiolysis*.

I have known Professor Jin-Woo Shin for a while now. In 2001, during Professor Shin's Ph.D. program at the University of Ulsan, I was able to get an up-close look at Professor Shin's academic accomplishments and competency as a journal reviewer.

I watched with keen interest every time Professor Jin-Woo Shin made a presentation at various conferences and always admired how dedicated he was to his research work, despite being one of the busiest people around due to his teaching and clinical practice; this clearly yielded many creative, original products of useful application to clinical practice. Indeed, it is no surprise at all that he developed and systemized spinal epidural balloon decompression and adhesiolysis and genicular nerve radiofrequency ablation procedures as a result of such industry.

As a university professor who gives his best effort into research and teaching, it is not easy to develop something new. Especially in the field of medicine that deals with people, both safety and efficacy must be considered. Consequently, it is very difficult to develop new equipment or procedures with a recognized academic basis that can be applied to actual clinical practice. However, Professor Shin developed a novel procedure despite his busy schedule and received recognition for its clinical and academic basis through continued research, which ultimately culminated in the publication of *Spinal Epidural Balloon Decompression and Adhesiolysis*: a compilation of his experience and research to date. Once again, I extend my sincerest congratulations to Professor Jin-Woo Shin for his hard work and achievements.

When treating patients, different outcomes may be observed depending on the determination and ability of the operator. Therefore, the operator must have an accurate understanding of not only the disease itself but also the procedural methods and equipment involved. This book, *Spinal Epidural Balloon Decompression and Adhesiolysis*, by Professor Jin-Woo Shin contains everything in this field, including the methods by which to accurately identify the site of procedure and methods for selecting the right equipment for the procedure. I therefore highly recommend anyone who is interested in this procedure to read this book.

Genicular nerve radiofrequency ablation is a well-known procedure that has already been introduced overseas and has been cited in numerous articles. I hope that the equipment for spinal epidural balloon decompression and adhesiolysis could pass the overseas certification process without further delay so that this procedure can be employed overseas and gain global recognition as an established procedure.

Yong-Chul Kim
Seoul National University
College of Medicine
Seoul, South Korea

Pain Center at Seoul National
University Hospital
Seoul, South Korea

International Congress of Spinal Pain
Seoul, South Korea

Letter of Recommendation

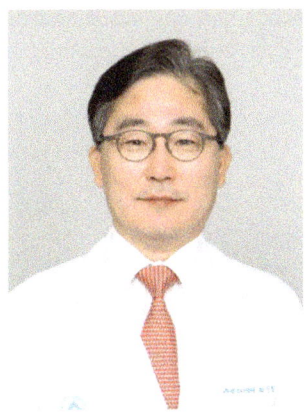

I would like to extend my sincere congratulations to Professor Jin-Woo Shin on the publication of his book, *Spinal Epidural Balloon Decompression and Adhesiolysis*.

Professor Jin-Woo Shin, who has labored tirelessly to publish this book, worked as a fellow and professor in the Department of Anesthesiology and Pain Medicine at Asan Medical Center after having completed his residency there. What I had noticed while working together with Professor Shin was that he exhibited peerless talent and passion. With his pleasant disposition, he has grown into someone who is irreplaceable in our world of medicine. In particular, even as a resident, he was very interested in the field of pain medicine and has continued to make significant sacrifices for the field of pain medicine in Korea while training many students. Because of his strong dedication to his patients, he treats not only their disease but their heart and mind as well. He is one among few clinicians to whom I would not hesitate recommending a patient.

I believe spinal epidural balloon decompression and adhesiolysis is a product of Professor Shin's commitment to his patients. As he deliberated over ways to ease the suffering of patients who are difficult to treat due to spinal stenosis and studied novel therapeutic modalities, he came across an idea by chance in 2010, which he had persistently elaborated until the actual development of the spinal epidural balloon catheter. After 2 years of development, the ZiNeu catheter was completed and was used to conduct a clinical trial, which demonstrated excellent therapeutic results. Since then, related research articles have been published in world-renowned journals, whereby the excellence of the ZiNeu catheter has gained global recognition. Through subsequent lectures at many academic conferences, it has drawn interest from physicians in Korea and throughout the world. We have even requested a training opportunity at our own hospital.

There are many medical books that have been published in Korea, but most of these books are devoted to introducing techniques that were developed overseas or summarize findings of studies conducted overseas. Spinal epidural balloon decompression and adhesiolysis were developed in Korea from an original idea by Professor Jin-Woo Shin, and this book summarizes the unprecedented experiences and know-how accumulated through clinical trials, which clearly differentiates this book from others.

I hope that the clinical acumen of many practitioners will be upgraded by this book and that it will serve as an opportunity to lessen the suffering of many patients.

Once again, I would like to congratulate Professor Jin-Woo Shin on the publication of his book, and I eagerly anticipate more advanced research and writings from Professor Jin-Woo Shin.

In-Chul Choi
Korean Society of Anesthesiologists
Seoul, South Korea

Department of Anesthesiology and
Pain Medicine at Asan Medical Center
Seoul, South Korea

Acknowledgments

There are many people who have contributed to the development of the ZiNeu catheter and balloon decompression procedure as well as the establishment of a protocol for genicular nerve radiofrequency ablation. While I should personally visit each and every person to thank them for their contribution, I first wish to extend my gratitude through these pages.

Since 2011, I had spent countless laborious hours researching and developing the balloon decompression procedure. I often regretted the fact that I could not spend enough time with my family, and for that, I am always grateful to my wife and children who have been steadfast in their support. I want to especially thank my wife for raising our kids so well while staying in the US during difficult times.

I would like to further extend my gratitude to Professors Sang-Chul Lee, Yong-Chul Kim, and Pyung-Bok Lee from Seoul National University; Professor Chung Lee from Korea Cancer Center Hospital; Professor Young-Ki Kim from Gangneung Asan Hospital; Professor Hahck-Soo Park from Ewha Woman's University Medical Center; Dr. Choon Keun Park from Wills Memorial Hospital; and Dr. Do-Hyung Kim from Thomas Hospital. Thank you for all your advice on performing the balloon decompression procedure.

I would also like to thank Professor Jae-Chol Shim from Hanyang University who taught me about retrograde interlaminar ventral approach when I was struggling with patients in entering the intervertebral foramen by the transforaminal approach that had proven difficult.

Clinical trials are very important for establishing the medical basis of balloon decompression. I am thankful for Professor Seong-Soo Choi from Asan Medical Center who supervised most of the clinical trials and continues to conduct research and education on balloon procedures.

To Dr. Jae-Do Lee from Central Veterans Hospital; Professor Jae-Hang Shim from Hanyang University; Professor Doo-Hwan Kim and Jun-Young Park and all other pain medicine fellows from Asan Medical Center, thank you for your efforts in the clinical trial on balloon decompression procedure. I would also like to express my gratitude for Professor Seong-Hun Kim from Asan Medical Center who named the ZiNeu catheter and helped to write an excellent paper that included the implementation of the 3D reconstruction view method.

We have recently conducted a multidisciplinary, multicenter study with a study population of 500 patients. This is indispensable to the establishment of the academic basis of the balloon decompression procedure. I would like to thank those who participated in this study, including Professor Dong-Ah Shin from Yonsei Severance Hospital; Dr. Sang-Won Lee from Yonsei Barun Hospital; Dr. Gyu-Yeul Ji from Guro Cham Tn Tn Hospital; Dr. Jin-Kyu Park from Bupyeong Himchan Hospital; Dr. Dong-Won Ha and Dr. Young-Mok Park from the Baro Hospital; and Dr. Sang-Ho Moon from Seoul Sacred Heart Hospital.

The genicular nerve radiofrequency ablation technique was presented for the first time in the Conference of the Korean Pain Society by Dr. Yong-Up Kang from Chung Sol Pain Clinic. Thank you for your graciousness in granting your permission to conduct our study at the Asan Medical Center for the systematization of the procedure, the results of which were published in *Pain*.

Very little was known about the genicular nerve, and there was no assurance that such a nerve even existed. We conducted a cadaveric dissection with Professor Seung-June Hwang from the Department of Anatomy at Asan Medical Center, and the existence of the genicular nerve was thereby confirmed. The cadaveric dissection results on the genicular nerve have helped to augment the reliability of the paper, which ultimately allowed for its publication in a renowned journal such as *Pain*. Once again, I thank Professor Seung-June Hwang.

I would like to express my gratitude to Professor Woo-Jong Choi from Asan Medical Center who actually published the paper on genicular nerve radiofrequency ablation in *Pain*.

I also wish to thank Professor Yul Oh, a full-time lecturer in pain medicine from Asan Medical Center, who helped with editing and revising this book.

I thank the generosity of many people: balloon decompression and genicular nerve radiofrequency ablation procedures were systematized and fully established because of you.

Lastly, I would like to express my gratitude to my son, Hojin Shin, and my daughter, Hyowon Shin, for translating many parts of this book in Korean to publish in English.

Once again, my sincerest gratitude to everyone for their support and interest.

March 1, 2020

Jin-Woo Shin

Introduction

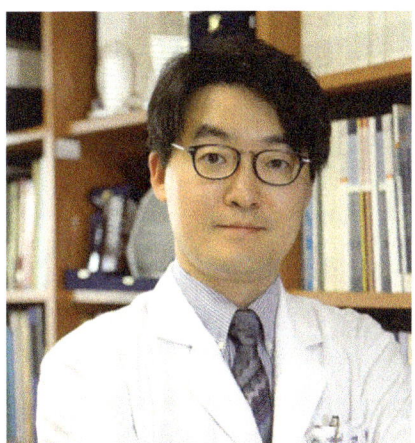

History

1. Bachelor's from Chung Ang University School of Medicine
2. Intern, Chung Ang University School of Medicine
3. Master's, Department of Anesthesiology and Pain Medicine, University of Ulsan College of Medicine
4. Doctoral, Department of Anesthesiology and Pain Medicine, University of Ulsan College of Medicine
5. Completion of residency and fellowship, Department of Anesthesiology and Pain Medicine, Asan Medical Center
6. Assistant and associate professor, Department of Anesthesiology and Pain Medicine, Asan Medical Center
7. Visiting Scholar at Harvard Medical School Brigham and Women's Hospital and Children's Hospital Pain Center
8. Current professor of Anesthesiology and Pain Medicine, Asan Medical Center
9. Current regular member of the Korean Society of Anesthesiologists
10. Current regular member of the Korean Pain Society
11. Current editor and journal reviewer, the Korean Pain Society
12. Current director of Academic Affairs, the Korean Spinal Pain Society

Accomplishments

1. First in the world to develop a spinal epidural balloon apparatus (ZiNeu catheter) and the procedure for its use
2. Received the New Medical Technology Certification from the National Evidence-based Healthcare Collaborating Agency for the spinal epidural balloon procedure
3. First in the world to systematize a genicular nerve radiofrequency ablation technique for the treatment of chronic knee pain
4. Publication in SCI or SCIE level journals—24 articles, Domestic journals—48 articles

Academic Awards

20.11.2010—Award from the Korean Pain Society. Effect of perioperative perineural injection of dexamethasone and bupivacaine on a rat spared nerve injury model. Korean J Pain. 2010;23(3):166–171.
5.11.2011—Award from the Korean Society of Anesthesiologists. Radiofrequency treatment relieves chronic knee osteoarthritis pain: a double-blinded randomized controlled trial. Pain. 2011;152(3):481–7.
19.11.2011—Award from the Korean Pain Society. Value of bone scintigraphy and single photon emission computed tomography in lumbar facet disease and prediction of short term outcome of ultrasound guided medial branch with bone SPECT. Korean J Pain. 2011;24:81–6.

Sample Articles

1. Choi WJ, Hwang SJ, Song JG, Leem JG, Kang YU, Park PH, Shin JW. Radiofrequency treatment relieves chronic knee osteoarthritis pain: a double-blind randomized controlled trial. Pain. 2011;152(3):481–7.
2. Kim SH, Choi WJ, Suh JH, Hwang CJ, Koh WU, Lee C, Leem JG, Lee SC, Shin JW. Effects of transforaminal balloon treatment in patients with lumbar foraminal stenosis: a randomized, controlled, double-blind trial. Pain Physician. 2013;16:213–24.
3. Koh WU, Choi SS, Park SY, Joo EY, Kim SH, Lee JD, Shin JY, Suh JH, Leem JG, Shin JW. Transforaminal hypertonic saline for the treatment of lumbar lateral canal stenosis: a double-blinded, randomized, active-control trial. Pain Physician. 2013;16:197–211.
4. Kim DH, Cho SS, Moon YJ, Kwon K, Lee K, Leem JG, Shin JW, Park JH, Choi SS. Factors Associated with successful responses to transforaminal balloon adhesiolysis for chronic lumbar foraminal stenosis: retrospective study. Pain Physician. 2017;20(6):E841–E848.
5. Kim DH, Choi SS, Yoon SH, Lee SH, Seo DK, Lee IG, Choi WJ, Shin JW. Ultrasound-guided genicular nerve block for knee osteoarthritis: a double-blind, randomized controlled trial of local anesthetic alone or in combination with corticosteroid. Pain Physician. 2018;21(1):41–52.

Jin-Woo Shin

Translators

Hojin Shin and Hyowon Shin

Introduction

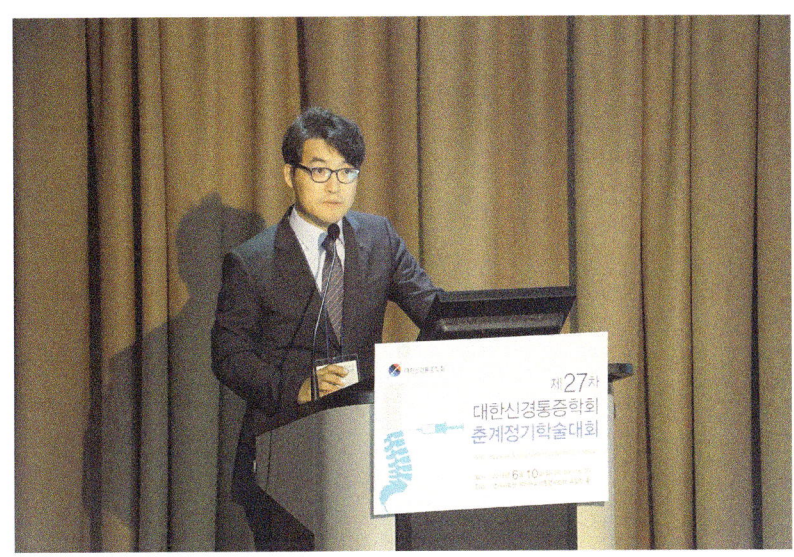

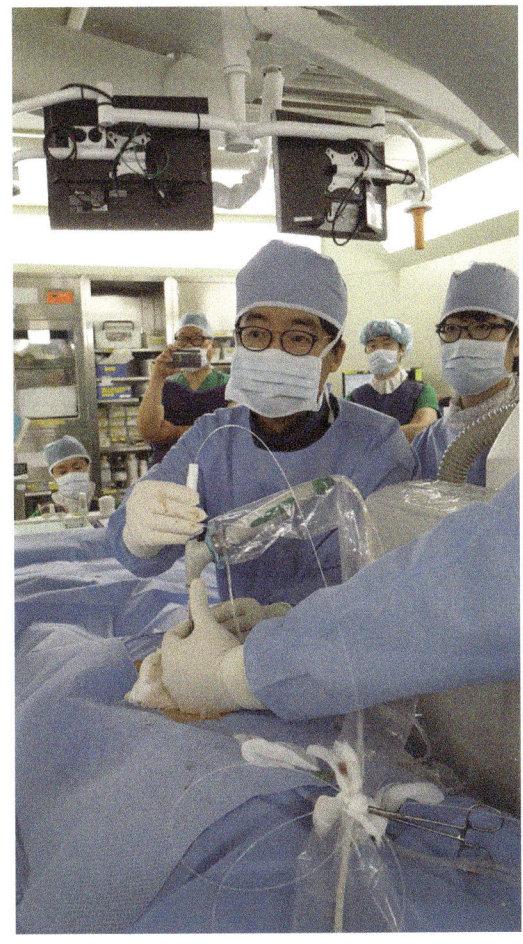

Contents

1 Introduction to Epidural Balloon Decompression 1
   1.1 Conventional Treatment Modalities for Patients
with Epidural Adhesion or Spinal Stenosis 1
   1.2 Academic Basis for Neuroplasty and Adhesiolysis 2
   1.3 Differences Between Neuroplasty and Adhesiolysis 4
   1.4 Theoretical and Academic Basis for Balloon
Decompression. 6
       1.4.1 Improved Blood Circulation by Expanding
the Free Space in the Area Affected by Stenosis 6
       1.4.2 Improved Adhesiolysis. 11
       1.4.3 Retrodiscal Decompression Theory 13
       1.4.4 Basis for Long-Term Improvements
Effected by Balloon Decompression 14
       1.4.5 Integration of Existing Procedural Techniques 20
       1.4.6 Other Relevant Articles 24
       1.4.7 Published Case Reports 29
   1.5 Lecture Video of Epidural Balloon Decompression
and Adhesiolsyis 30
   Bibliography 31

2 Types of ZiNeu Catheters and Their Features 33
   2.1 ZiNeu Series. 33
       2.1.1 ZiNeu01 33
       2.1.2 ZiNeuS 33
       2.1.3 ZiNeu02 34
   2.2 ZiNeuF Series 34
       2.2.1 ZiNeuF 34
       2.2.2 ZiNeuF03 35
   2.3 Differences Between Elastic and Inelastic Balloons 35
       2.3.1 Differences Between the Role of Elastic
and Inelastic Balloons According to the Degree
of Foraminal Stenosis or Adhesion 35
       2.3.2 Differences Between the Role of Elastic
and Inelastic Balloons in Cases Involving
Central Stenosis or Adhesion. 36

3	**Pre-Procedural Preparation and Precautions**		43
	3.1 Before the Procedure		43
	3.2 Drugs Used		43
		3.2.1 Dexamethasone	43
		3.2.2 Lidocaine and Contrast Dye	44
		3.2.3 Hyaluronidase	45
		3.2.4 Normal Saline	45
		3.2.5 Hypertonic Saline	46
	3.3 Procedure-Related Precautions		48
		3.3.1 Method for Preventing Balloon Rupture	48
		3.3.2 Method for Preventing Catheter Damage During the Procedure	50
		3.3.3 Method for Preventing Injection into the Intrathecal Space	50
		3.3.4 Method for Reducing Pain During the Procedure	50
	Bibliography		53
4	**Methods for Executing the ZiNeu Series Catheter Procedure**		55
	4.1 Target Diseases		55
		4.1.1 Best Indication	56
	4.2 Pre-Procedure Preparations		56
		4.2.1 Posture and Disinfection	56
		4.2.2 Removal of Air Inside the Catheter and Contrast-Dye Filling	57
		4.2.3 Connecting the Syringe for Balloon Decompression	57
		4.2.4 Balloon Expansion	58
	4.3 Recommended Procedure		59
		4.3.1 Guide Needle Insertion	59
		4.3.2 Epidurogram and Regional Anesthesia	61
		4.3.3 ZiNeu Series Catheter Insertion	66
		4.3.4 Method for Adjusting the Direction of the Catheter	68
		4.3.5 Entry into the Intervertebral Foramen	73
		4.3.6 Entry into the Central Area	85
		4.3.7 Contrast Dye Injection	93
		4.3.8 Irrigation	96
		4.3.9 Injection of Therapeutic Drug and Placement of the Drug-Injection Catheter	96
		4.3.10 Drug Administration After Admission	97
5	**Methods for Executing the ZiNeuF Catheter Procedure**		101
	5.1 Target Diseases		101
		5.1.1 Best Indications	101
	5.2 Pre-Procedure Preparation		102
	5.3 Recommended Procedural Methods		102
		5.3.1 Transforaminal Approach	102
		5.3.2 Interlaminar Approach	126
		5.3.3 Cervical Interlaminar Approach	135

Contents

6 Methods for Executing the ZiNeuF03 Catheter Procedure 141
- 6.1 Target Diseases 141
  - 6.1.1 Best Indications 141
- 6.2 Pre-Procedural Preparation 141
- 6.3 Recommended Procedural Methods 142
  - 6.3.1 Insertion of the Guide Needle 142
  - 6.3.2 Epidurogram and Regional Anesthesia 142
  - 6.3.3 Insertion of the ZiNeuF03 Catheter 143
  - 6.3.4 Balloon Decompression 144
  - 6.3.5 Contrast Dye Injection 147
  - 6.3.6 Irrigation 148
  - 6.3.7 Therapeutic Drug Injection 148
  - 6.3.8 Removal of the Needle or Sheath 148
  - 6.3.9 Drug Administration After Admission 148

7 Dural Puncture 151
- 7.1 Problems That Could Arise from a Dural Puncture 151
  - 7.1.1 Post-Dural Puncture Headache (PDPH) 151
  - 7.1.2 Drug Injection into the Punctured Area 151
- 7.2 Tips Concerning Dural Puncture 152
- 7.3 Findings Indicative of Dural Puncture 152
- 7.4 Characteristic Contrast Image Findings Indicative of Dural Puncture 155
- 7.5 Coping Strategies for Dural Puncture 160
  - 7.5.1 Performing the Procedure by a Different Path After Discovering Dural Puncture 161
  - 7.5.2 The Performance of an Alternative Procedure Following Dural Puncture 164
  - 7.5.3 Coping Strategies for When the Drug Is Administered to the Punctured Site 164
- Bibliography 170

8 Method for Catheter Selection 171
- 8.1 Catheter Selection Recommendations According to Case 171
  - 8.1.1 Selecting Between the ZiNeu01 and ZiNeuS Catheters 171
  - 8.1.2 Selecting the ZiNeu02 Catheter 173
  - 8.1.3 Selecting Between the ZiNeuF and ZiNeuF03 Catheters 175
- 8.2 Catheter Selection Recommendations According to the Procedural Approach 176
  - 8.2.1 Transforaminal Approach 176
  - 8.2.2 Interlaminar Approach 176
  - 8.2.3 Caudal Approach 176
  - 8.2.4 Simultaneous Application of Two Approaches 177

9	Methods for Determining the Site of Procedure According to Case	181
	9.1 Cases Involving Procedures in the Retrodiscal Area at the Level Immediately Above the Intervertebral Foramen	181
	9.2 Cases Involving Procedures in the Intervertebral Foramen	186
	9.3 Cases Involving Procedures in the Retrodiscal Area	188
	9.4 Cases Involving Procedures in Filling Defect Areas	203
	9.5 Cases Involving Procedures in Both the Anterior and Posterior Epidural Spaces	205
	9.6 Procedure for Patients with Bertolotti's Syndrome (Lumbosacral Transitional Vertebrae)	212
	9.7 Procedure for Patients Who Are Not Expected to Benefit from Balloon Decompression	214

10	Post-Procedural Care and Prognosis	219
	10.1 Post-Procedural Care	219
	10.2 Prognosis	220
	10.3 General Questions About the Procedure	225
	10.3.1 If the Balloon Compresses a Nerve, Could It Cause Nerve Damage or Dysfunction?	225
	10.3.2 Can the Intervertebral Foramen Actually be Expanded With a Balloon?	226
	10.3.3 How Long Can the Expansion of the Balloon be Maintained?	226
	10.3.4 What Should the Patients be Told Concerning the Duration of Sustained Effect?	226
	10.3.5 Even Balloon-Less Catheters Allow for Good Contrast Dye Spread After the Procedure. How Are They Different Then from Balloon Catheters?	227
	10.3.6 How Many Times Can This Procedure be Performed in 1 Year on the Same Patient?	227
	Bibliography	231

11	Genicular Nerve Radiofrequency Ablation	233
	11.1 Indications and Contraindications	235
	11.1.1 Indications	235
	11.1.2 Contraindications	235
	11.2 Anatomy	235
	11.3 Techniques	238
	11.3.1 C-Arm-Guided Genicular Nerve RFA	238
	11.3.2 C-Arm-Guided Genicular Nerve Cooled RFA	241
	11.3.3 Diagnostic Genicular Nerve Block	245
	11.3.4 Ultrasound-Guided Genicular Nerve Block	246
	11.4 Comparison of Outcomes According to Procedure	247
	Bibliography	252

List of Videos

Video 1.1 3D-reconstruction view before and after balloon decompression
Video 1.2 Lecture on ZiNeu catheter (English voice)
Video 2.1 ZiNeu01 catheter
Video 2.2 ZiNeu02 catheter
Video 4.1 Adhesiolysis while pulling down from the spinal canal
Video 4.2 ZiNeu series catheter
Video 6.1 ZiNeuF03 catheter

Introduction to Epidural Balloon Decompression

1.1 Conventional Treatment Modalities for Patients with Epidural Adhesion or Spinal Stenosis

The point prevalence of low back pain in the adult population of the US is 37%, and its lifetime prevalence escalates to 60–85%. An approximate 12 to 90.6 billion dollars are spent on pain and disability related to low back pain each year in the US. Following angina, hypertension, and diabetes, low back pain thus accounts for the fourth-highest medical expenditure among American workers.

Treatment of degenerative spinal disease formerly entailed aggressive spinal surgery when the patient was nonresponsive to medication or physical therapy. However, spinal surgery is associated with much higher rates of recurrence and postoperative pain than are other types of surgery, reflecting the difficulty of resolving such cases. Nonsurgical interventional procedures have thus become increasingly popular and have reportedly helped to reduce the number of spinal surgery cases.

Among the various interventional procedures used to treat degenerative spinal diseases, the most typical include epidural block (transforaminal, caudal, and interlaminar), medial branch block, facet joint injection, sacroiliac joint block, nucleoplasty, neuroplasty, and radiofrequency ablation. The selection of the treatment modality is informed by the etiology of the low back and leg pain: the most common include disc herniation and spinal stenosis, which primarily induce neurogenic pain or nerve compression and subsequent perineural inflammation; increased neuronal excitability; and impaired blood and nutrient supply. Accordingly, epidural block performed with an injection of a local anesthetic/steroid mixture is the most common procedure used to reduce pain, resolve inflammation, and edema, and improve blood circulation.

An epidural block involves the injection of drugs directly into the lesion within the epidural space. Relative to oral or intravenous pharmacotherapeutic administration, an epidural block offers the advantage of achieving a maximal effect with a minimal amount of the injected drug. This procedure is therefore highly recommended for patients who show little improvement after the completion of first-line conservative treatment, such as oral drug administration or physical therapy. Although patients with obvious perineural or neurogenic inflammation can evince excellent improvements, they tend to last for only a short period among patients with spinal stenosis and limited evidence of inflammation. Despite differences between patients with spinal stenosis, as well as those with disc herniation, there is a general tendency for the therapeutic effects to

Electronic Supplementary Material The online version of this chapter (https://doi.org/10.1007/978-981-15-7265-4_1) contains supplementary material, which is available to authorized users. The videos can be accessed by scanning the related images with the SN More Media App.

© Springer Nature Singapore Pte Ltd. 2021
J. W. Shin, *Spinal Epidural Balloon Decompression and Adhesiolysis*,
https://doi.org/10.1007/978-981-15-7265-4_1

last for increasingly shorter periods with more repetitions of the procedure. Proposed explanations for this tendency lack evidence in the literature, and it thus remains an object of controversy. However, possible causes are summarized below:

First, it is according to the nature of degenerative diseases that they worsen over time.

Second, fibrosis or adhesion associated with chronic degenerative spinal diseases deteriorate over time and thus progressively diminish the effectiveness of the epidural procedure by interfering with drug dispersion.

Third, repeated performance of the epidural block or steroid administration may actually promote adhesion in the epidural space.

These causes may lead to a tendency for the effectiveness of the procedures to be reduced as they are repeated. In particular, repeated use of particulated steroids, such as triamcinolone, into the epidural space may be slightly more effective than using non-particulated steroids, but particulated steroids may further promote epidural adhesion.

The aforementioned causes are equally applicable to all epidural procedures, not just epidural block; hence, the prevention of recurrence and removal of adhesion are significant to the prognosis of the patient regardless of the treatment selected. All interventions should therefore be performed according to a stepwise approach based on accurate criteria that include a consideration of the detriment of repeating procedures: if the patient shows sufficient response to medication, exercise therapy, and/or physical therapy and can exercise without discomfort, more aggressive interventional procedures should not be performed. However, if the patient shows little improvement from such conservative treatment, decline in their quality of life, and difficulty in walking, the exact cause should be reconfirmed, and an appropriate, simple therapeutic strategy should be attempted before more intensive alternatives are considered. With respect to the author, the same procedure is repeated if the improvement effected by a simple interventional procedure, such as epidural block, is sustained for 3 months or longer. On the other hand, more involved, complex procedures should only be considered when the simple alternative is ineffectual or does not achieve an effect for longer than 3 months.

Neuroplasty or adhesiolysis have traditionally been performed when degenerative spinal disease is not resolved by epidural block. With these procedures, if the effect is sustained for 2–3 months or longer, repeating the procedure in combination with drug and exercise therapy is recommended. On the other hand, if the procedures yield improvements that last less than 3 months, endoscopic lesion removal, open surgery, and pulsed radiofrequency ablation may be considered.

Balloon decompression, the procedure described at length in this book, entails the performance of balloon dilation in tandem with the functions achieved by neuroplasty or adhesiolysis. Hence, balloon decompression may be considered instead when neuroplasty or adhesiolysis are indicated.

1.2 Academic Basis for Neuroplasty and Adhesiolysis

The effect of epidural block tends to last for shorter periods or become less effective with repetition. In such cases, neuroplasty or adhesiolysis are often considered as an alternative means of addressing the patient's condition. The basis for these procedures is that patients with chronic degenerative spinal disease or postspinal surgery pain often exhibit epidural adhesion. This adhesion prevents epidural block from effecting any improvements. To resolve this, neuroplasty or adhesiolysis are used to allow accurate injection of the drug into the lesion.

Since its first documentation in 1989 by Racz, neuroplasty has become one of the most widely used spinal procedures in the world and has garnered much attention in the literature. However, despite the considerable establishment of the academic basis for neuroplasty, whether epidural adhesion present and adhesions or fibrosis actually account for the pain in patients who have not undergone surgery remains controversial.

To summarize multiple reports, adhesion was found in approximately 95% of the patients who underwent spinal surgery and was determined as the cause of pain in 20–36% of the patients with postspinal surgery pain syndrome. However, because filling defects were found in the epidurograms of a significant number of patients with chronic degenerative spinal disease who had not undergone surgery (Figs. 1.1 and 1.2) and adhesion was found on epiduroscopic examination in these patients (Fig. 1.3) It is clear that adhesion and fibrosis occur in patients with degenerative spinal disease regardless of the receipt of surgery.

Adhesion in patients who have not undergone surgery is most commonly found in the retrodiscal area, especially in the anterior epidural space of the L4–5 retrodiscal area (Fig. 1.4). This accounts for why balloon decompression on the spinal column should focus on the retrodiscal area of L4–5 and L5–S1.

The literature features no reports of pain directly attributable to adhesion or fibrosis. However, various studies have reported that pain may be caused or worsened when adhesion occurs around nerves or structures related to movement—i.e., fibrosis may cause hypertrophy of facets joint as well as adhesion that could subsequently induce stenosis and nerve impingement that could further restrict movement or induce neurogenic inflammation. Concurrently, the blockage of blood flow and consequent lack of nutrient supply from the cerebrospinal fluid may induce nerve hypoxia. Adhesion or fibrosis is thus often associated with pain or neurogenic claudication through diverse mechanisms, and the theoretical basis for using neuroplasty or adhesiolysis to alleviate as much pain as possible is therefore valid if the adhesion is suspected to be associated with the pain.

Surgeons who perform spinal surgery encounter many cases of scars, adhesion, and fibrosis in patients who receive repeated spinal surgeries. Thus, adhesion caused by a hard scar or fibrosis tend to be considered separately from the weak type of adhesion found in chronic degenerative spinal diseases. Because of this tendency, they would often rebut by questioning "What is the correlation between adhesion and pain?" and stating "It is ridiculous to say that adhesion could be removed with such a thin catheter" when they encounter neuroplasty or adhesiolysis for the first time. Alleviating adhesion of firm scar tissue would undoubtedly be difficult. However, the goal of adhesion mitigation via neuroplasty or adhesiolysis is to attenuate the adhesion as much as possible by only approaching and administering the drugs at the lesion associated with the pain—the goal is not and should not be to remove all adhesion in the spine.

The adhesion exhibited by patients who have not undergone surgery is weak in most cases and can thus be alleviated with a catheter without difficulty. Furthermore, the level of improvement achieved with adhesiolysis or neuroplasty is generally superior in patients with chronic degenerative spinal disease than in those with postoperative pain.

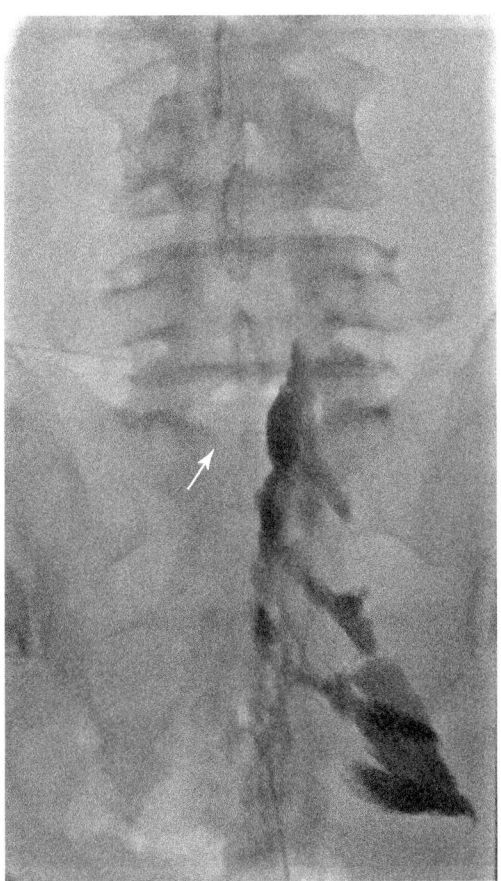

Fig. 1.1 An adhesion-induced left filling defect on the epidurogram of a patient with spinal stenosis who did not receive surgery. Arrow: filling defect

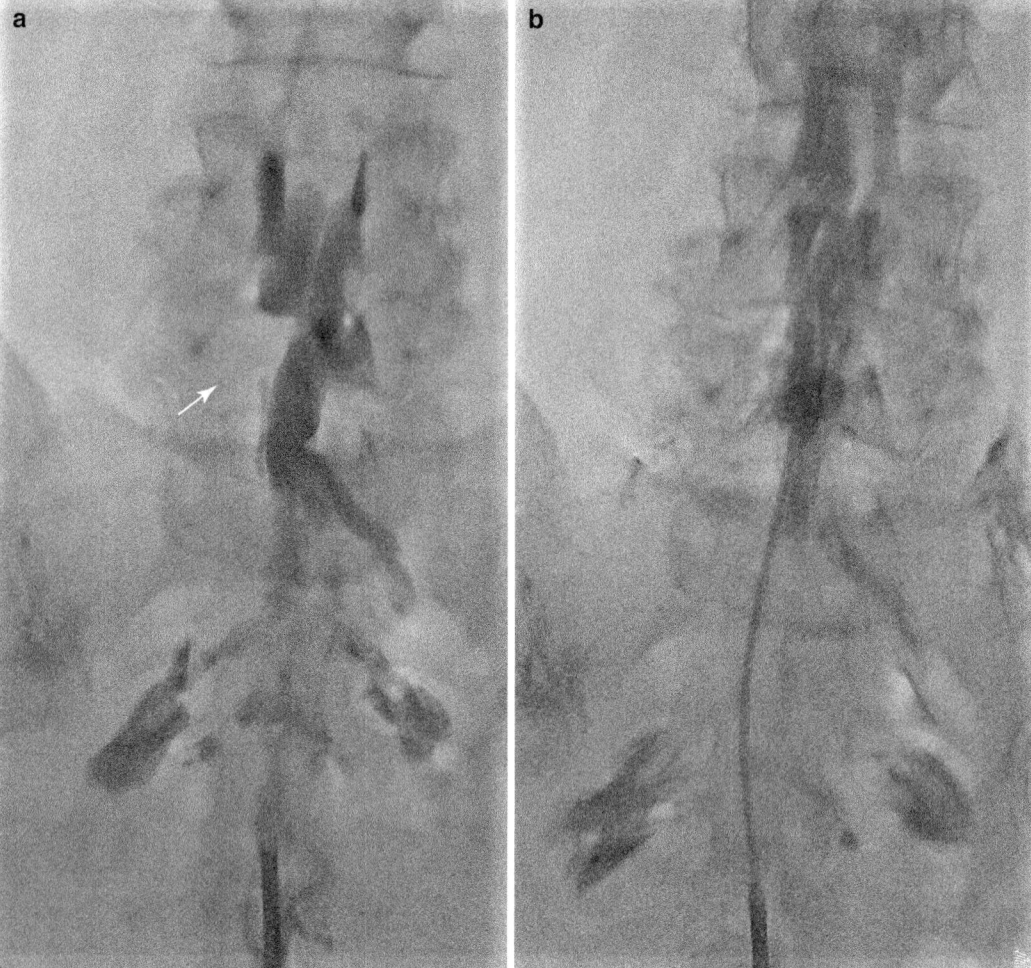

Fig. 1.2 (**a**) Left filling defect on the epidurogram of a patient with degenerative spinal disease who did not receive surgery. (**b**) Resolution of the filling defect with the removal of adhesion by balloon decompression in the same patient. Arrow: filling defect

1.3 Differences Between Neuroplasty and Adhesiolysis

The concepts of neuroplasty and adhesiolysis are often confusing. In Korea, there are many instances where discussions of neuroplasty involve all adhesiolysis-related procedures, including those that use balloon decompression. However, these two techniques are not the same. Neuroplasty is a method that involves approaching the lesion site with a thin catheter through the caudal epidural space to administer a hypertonic (5–10%) saline solution as well as steroids across 2–3 days; adhesiolysis entails using the catheter to directly remove the adhesion at the lesion site with the force used to move the catheter tip.

With respect to neuroplasty, numerous articles have reported that improvement was achieved after using a hypertonic saline solution in patients with spinal stenosis or pain developed following spinal surgery. These findings have led to suppositions that hypertonic saline solution can help to mitigate pain by reducing adhesion. However, there is no evidence for the efficacy of reducing adhesion with hypertonic saline solution.

1.3 Differences Between Neuroplasty and Adhesiolysis

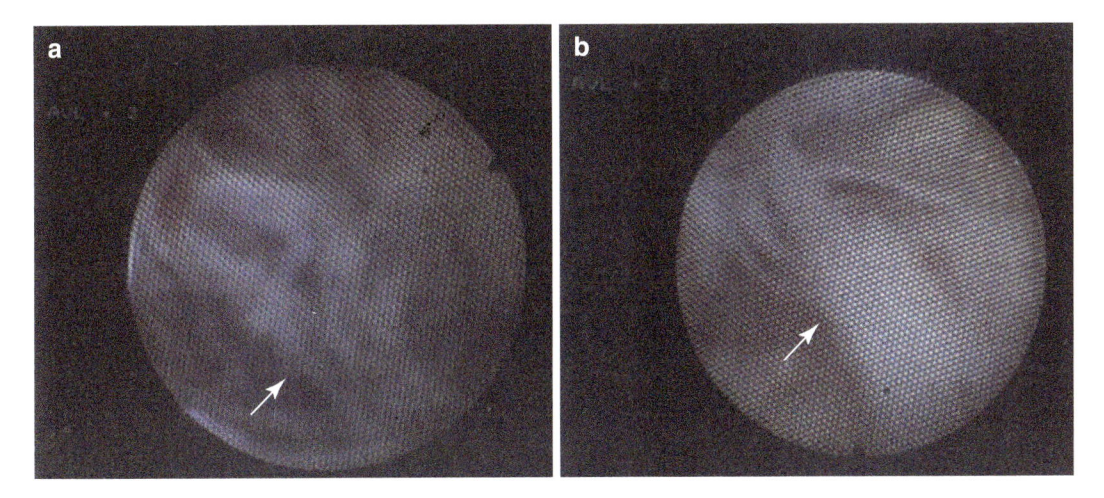

Fig. 1.3 Epiduroscopic findings. (**a**) Adhesion. (**b**) Fibrosis

Fig. 1.4 Cadaveric study of a patient with spinal stenosis who did not receive spinal surgery. (**a**) Adhesion at the L4–5 retrodiscal area was unresolved even when the anterior dura was lifted using a thread with 60 g of force. (**b**) Percentage of adhesion found in each retrodiscal area of the anterior epidural space. Adhesion was most commonly found at the L4–5 level, with the L5–S1 level being the second most common

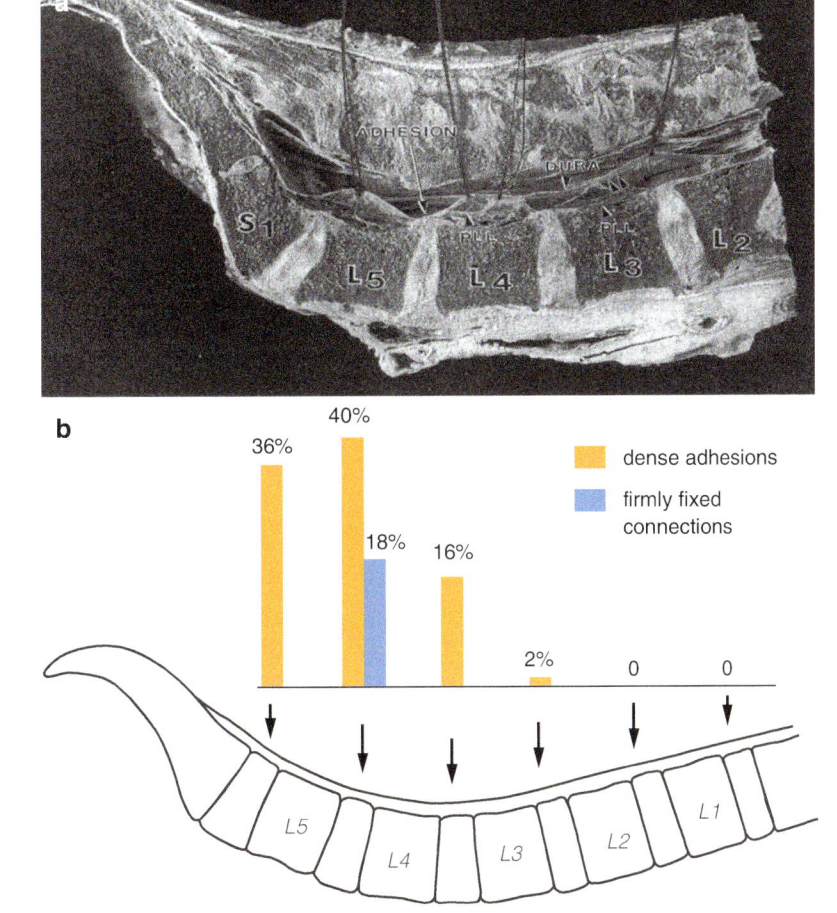

Mechanisms by which it is posited that hypertonic saline solution may help to reduce pain include the reduction of cell edema and inflammation, a decrease in neuronal excitability mediated by hyperosmolarity and highly concentrated chloride content, and the inhibition of C-fiber conduction.

Neuroplasty has reportedly induced pain reduction superior to that achieved through conservative treatment and epidural block in patients with chronic degenerative spinal disease. It has thus become relatively well-established in medical practice. However, when the hypertonic saline solution is injected into the nerves, it may cause pain, tremor, and partial weakness, while the injection of a large volume of the solution into the intrathecal area could cause serious adverse events, including as arachnoiditis, hypertension, tachycardia, and pulmonary edema. Therefore, it is important to check the contrast dye before injecting the drug as well as to use only a small volume of the hypertonic saline solution.

Adhesiolysis is a technique that uses a catheter to approach the lesion through the caudal epidural space for physically detaching the adhesion using the force of the catheter moving from side to side and administering the drug. It may be used with epiduroscopy when deemed appropriate.

Studying patients with postoperative pain, Manchikanti et al. compared those who received epiduroscopy to those whose procedures employed the Racz catheter. Therapeutic effects were sustained for longer periods among those who received epiduroscopy, and the average period before a second operation was needed was 5 and 3 months for the epiduroscopy and Racz groups, respectively. This finding further indicated the differential sustainment of the procedures' therapeutic effects. Of note, however, the use of the Racz catheter was found to be more cost-effective.

Neuroplasty and adhesiolysis could be excellent treatment modalities capable of overcoming the limitations of the conventional epidural block. However, they are recognized only for inducing short-term pain alleviation; their ability to effect function is reportedly insufficient. This may be ascribed to the inability of either method to mitigate stenosis or remove adhesion. Moreover, as the insufficient removal of adhesion can easily lead to readhesion, it would be difficult to expect neuroplasty or adhesiolysis to achieve long-term effects. There has been thus been a persistent demand for safe nonsurgical procedures that can remove adhesion and even provide mitigate stenosis with greater efficacy. To a certain degree, balloon decompression can satisfy this demand.

1.4 Theoretical and Academic Basis for Balloon Decompression

1.4.1 Improved Blood Circulation by Expanding the Free Space in the Area Affected by Stenosis

Characterized by severe pain, numbness, or weakness, neurogenic claudication refers to a phenomenon in which stenosis at two or more sites causes congestion and poor blood circulation to the nerves, consequently restricting the blood supply needed for walking. Although the condition prohibits a patient from walking for an extended period, the patient may be able to walk again when normal blood circulation resumes, and stenosis from bending at the waist or sitting is alleviated (Fig. 1.5).

When stenosis occurs at two levels of the central canal (Fig. 1.5a), claudication may occur due to symptoms that manifest in the lower back or both legs. On the other hand, when blood flow is impaired by stenosis in the central canal and intervertebral foramen (Fig. 1.5b), claudication may occur due to symptoms that occur in just one leg. While claudication may not be fully explained by impaired blood circulation, it is recognized as one of the key mechanisms.

This postulated mechanism suggests that circulatory congestion can be restored and claudication resolved by alleviating stenosis in either of the two sites. Balloon decompression was developed based on this supposition.

It is natural that the idea of expanding stenosed areas with a small balloon would meet with skepticism. Indeed, it would be impossible for the balloon to expand the stenosed areas

1.4 Theoretical and Academic Basis for Balloon Decompression

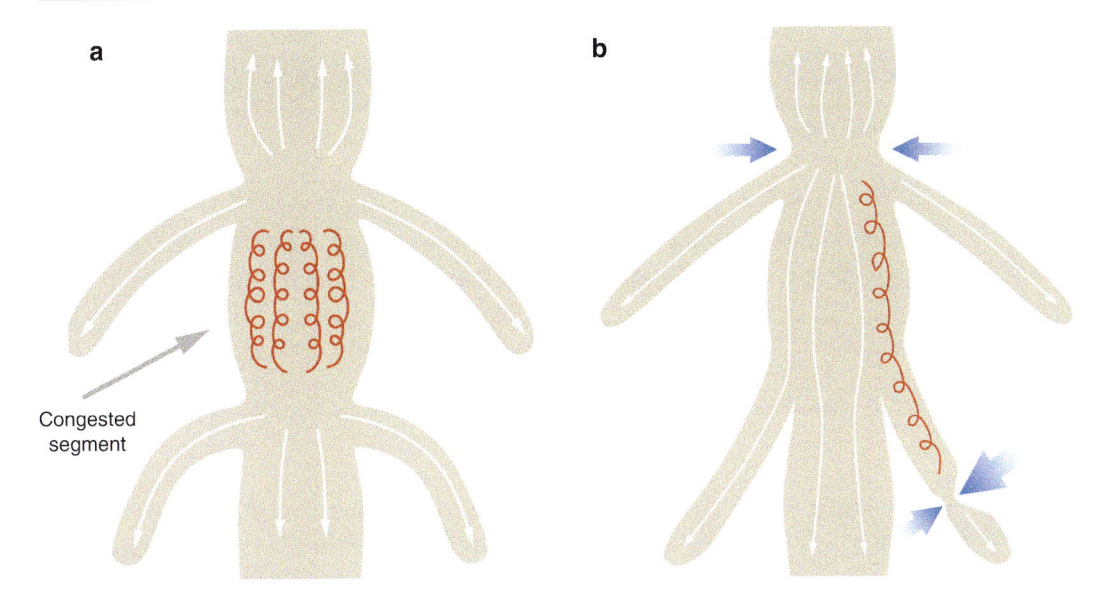

Fig. 1.5 Mechanism of claudication. (**a**) Impaired blood circulation caused by stenosis at two levels of the central canal. Claudication develops in both legs. (**b**) Impaired blood circulation caused by stenosis in the central canal and intervertebral foramen. Claudication develops in the leg with the lesion

Fig. 1.6 When the pressure in the blood pressure manometer cuff is raised to create circulatory congestion, and the pressure is subsequently relaxed slowly, blood circulation improves even while the cuff remains tightened

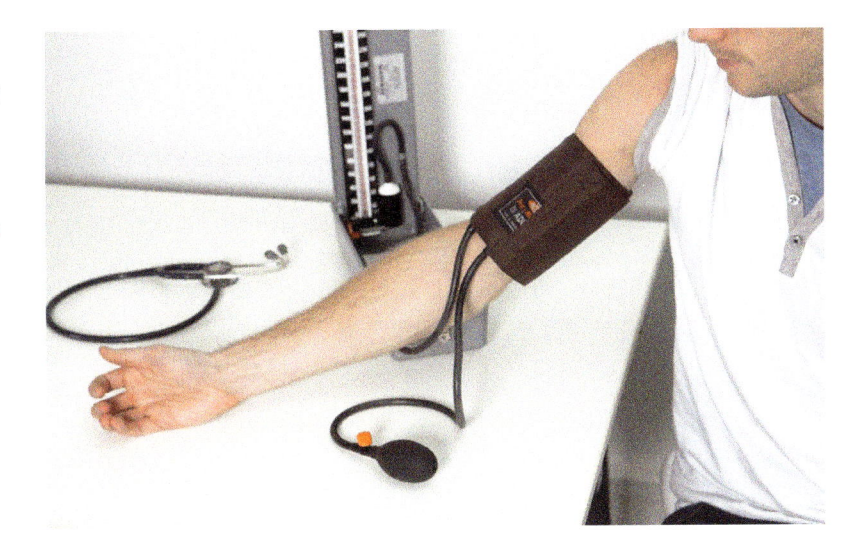

as much as would be possible in a surgical operation. To alleviate stenosis with a balloon means to create more free space by pushing, compressing, and reorganizing the surrounding tissues, similar to cleaning a hard drive to create more storage space in a computer. Balloon decompression can attain a certain level of stenosis alleviation and thereby significantly improve blood circulation.

As shown below in Fig. 1.6, when blood pressure is raised with a manometer cuff to create circulatory congestion and is then slowly relaxed, blood circulation improves even while the cuff remains tightened. Similarly, enlarging free space without completely alleviating stenosis can improve blood circulation, pain, and claudication.

These principles informed an investigation of the effect of balloon treatment for foraminal stenosis. Published in *Pain Physician* in 2013, the details of this study were as follows:

Randomized Trial

Effects of Transforaminal Balloon Treatment in Patients with Lumbar Foraminal Stenosis: A Randomized, Controlled, Double-Blind Trial

Sung-Hoon Kim, MD[1], Woo-Jong Choi, MD[1], Jeong Hun Suh, MD[1], Sang-Ryong Jeon, MD, PhD[2], Chang Ju Hwang, MD[3], Won-Uk Koh, MD[1], Chung Lee, MD, PhD[4], Jeong Gil Leem, MD, PhD[1], Sang Chul Lee, MD, PhD[5], and Jin-Woo Shin, MD, PhD[1]

The study included patients with intractable unilateral foraminal stenosis without a sustained improvement effect of ≥50% across the month following treatment with conventional transforaminal epidural block. The balloon group received balloon decompression: a balloon catheter was inserted into the intervertebral foramen, the catheter was removed, and the drug was administered. Balloon decompression was performed by withdrawing the balloon slowly from the middle of the spinal canal to the lateral aspect of the intervertebral foramen while repeating balloon inflation and deflation (Fig. 1.7). The balloon catheter was similarly inserted into the patients in the sham group but was removed without being inflated; the drug was subsequently administered to this group as well. Hence, the only difference between the two groups was whether the balloon was inflated prior the removal of the catheter.

At the 3-month follow-up of the procedure, the balloon group showed significant improvements in leg pain, low back pain, Oswestry Disability Index score, and claudication distance relative to the sham group. At the 1-year follow-up, approximately 20% of the patients in the balloon group retained ≥50% improvement in pain; no patient in the sham group sustained any gained improvements (Figs. 1.8 and 1.9).

In the sham group, a balloon catheter was inserted into the intervertebral foramen and subsequently withdrawn—without being inflated—before the drug was administered. Hence, this procedure is practically equivalent to adhesiolysis, which achieves therapeutic benefits with more efficacy than does conventional transforaminal epidural block: In patients with severe foraminal stenosis or adhesion, a conventional transforaminal epidural block does not allow for the efficient administration of the drug into the medial epidural space. However, in the shame group of this study, the drug can spread well to epidural space through the path created by the catheter as it is inserted and withdrawn even in the patient with sever foraminal stenosis or adhesion. This is the same as injecting the drug after inserting a balloon-free catheter into the intervertebral foramen in the epidural adhesiolysis. Hence, this study is equivalent to comparing the effects of balloon decompression and conventional balloon-free adhesiolysis. The balloon group achieved significant differences in all measured variables across treatment relative to the sham group, indicating that balloon decompression is a technique superior to conventional adhesiolysis (Fig. 1.10).

This study is unique in that it directly measured the claudication distance of patients using a treadmill in an outpatient setting. More objective than self-reports, this method increases the reliability of the data.

As aforementioned, while existing treatment modalities for spinal stenosis exert beneficial short-term effects on relieving pain, they have a limited impact on motor function and claudication. By contrast, balloon decompression demonstrably improved motor function and claudication as predicted.

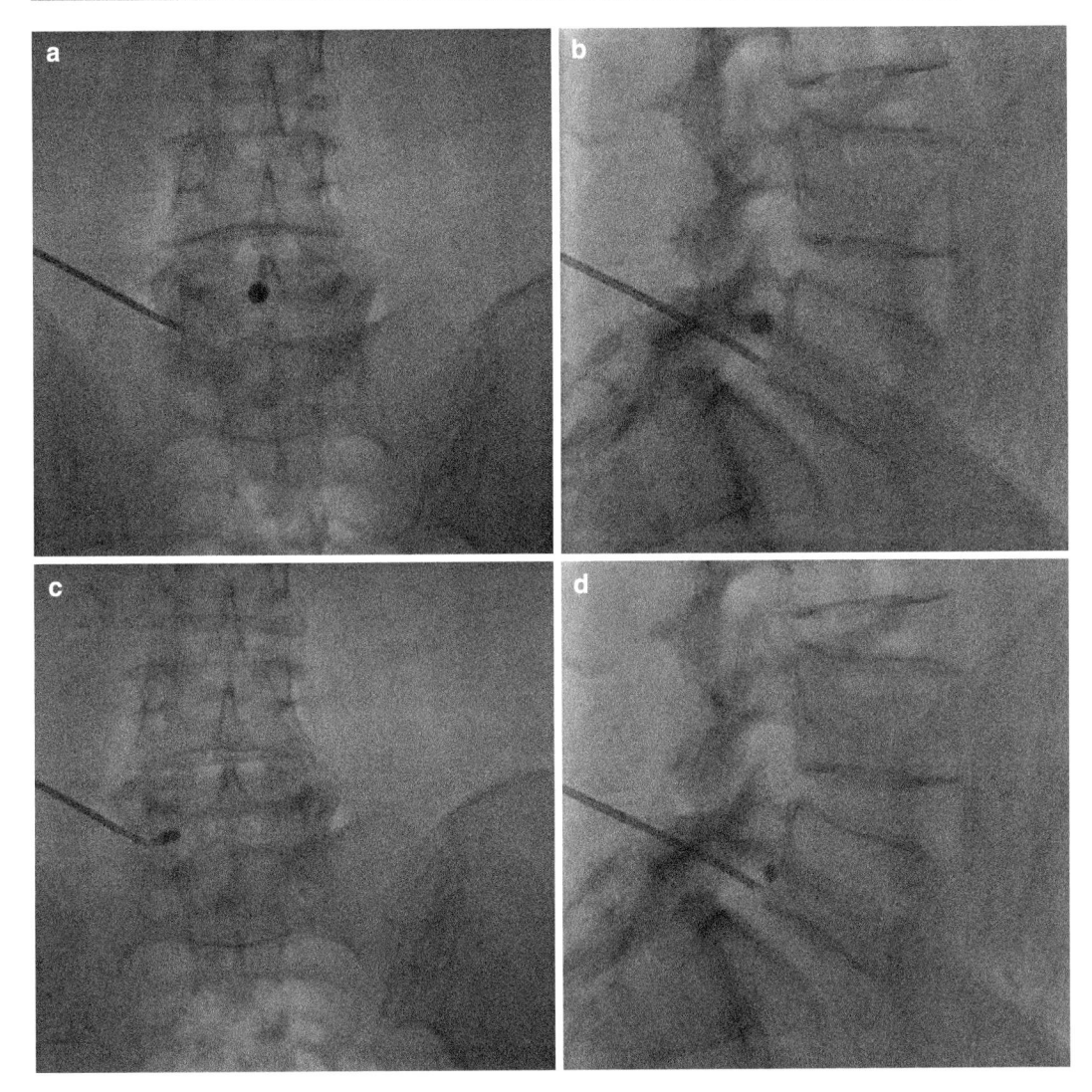

1.4 Theoretical and Academic Basis for Balloon Decompression

Fig. 1.7 (**a**, **b**) AP and lateral images of balloon decompression after the balloon catheter was inserted into the midline through the intervertebral foramen. (**c**, **d**) AP and lateral images of repeated inflation and deflation of the balloon while it is slowly withdrawn. The last repetition of the inflation of the balloon was at the end of the intervertebral foramen

This study further constructed three-dimensional reconstruction views of the spread of the contrast dye to measure changes in volume and diameter of the intervertebral foramen across balloon decompression. This additional step helped to determine whether the observed improvement was attributable to the expansion of the free space in the stenosed intervertebral foramen and, if so, by how much such the space had increased: the diameter and volume increased by 28% and 98%, respectively (Fig. 1.11), indicating that the free space of the intervertebral foramen is increased and blood circulation is improved. In other words, this proved that although the balloon was small and thin, it was capable of expanding the free space in the intervertebral foramen enough to improve blood circulation and facilitate drug administration. This benefit may apply to cases involving spinal central stenosis.

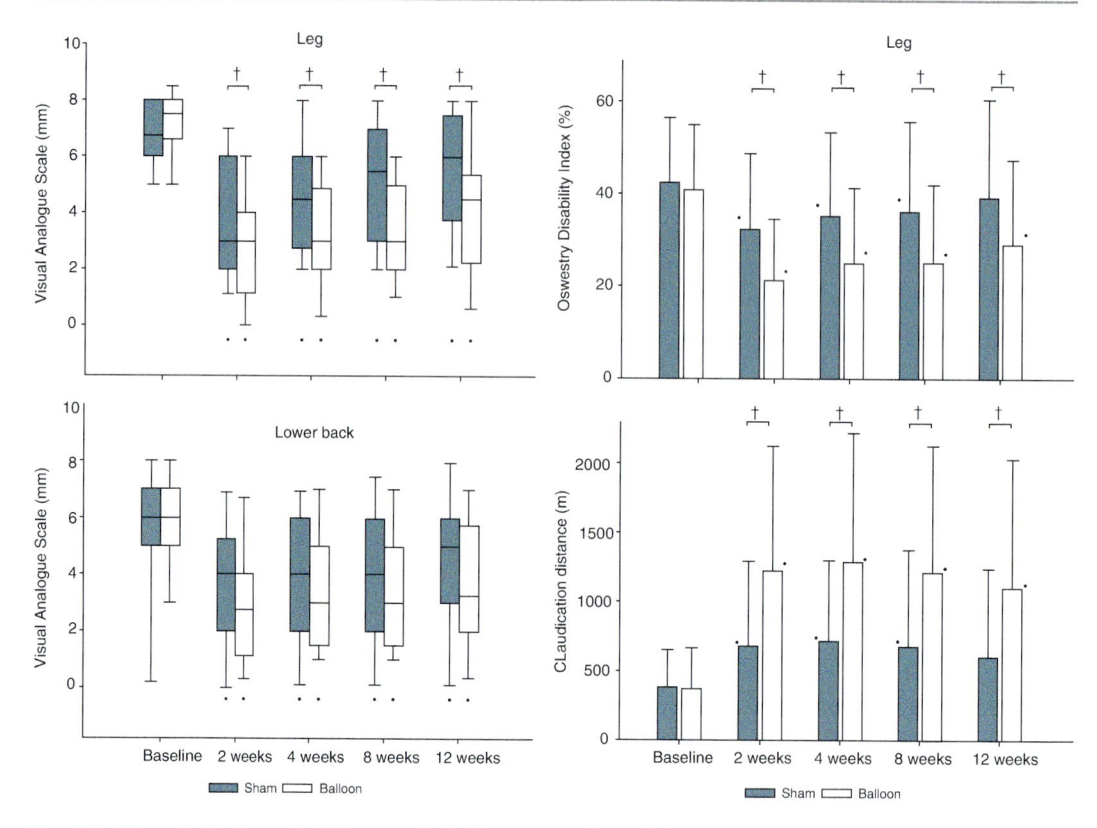

Fig. 1.8 Through the 3-month follow-up, the balloon group showed significant improvement in leg pain, low back pain, Oswestry Disability Index score, and claudication distance relative to the sham group

Fig. 1.9 At the follow-up performed over a year following the procedure, an approximate of 20% and 0% of the patients in the balloon and sham groups, respectively, retained ≥50% improvement in pain

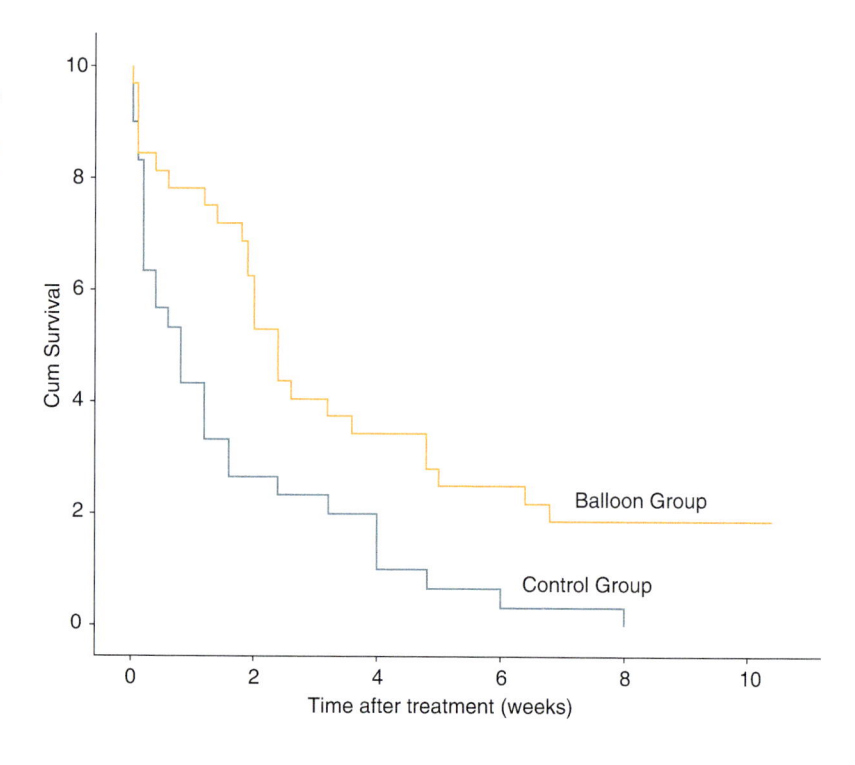

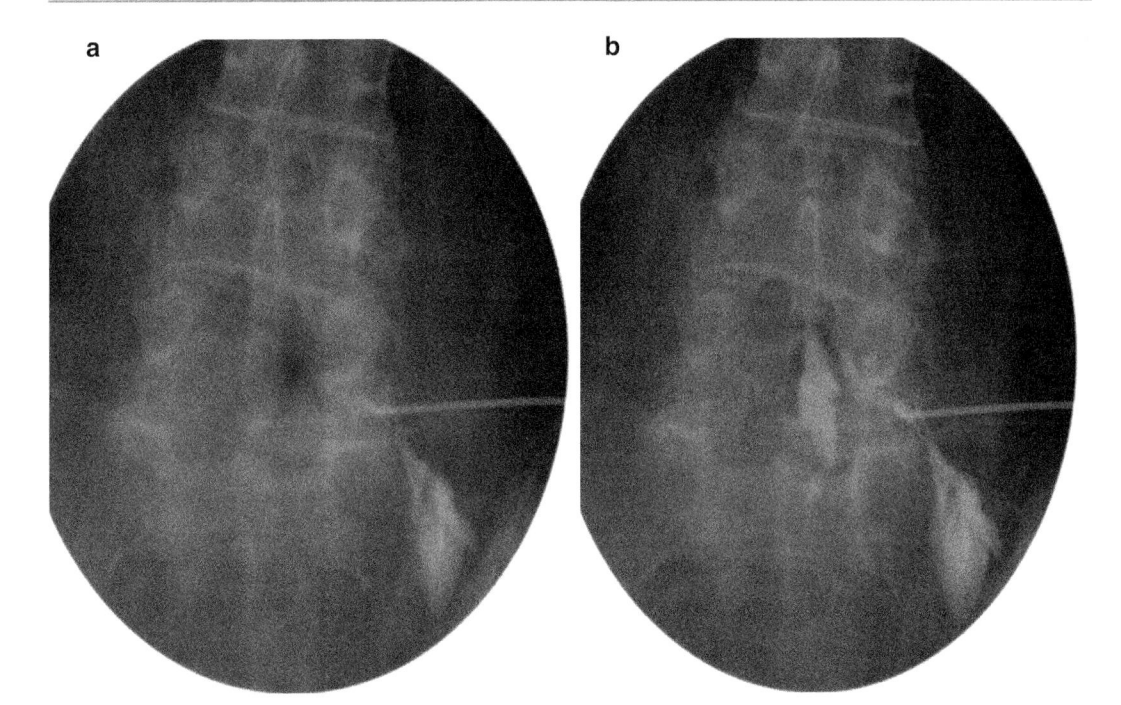

1.4 Theoretical and Academic Basis for Balloon Decompression

Fig. 1.10 (**a**) While general transforaminal epidural block was performed in patients with severe stenosis or adhesion, the drug did not spread into the preganglionic or medial epidural space. (**b**) Image of the drug spreading into the preganglionic and medial epidural space in the same patient when the drug was administered after the insertion and withdrawal of the catheter in the intervertebral foramen. This indicated that inserting and withdrawing the catheter is more effective for drug dispersion than is general transforaminal epidural block. This article compared balloon decompression with the procedure indicated in **b**

1.4.2 Improved Adhesiolysis

The importance of the mechanical adhesiolysis offered by epidural adhesiolysis was previously described in the section on the fundamentals of neuroplasty and adhesiolysis. However, conventional neuroplasty has little adhesion removal. Conventional adhesiolysis cannot remove adhesions effectively, as its efficacy relies solely on the force exerted through the catheter. A common problem when removing adhesions using catheter movement is that the catheter creates a path upon its first is insertion; as the catheter tends continue following this path upon subsequent insertions, it is difficult to detach the surrounding adhesions. However, similar to lifting a thin board, expanding the target area with a balloon increases the range of the extent of adhesion that can be detached and facilitates the maneuverability of the catheter when the procedure progresses onto a different lesion (Fig. 1.12). The extensive adhesion removal enabled by using the balloon might account for the relatively lower recurrence rate after the procedure. In addition, balloon decompression is associated with a relatively lower risk of dural damage relative to the use of the force of the catheter alone and requires less irrigation with normal saline.

Generally, efforts to remove adhesion tend to focus on the spinal canal. However, cases of foraminal stenosis may induce prolonged contact with the surrounding nerve tissues, causing adhesion and compression; hence, such cases demand the removal of adhesion, as well as perineural decompression in the intervertebral foramen (Figs. 1.13 and 1.14).

Most procedures or surgeries for alleviating foraminal stenosis tent to attempt expansion by approaching the inferior aspect of the intervertebral foramen—through Kambin's triangle—to avoid nerve damage. However, in such cases, the direct removal of perineural adhesion may not be achieved on account of its excessive distance from the nerve path (Fig. 1.14).

On the other hand, balloon decompression involves the insertion of the catheter close to the nerve path and the subsequent inflation of the balloon. As a result, balloon decompression offers the important advantage of allowing for the removal of perineural adhesion while also alleviating nerve compression.

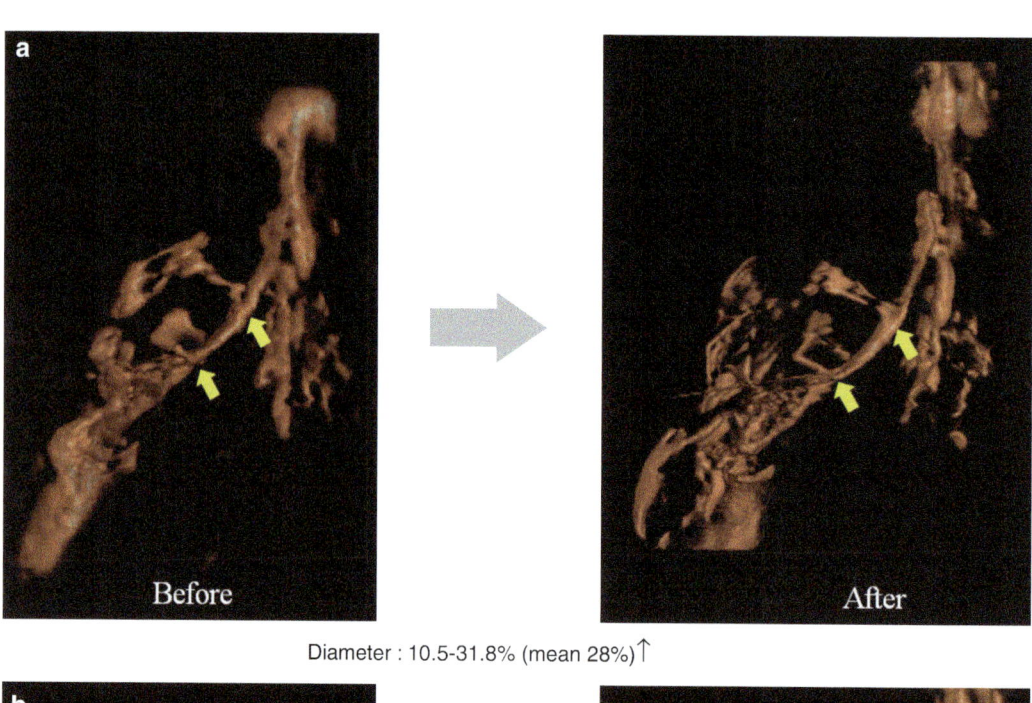

Fig. 1.11 Three-dimensional reconstruction views of the spread of the contrast dye across balloon decompression. (**a**) Dye spread across balloon decompression. Yellow arrows: intervertebral foraminal area. (**b**) The diameter of contrast dye spread increased by approximately 28% across balloon decompression. (**c**) The volume of the contrast dye spread increased by approximately 98% across balloon decompression

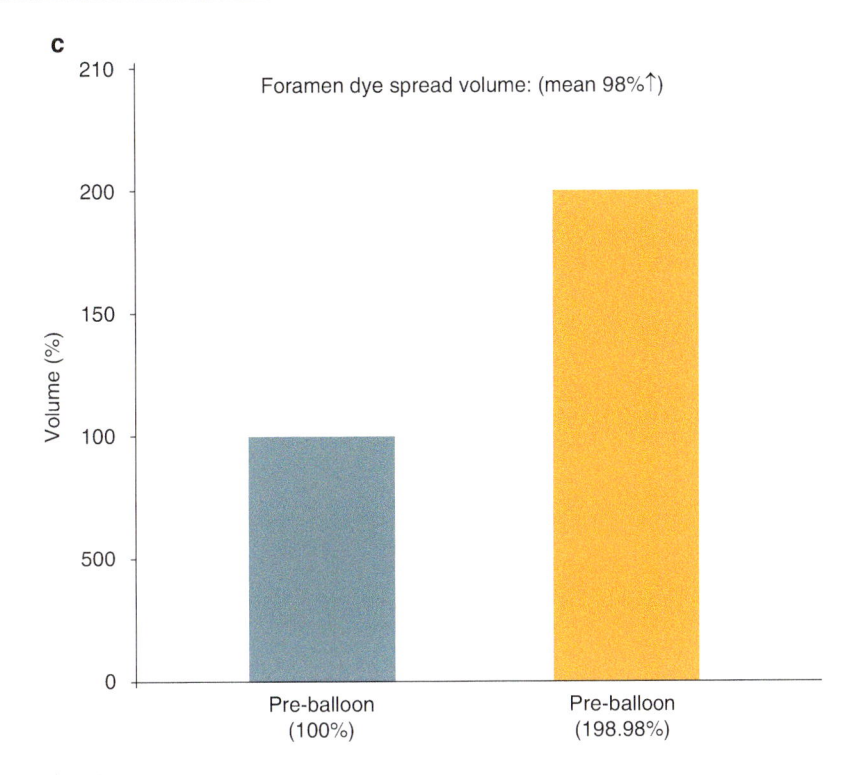

1.4 Theoretical and Academic Basis for Balloon Decompression

Fig. 1.11 (continued)

1.4.3 Retrodiscal Decompression Theory

Basaran et al. proposed that when disc herniation induces nerve compression in the retrodiscal area, inserting and inflating a balloon could allow the compressed nerve to be released to the side to relieve the compression (Fig. 1.15). Although ZiNeuF or ZiNeu catheters have been used on multiple occasions for such procedures, whether the operative course and outcome reflected the theory of Basaran et al. cannot be determined. However, the significant improvement of the patients' symptoms partially validates the theory.

The two procedures that used the method described by this theory are outlined as follows.

Case 1 The patient had developed lower right leg pain due to S1-root compression in the L5–S1 retrodiscal area. As the foraminal approach was difficult due to high iliac crest, the ZiNeu catheter was inserted into the caudal epidural space to approach the right L5–S1 retrodiscal area of the anterior epidural space. The balloon was then inflated to decompress the S1 root. The improvement in the patients' symptoms following the procedure was maintained for approximately 1 year (Fig. 1.16).

Case 2 The patient had developed left L5 traversing root compression due to L4–5 disc sequestration. The ZiNeuF catheter was inserted into the Lt. L4–5 retrodiscal area through the intervertebral foramen to alleviate L5 root compression. The patients' symptoms improved across follow-ups conducted for over a year (Fig. 1.17).

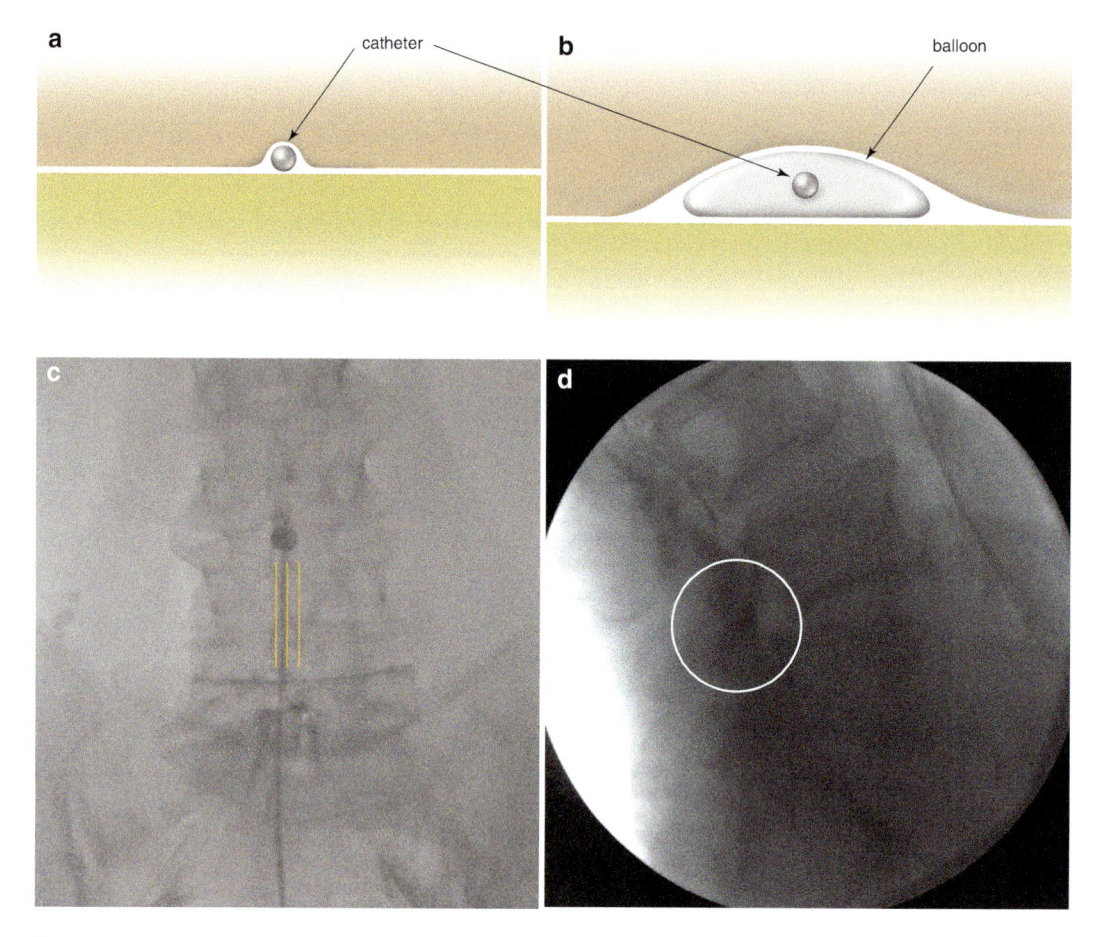

Fig. 1.12 (**a**) Cross-sectional view of the removal of adhesion with only the catheter. (**b**) Cross-sectional view of the removal of adhesion with balloon decompression, which allows for the removal of adhesion from a wider area. (**c**) An image showing how the balloon catheter expands at once what would take a regular catheter three places. (**d**) Removal of adhesion in the retrodiscal area of the patient by relieving stenosis and lifting the dura with the balloon. Circle: Inflated balloon

1.4.4 Basis for Long-Term Improvements Effected by Balloon Decompression

While the capacity of a thin balloon to alleviate stenosis, improve blood circulation, and remove adhesions with greater efficacy has been demonstrated, the certainty that the site of the procedure will eventually redevelop stenosis and adhesion might augment skepticism of the balloon decompression. However, no currently available surgery or procedure can cure degenerative spinal diseases or completely preclude recurrence, and successfully performed balloon decompression lowers the recurrence rate and achieves a more sustained therapeutic effect relative to conventional procedures on account of its superior stenosis alleviation and adhesion removal. As mentioned previously, this relative outperformance can be particularly ascribed to the unique

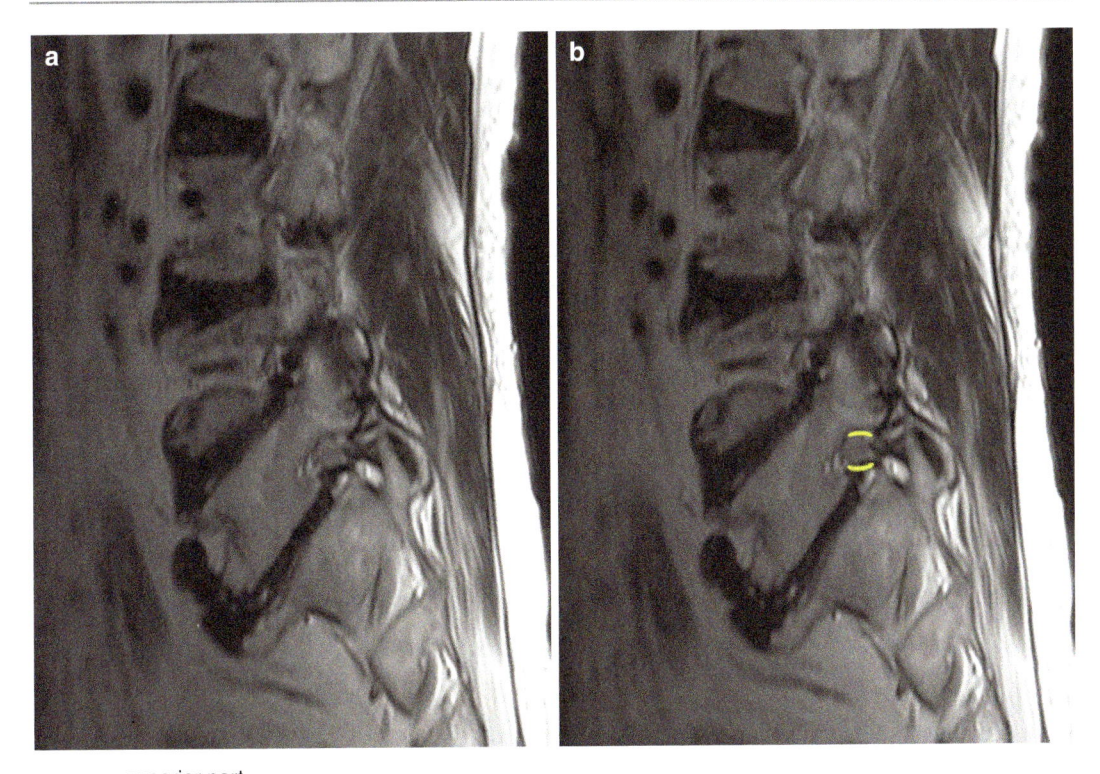

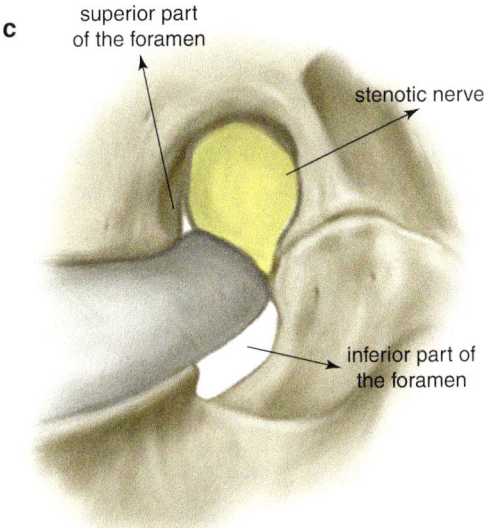

1.4 Theoretical and Academic Basis for Balloon Decompression

Fig. 1.13 (**a**) L5 intervertebral stenosis. (**b**) Adhesion area in the same patient. (Yellow line: are of stenosis-induced contact—i.e., the adhesion area). (**c**) Magnified view of the MRI findings in the intervertebral foraminal area. Despite the presence of stenosis at the superior aspect of the intervertebral foramen, the removal of adhesion (yellow line) is impossible if the procedure is performed by approaching the inferior aspect of the intervertebral foramen through Kambin's triangle

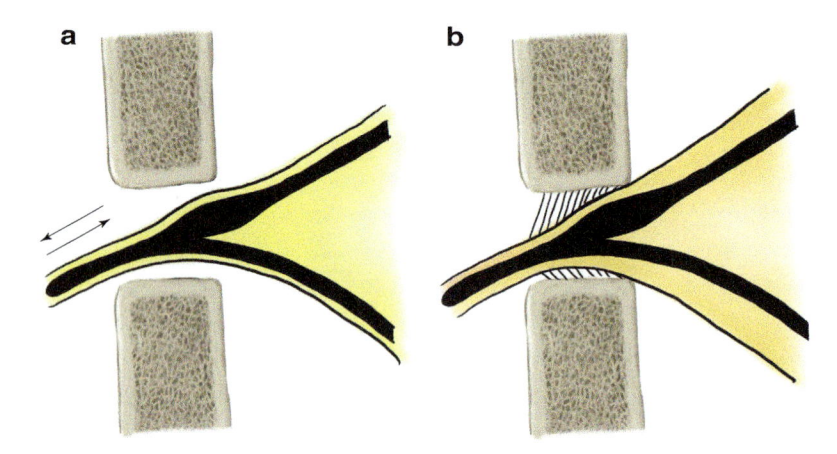

Fig. 1.14 (**a**) When adhesion is absent from the intervertebral foramen, there is no limitation to nerve movement within the intervertebral foramen. (**b**) When perineural adhesion is present in the intervertebral foramen, it may cause limitations in mobility, impaired blood circulation, inflammation, and stretching injury

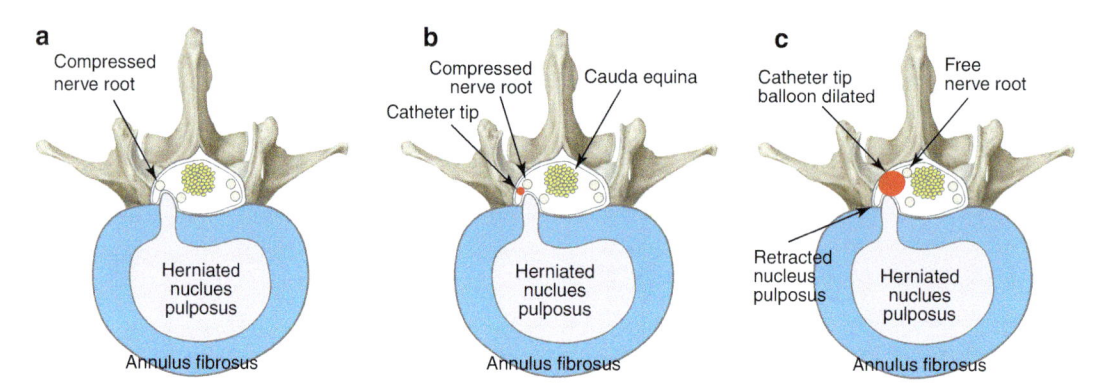

Fig. 1.15 (**a**) Nerve compression in the retrodiscal area caused by disc herniation. (**b**) Image of the catheter inserted adjacent to the compressed nerve. (**c**) Image of relieving compression by pushing the compressed nerve to the side by inflating the balloon

capacity of balloon decompression among procedures that do not employ balloons to remove adhesion from wide areas.

Other evidence of the long-term improvements associated with balloon decompression includes the following.

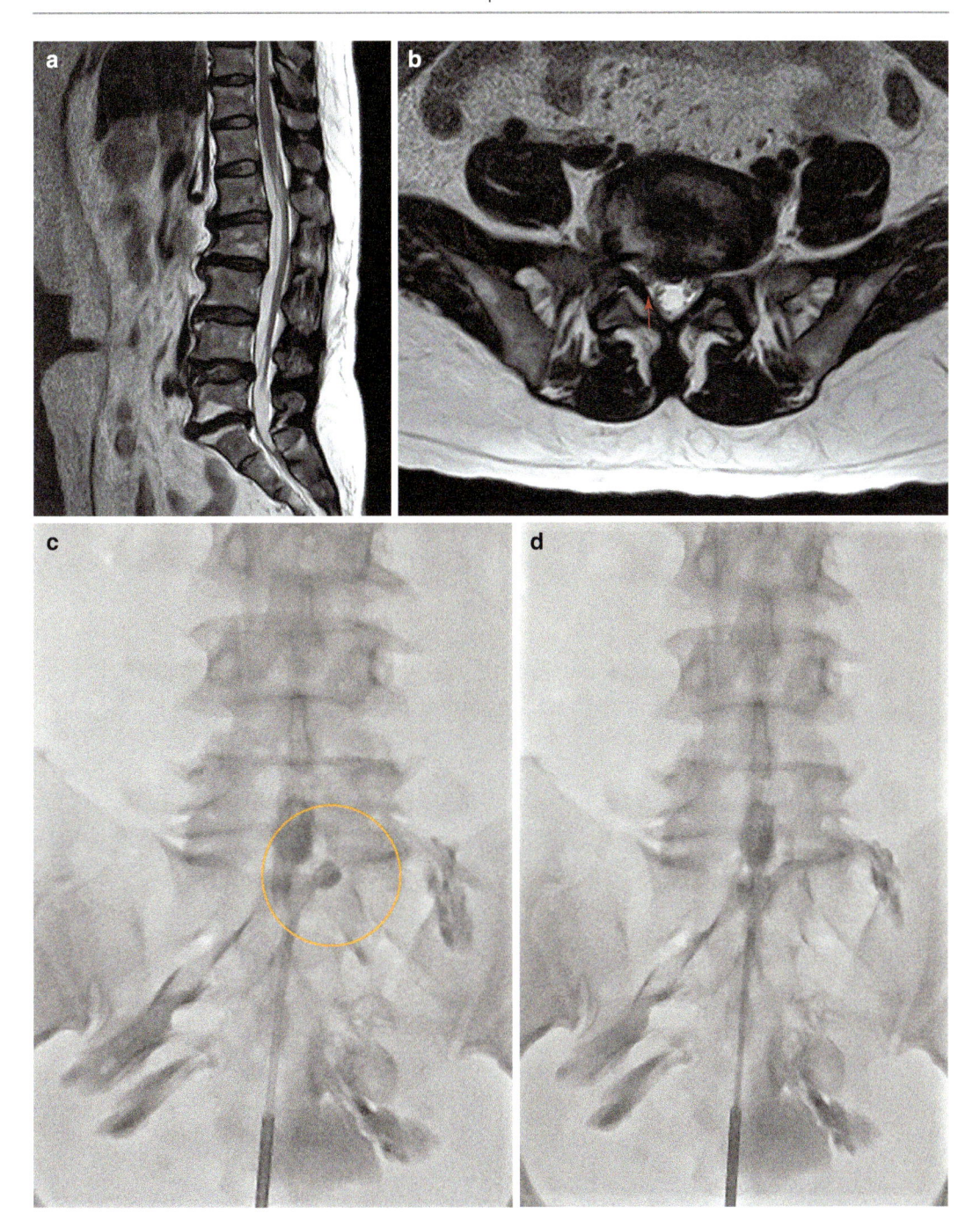

1.4 Theoretical and Academic Basis for Balloon Decompression

Fig. 1.16 (**a**, **b**) MRI findings. Image of Rt. S1 root compression in the L5–S1 retrodiscal area. Arrow: Rt. S1 root. (**c**) Image of the insertion of the ZiNeu catheter into the Rt. L5–S1 retrodiscal area and the inflation of the balloon near the compressed nerve. (**d**) Contrast dye injected after the deflation of the balloon confirmed that the drug was accurately administered to the lesion

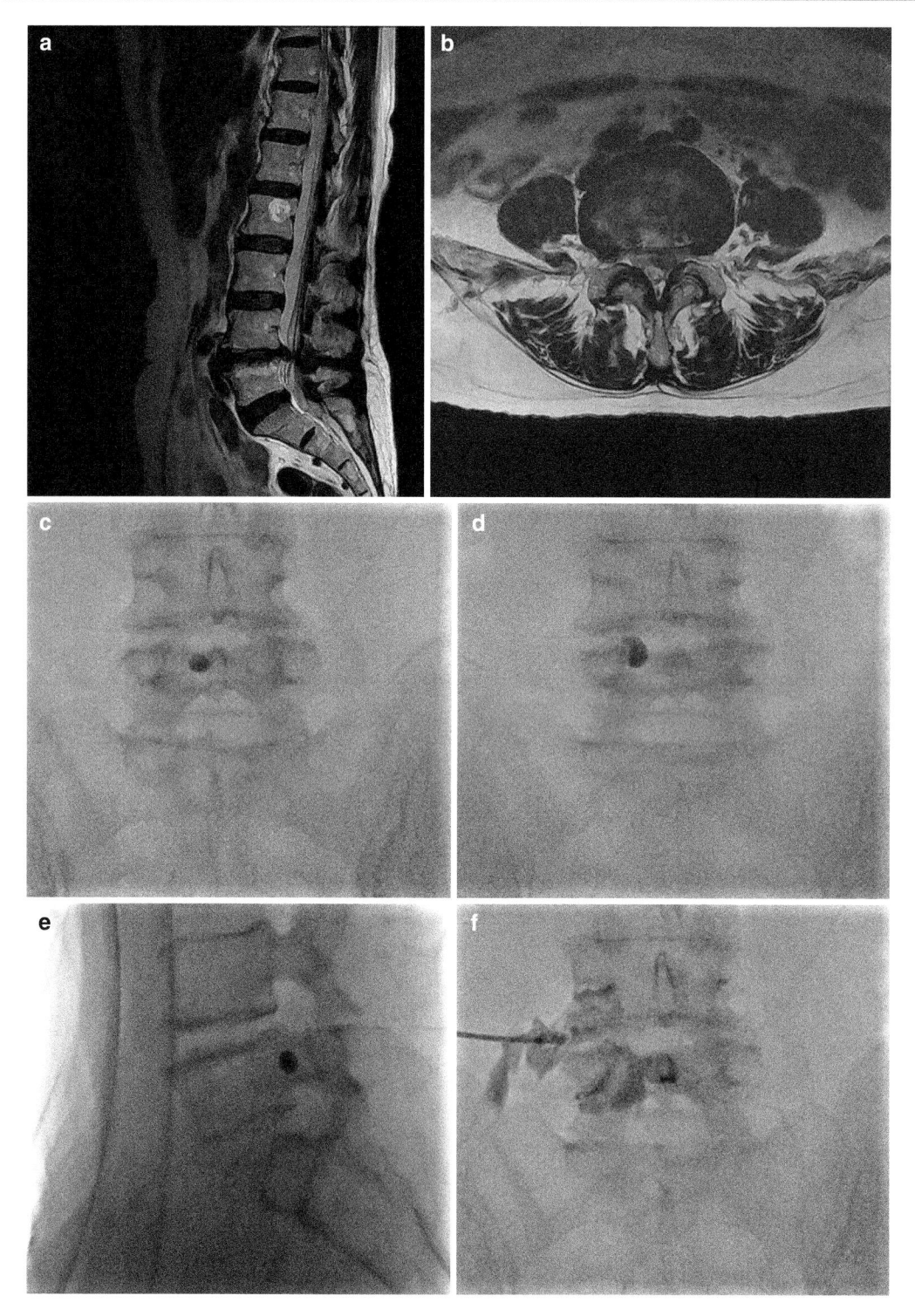

Fig. 1.17 (**a**, **b**) MRI findings. Lt. L5 traversing root compression due to L4–5 disc sequestration. Arrow: Lt. L5 root. (**c**) Image of procedure involving the insertion of the ZiNeuF catheter into the Lt. L4–5 retrodiscal area, followed by its slow withdrawal and the repeated inflation and deflation of the balloon. (**d**) The inflation of the balloon at the site of Lt. L5 root compression. (**e**) Lateral image of **c**. The inflation of the balloon in the anterior epidural space. (**f**) The contrast dye accurately spreads into the lesion area after balloon decompression

1.4.4.1 Pain Reduction and Motor Function Improvement

Pain Medicine 2016; 17: 476–487
doi: 10.1093/pm/pnv018

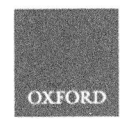

OXFORD

SPINE SECTION

Original Research Articles

Effectiveness and Factors Associated with Epidural Decompression and Adhesiolysis Using a Balloon-Inflatable Catheter in Chronic Lumbar Spinal Stenosis: 1-Year Follow-Up

A study conducted in the pain clinic at Seoul Asan Medical Center and published in *Pain Medicine* prospectively observed 61 patients with degenerative spinal disease for a year after they underwent balloon decompression with the ZiNeu catheter. Specifically, the study population only included patients who had previously undergone epidural block and whose improvement effect of ≥50% did not last for more than a month. The patients attended follow-up immediately after receiving only one balloon decompression procedure.

Improvements in leg/low back pain and function were sustained for a year. In particular, functional improvement tended to increase over time (Fig. 1.18). Relative to most conventional procedures characterized by the difficulty in achieving sustained improvements for more than 3 months, balloon decompression yielded a relatively longer duration of sustained effects and greater improvements over time. This enhancement in therapeutic benefit tended to result from increased exercise, such as walking, which can be attributed to the superior mitigation of claudication effected by balloon decompression. Accordingly, the present author always instructs patients to walk regularly—for about 1 h a day—as soon as the symptoms improve after the procedure. Such exercise helps to reduce the likelihood of recurrence as well as enhance functional improvement.

The aforementioned study subsequently performed multivariate logistic regression analysis of the study population for reference. They found that patients with diabetes had a significantly lower likelihood of attaining sustained improvement for over a year than did patients without diabetes. If patients are screened for diabetes before undergoing balloon decompression, this observation recommends that patients should be informed of the possible diminished therapeutic benefit of the procedure.

The investigation also presented 3D-reconstructed images of the spread of the contrast dye before and after transforaminal balloon decompression. These images confirmed that the volume of the spread increased significantly across balloon decompression, indicating that the procedure can improve blood circulation as well as the delivery of the drug to the lesion (Fig. 1.19), (Video 1.1).

1.4.4.2 Facilitation of Spontaneous Resorption

While spontaneous resorption occurs more readily in cases of disc herniation with high interver-

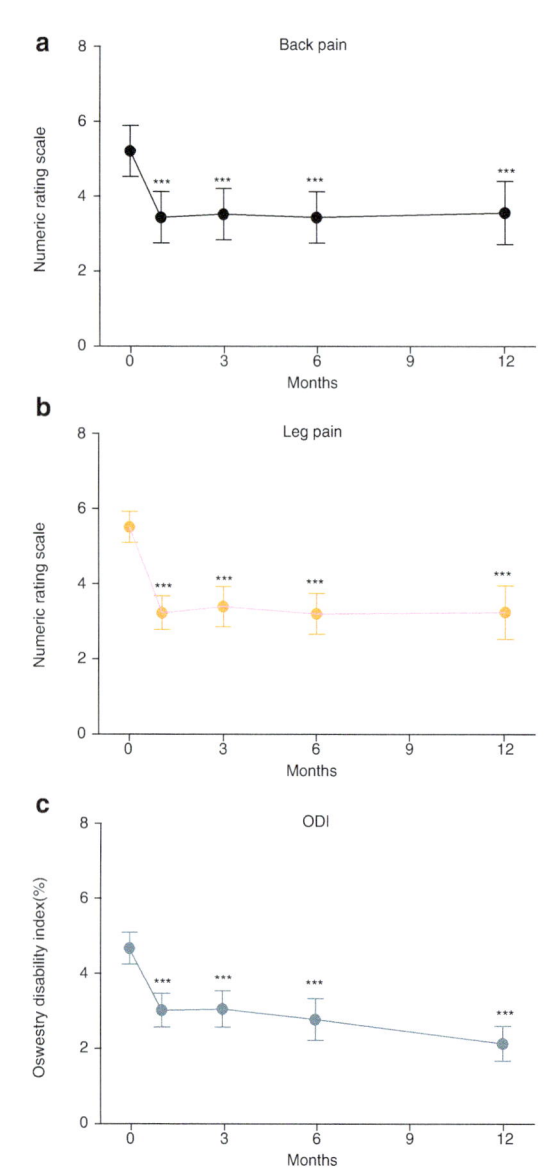

Fig. 1.18 One-year follow-up results following balloon decompression. (**a**) Low back pain. (**b**) Leg pain. (**c**) Oswestry Disability Index (ODI). Improvements over time were observed

tebral disc water content, a large degree of disc herniation, and severe sequestration, these benefits depend on the patient's capacity to walk with good posture and without pain. If the patient has developed the habit of adopting a bad, painful posture, the herniation may worsen, and the probability of the herniated disc being resorbed may decrease. Various procedures for alleviating the symptoms of intervertebral disc diseases, such as epidural block, can reduce pain and enhance the probability of the spontaneous resorption of the herniated disc.

The cases shown in Figs. 1.20, 1.21 and 1.22 involve patients with severe disc herniation whose pain reduction was achieved after a single round of transforaminal epidural block, and MRI obtained at the 4-month and 1-year follow-ups showed that spontaneous resorption had resolved their disc herniations. Hence, even in cases of severe intervertebral disc disease—as identified on MRI—spontaneous resorption can be expected if the pain is well-managed. Accordingly, if conservative treatment (e.g., epidural block) does not satisfactorily improve pain and motor functions, balloon decompression is recommended for facilitating spontaneous resorption.

Balloon decompression may provide long-term improvements lasting over a year. This may be attributable to relatively more patients having achieved spontaneous resorption because of an increased amount of exercise and improvements in pain and claudication relative to other nonsurgical procedures.

1.4.5 Integration of Existing Procedural Techniques

As a combination of balloon dilation, conventional neuroplasty, and adhesiolysis, balloon decompression is a three-in-one procedure that can enhance the efficacy and sustainability of existing treatment modalities. As in conventional adhesiolysis, additional balloon dilation is performed during balloon decompression after adhesion is broken with the force of the catheter. Thus, balloon decompression is more effective and results in less recurrence than does conventional adhesiolysis. In addition, this technique could be performed in conjunction with neuroplasty by accurately placing a regular drug-injection epidural catheter on the lesion after balloon decompression and using the catheter to inject hypertonic saline for 2–3 days. While neuro-

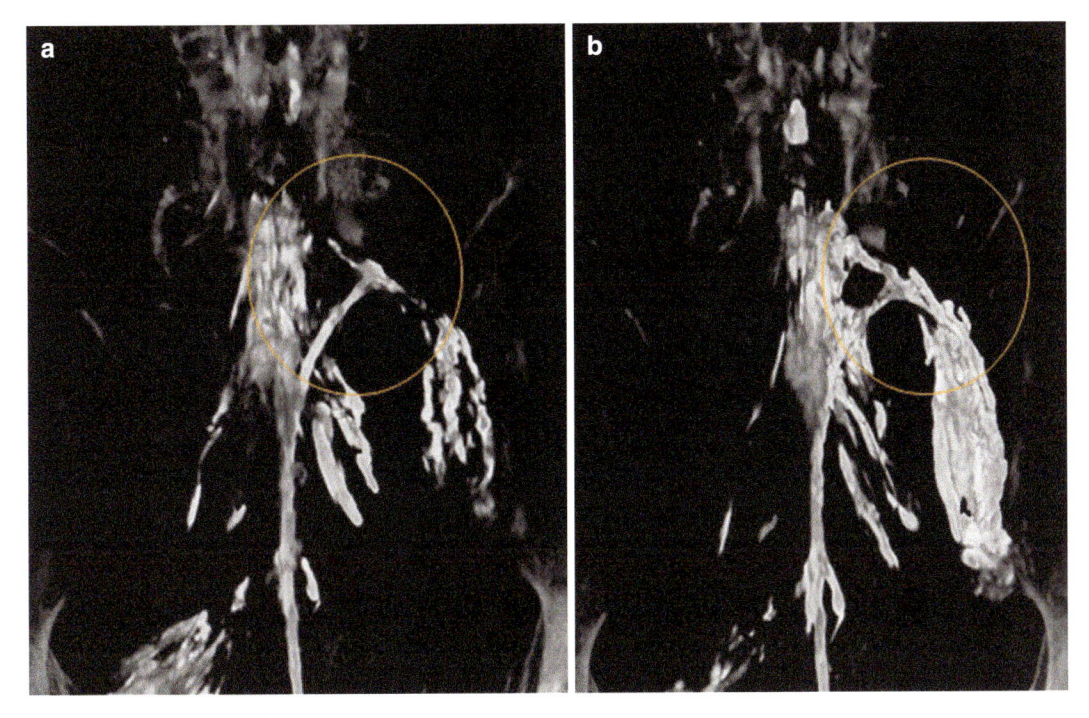

1.4 Theoretical and Academic Basis for Balloon Decompression

Fig. 1.19 (**a**) The spread of the contrast dye before balloon decompression. (**b**) The spread of the contrast dye after the balloon decompression with the ZiNeu catheter. The volume of the spread increased significantly across the procedure. Circle: Intervertebral foramen area

F/69, 2 years later

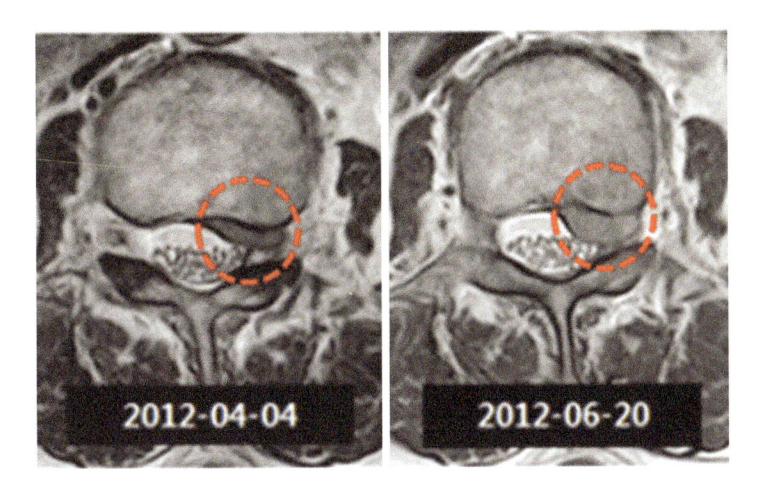

Fig. 1.20 A 69-year-old female patient experienced no pain after a single round of transforaminal epidural block. Radiological images obtained at the 2-year follow-up showed the resolution of the disc protrusion

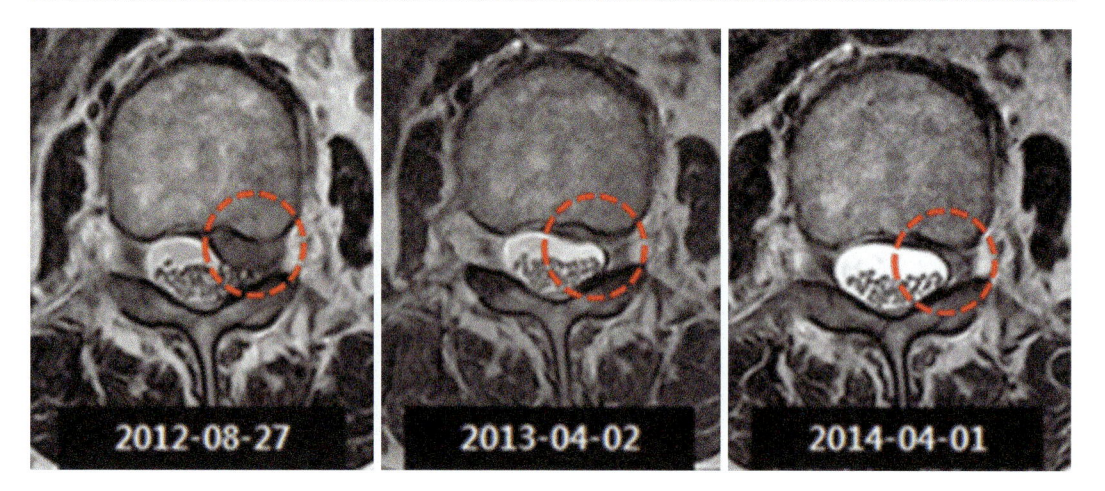

Fig. 1.20 (continued)

Fig. 1.21 A 68-year-old female patient experienced no pain after a single round of transforaminal epidural block. Radiological images obtained at the 1-year follow-up showed the resolution of the extruded disc

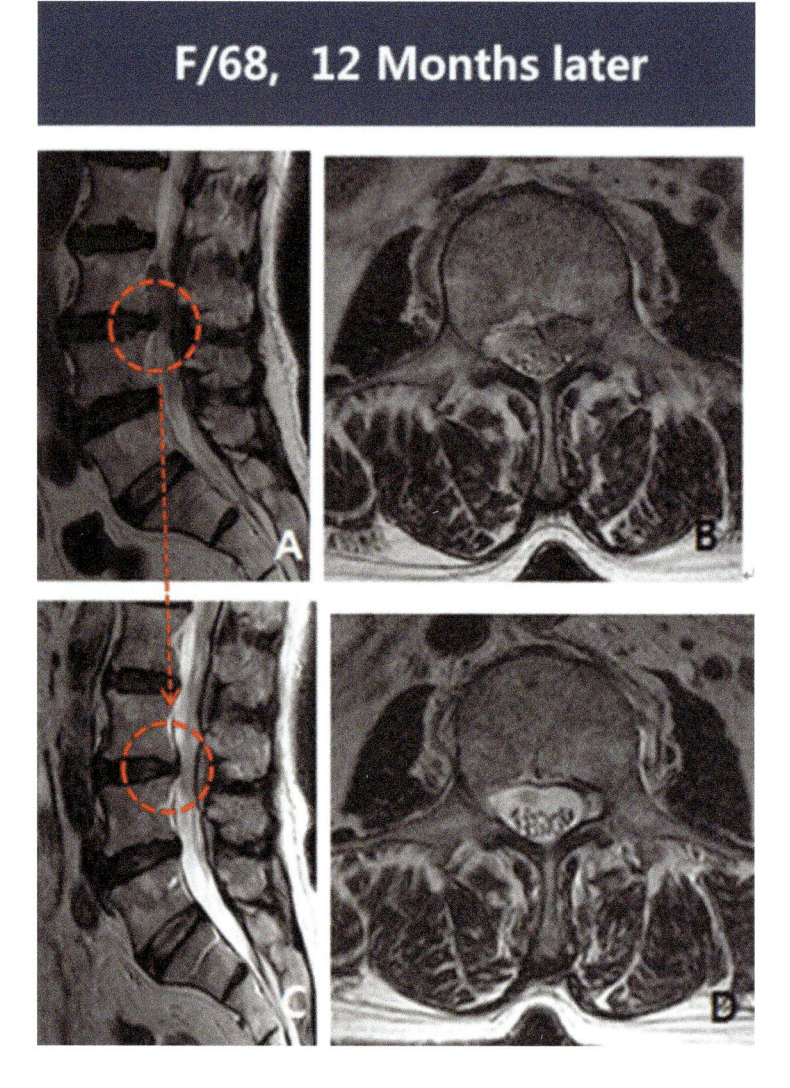

1.4 Theoretical and Academic Basis for Balloon Decompression

Fig. 1.22 A 44-year-old female patient. Radiological images taken at the 4-month follow-up after a single round of transforaminal epidural block showed that the extruded disc had been resolved

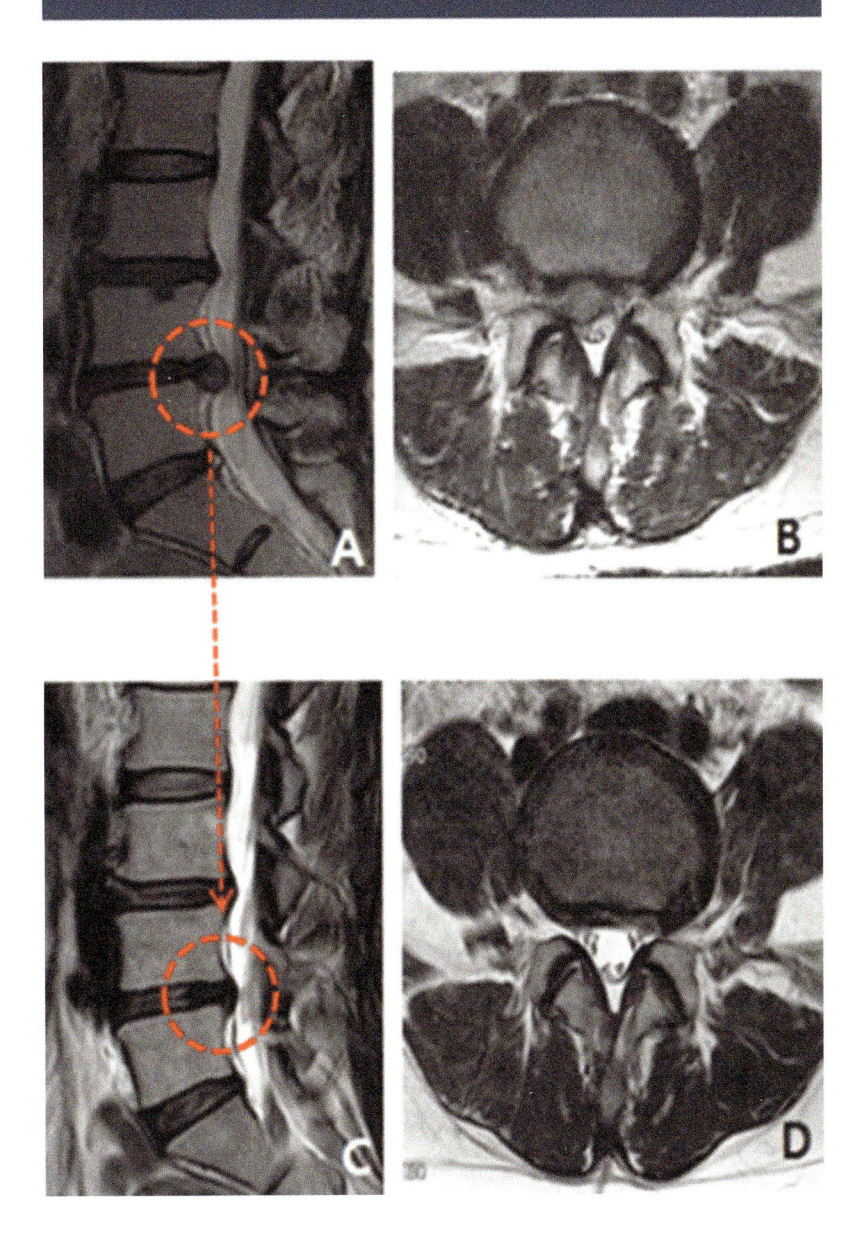

plasty performed with hypertonic saline has already gained recognition in the literature, injecting hypertonic saline following the attainment of a more accurate approach to the lesion and the removal of adhesion with balloon dilation instead of with the existing Racz catheter would undoubtedly be more effective than conventional neuroplasty.

1.4.6 Other Relevant Articles

Pain Physician 2017; 20:E841-E848 • ISSN 2150-1149

Retrospective Study

Factors Associated with Successful Responses to Transforaminal Balloon Adhesiolysis for Chronic Lumbar Foraminal Stenosis: A Retrospective Study

Doo Hwan Kim, MD[1], Seong-Sik Cho, MD[2,3], Yeon-Jin Moon, MD[1], Koo Kwon, MD[1], Kunhee Lee, MD[1], Jeong-Gil Leem, MD, PhD[1], Jin-Woo Shin, MD, PhD[1], Ji Hyun Park, MD[4], and Seong-Soo Choi, MD, PhD[1]

A retrospective analysis of 199 patients with chronic lumbar foraminal stenosis that underwent transforaminal balloon adhesiolysis found an association between stenosis caused by degenerative disc herniation and good outcomes at 3 months following the procedure; i.e., patients with soft stenosis caused by disc herniation tended to respond better to treatment than did those with hard stenosis attributable to other factors. Hence, factors such as the patient's exact condition and its underlying causes should be considered when selecting balloon compression, and sufficient explanation should be provided to the patient and guardian(s) in cases of hard stenosis.

In order to establish the medical basis and the foundational procedural techniques of balloon decompression, we conducted a randomized controlled study from the initial stage of apparatus development. As aforementioned, the results of this study have been published in several renowned journals. However, because most of the published articles reported on procedures performed at Asan Medical Center, with which the author of this book is affiliated, the implications of these findings may meet with skepticism. While the author maintained objectivity by abstaining from data collection and statistical analysis—these were instead performed by Dr. S. S. Choi, who only performed procedures and did not directly participate in their development—doubt concerning the reliability of the aforementioned findings could persist. Hence, a subsequent multidisciplinary, multicenter study was conducted.

Journal of *Clinical Medicine*

MDPI

Article

Relationship of Success Rate for Balloon Adhesiolysis with Clinical Outcomes in Chronic Intractable Lumbar Radicular Pain: A Multicenter Prospective Study

Jun-Young Park [1,†], Gyu Yeul Ji [2,†], Sang Won Lee [3], Jin Kyu Park [4], Dongwon Ha [3,‡], Youngmok Park [3,‡], Seong-Sik Cho [5], Sang Ho Moon [6], Jin-Woo Shin [1], Dong Joon Kim [1], Dong Ah Shin [7,*] and Seong-Soo Choi [1,*]

1.4 Theoretical and Academic Basis for Balloon Decompression

Including a study population of 317 patients, this study features a collaboration among numerous hospitals (Seoul Asan Medical Center, Yousei Severance Hospital, Himchan Hospital, Guro Cham Teun Teun Hospital, Yonsei Barun Hospital, Yonsei TheBaro Clinic, Seoul Sacred Heart General hospital) as well as among departments (anesthesiology and pain medicine, neurosurgery, and orthopedic surgery). The procedures were performed using the ZiNue catheter in the caudal epidural space, and changes in lower back and leg pain as well as the Oswestry Disability Index scores were recorded for 6 months following the operation. We published this study in *Journal of Clinical Medicine*.

The nature of multidisciplinary, multicenter studies risks variance in the procedural methods or tendencies of the participating institutions that could significantly influence the study outcomes. To minimize this possibility and maintain objectivity, the study was conducted in a novel way: once the target site of the operation was determined, balloon dilation was performed at every possible site. Upon the completion of the operation, the success or failure of the procedure was marked as shown in Fig. 1.23 by the operator directly for comparisons of procedure success rates and degrees of improvement: the operated area was marked with the letter "B" (balloon) if ballooning was achieved and with the letter "F" (fail) if not. The success rate of ballooning was then calculated based on the markings. Collected in this manner for the first time in a procedure-related study, the data allowed for patient- and physician-associated factors to offset each other and, as a result, helped to enhance its reliability and objectivity.

Similar to the observations of previous studies, when the success rate of the procedure was high—i.e., and when the success rate was ≥50%—long-term pain and functional improvements were demonstrably superior at the 6-month follow-up. However, when the success rate was <50%, the rate of improvement tended to decrease over time (Fig. 1.24).

The analysis of MRI findings showed no statistically significant association between the degree of stenosis and the success rate of the procedure—i.e., the severity of stenosis did not decrease the success rate of the operation and thus could not account for the aforementioned results. Hence, regardless of the degree of stenosis, the success rate of the procedure was found to influence the level and sustainment of symptom attenuation.

In conclusion, the multicenter study of 317 patients demonstrated that balloon decompression achieved sustained, superior effects across 6 months. However, these 6-month outcomes were only observed in cases of a success rate of ≥50%. It is paramount that the operative team makes their best effort to perform a successful procedure in the lesion area.

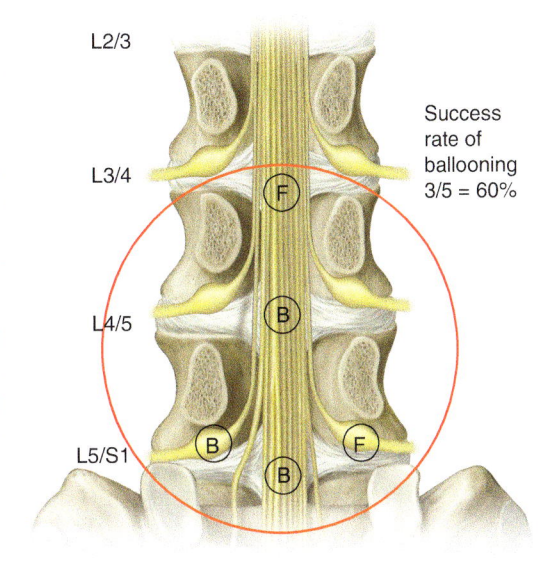

Fig. 1.23 Example of markings indicating the success or failure of the procedure. Target areas were set around the site of the procedure in every patient and were marked based on successful ballooning (B) and failed ballooning (F). The markings were then used to calculate the success rate

Fig. 1.24 Changes in lower back pain, leg pain, and ODI according to the success rate of balloon decompression. When the success rate of balloon decompression was ≥50%, continued improvement was observed for over 6 months. (**a**) Lower back pain. (**b**) Leg pain. (**c**) Oswestry Disability Index (ODI). ** $P < 0.01$ vs. baseline. *** $P < 0.001$ vs. baseline. † $P < 0.05$ vs. <50% group at each time point. †† $P < 0.01$ vs. <50% group at each time point. ††† $P < 0.001$ vs. <50% group at each time point. The data are presented as estimated mean ± 95% confidence interval

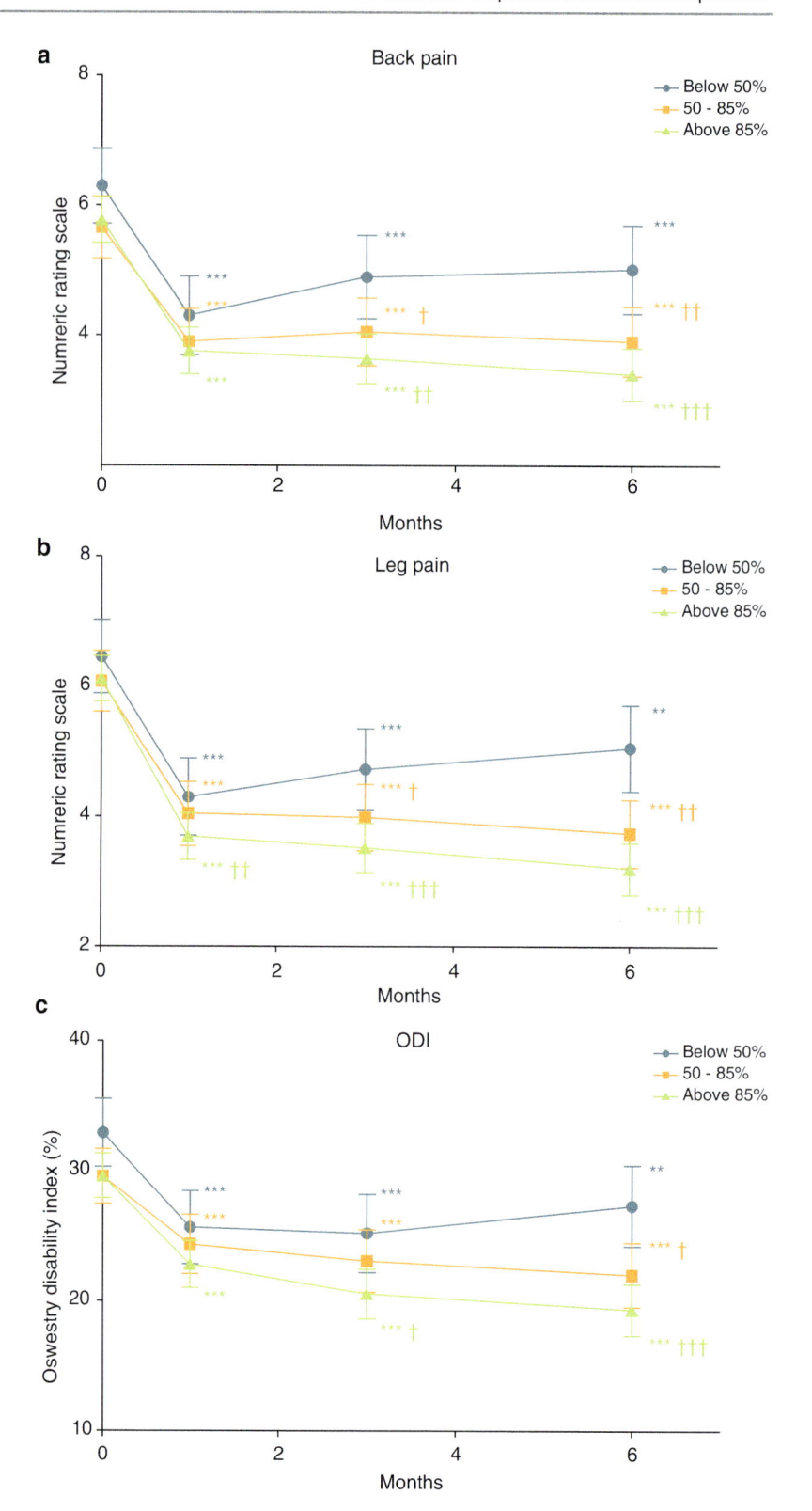

1.4 Theoretical and Academic Basis for Balloon Decompression

> Pain Physician 2018; 21:593-605 • ISSN 1533-3159
>
> **Randomized Trial**
>
> ### Percutaneous Epidural Adhesiolysis Using Inflatable Balloon Catheter and Balloon-less Catheter in Central Lumbar Spinal Stenosis with Neurogenic Claudication: A Randomized Controlled Trial
>
> Myong-Hwan Karm, MD[1], Seong-Soo Choi, MD, PhD[2], Doo-Hwan Kim, MD[2], Jun-Young Park, MD[2], Sukyung Lee, MD[2], Jin Kyu Park, MD[3], Young joong Suh, MD[2], Jeong-Gil Leem, MD, PhD[2], and Jin Woo Shin, MD, PhD[2]

In a study of 60 patients with central spinal stenosis comorbid with neurogenic claudication, half of the participants received balloon decompression with the ZiNeu catheter, while the other half underwent neuroplasty with the Racz catheter.

Following the procedures, the patients were followed up for 6 months, and the findings were reported.

The investigation found that neuroplasty resulted in decreased degrees of improvements over time, whereas balloon decompression effected the sustained improvement of pain and motor function across the 6 months. In addition, balloon decompression was associated with a significantly higher level of satisfaction and successful responses than was neuroplasty (Fig. 1.25).

This direct comparison confirmed that balloon decompression is more effective and achieves a longer duration of sustained effects than does neuroplasty.

Fig. 1.25 Neuroplasty (Racz) tended to show decreased degrees of improvements over time, whereas balloon decompression (ZiNeu) achieved sustained improvements of pain and function across the 6 months. Prediction of values ±95% confidence interval. P values of interaction between group and time for back pain, leg pain, and ODI were 0.156, 0.001, and 0.074, respectively.
*$P < 0.05$ vs. baseline in Racz catheter group.
*$P < 0.05$ vs. Baseline in ZiNeu catheter group

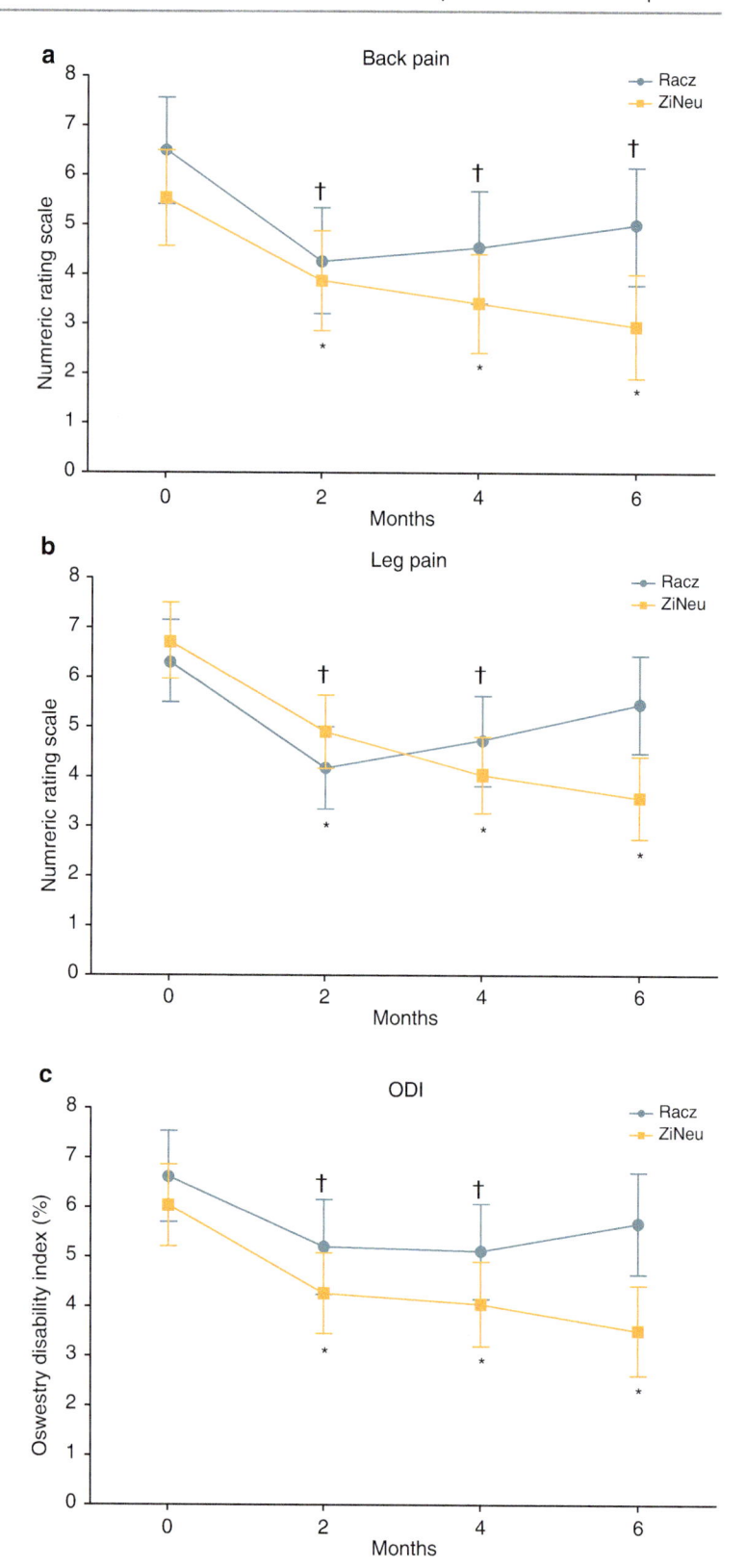

1.4.7 Published Case Reports

Other balloon decompression-related case reports that have been published include the following.

Reading these articles should help to facilitate understanding of this procedure.

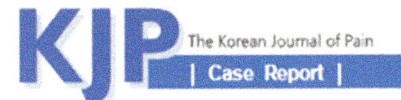

Korean J Pain 2012 January; Vol. 25, No. 1: 55-59
pISSN 2005-9159 eISSN 2093-0569
http://dx.doi.org/10.3344/kjp.2012.25.1.55

KJP The Korean Journal of Pain
| Case Report |

Clinical Experiences of Transforaminal Balloon Decompression for Patients with Spinal Stenosis

Department of Anesthesiology and Pain Medicine, University of Ulsan College of Medicine, Asan Medical Center, Seoul, Korea

Sung Hoon Kim, MD, Won Uk Koh, MD, Soo Jin Park, MD, Woo Jong Choi, MD, Jeong Hun Suh, MD, Jeong Gil Leem, MD, Pyung Hwan Park, MD, and Jin Woo Shin, MD

Case Report

Korean J Anesthesiol 2014 February 66(2): 169-172
http://dx.doi.org/10.4097/kjae.2014.66.2.169

Clinical experiences of performing transforaminal balloon adhesiolysis in patients with failed back surgery syndrome -two cases report-

Bo-Young Hwang[1], Hong-Seok Ko[2], Jeong-Hun Suh[1], Jin-Woo Shin[1], Jeong-Gill Leem[1], and Jae-Do Lee[2]

Department of Anesthesiology and Pain Medicine, [1]Asan Medical Center, University of Ulsan Collage of Medicine, [2]Veterans Health Service Medical Center, Seoul, Koera

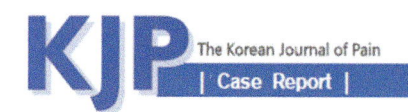

A Novel Balloon-Inflatable Catheter for Percutaneous Epidural Adhesiolysis and Decompression

Department of Anesthesiology and Pain Medicine, Asan Medical Center, University of Ulsan College of Medicine, Seoul, Korea

Seong Soo Choi, Eun Young Joo, Beom Sang Hwang, Jong Hyuk Lee, Gunn Lee, Jeong Hun Suh, Jeong Gill Leem, and Jin Woo Shin

1.5 Lecture Video of Epidural Balloon Decompression and Adhesiolsyis

A lecture video in ppt file format was prepared. This will help you understand the overall caudal and transforaminal approach of balloon procedure (Video 1.2).

In summary, while no existing nonsurgical treatment can directly alleviate spinal stenosis to the degree possible with surgical intervention, balloon decompression can secure free space and break adhesion to facilitate the delivery of therapeutic drugs to the lesion, thereby resolving blood circulation, pain, and functional problems such as claudication. In addition, although most existing nonsurgical treatment modalities are recognized for their short-term pain reduction effects, they do not induce lack long-term motor function improvements; by contrast, balloon decompression achieves long-term effects and improvements of motor function when used in tandem with neuroplasty and adhesiolysis, two therapeutic techniques that have already gained recognition in the literature.

Developed by the author, balloon decompression is a safe, highly effective therapeutic technique that is the first of its kind in the world to overcome the limitations of existing noninvasive procedures. In recognition of its safety and efficacy, this procedure has received the "New Medical Technology Certification" from the National Evidence-based Healthcare Collaborating Agency and was recognized by the Ministry of Health and Welfare Notification (number 2013–122) in August 2013. Currently, the ZiNeu got the CE certification and is awaiting US FDA. This new technique is expected to become a key procedure in clinical practices around the world.

Bibliography

Extraneous Knowledge 1

Extraneous knowledge 1   Spinal nerve

- Nerv root
- Dural sac
- Pedicle
- DRG
- Spinal nerve
- Extraforaminal zone
- Lateral recess zone
- Foraminal zone

Fig. E1 Intra-spinal anatomy

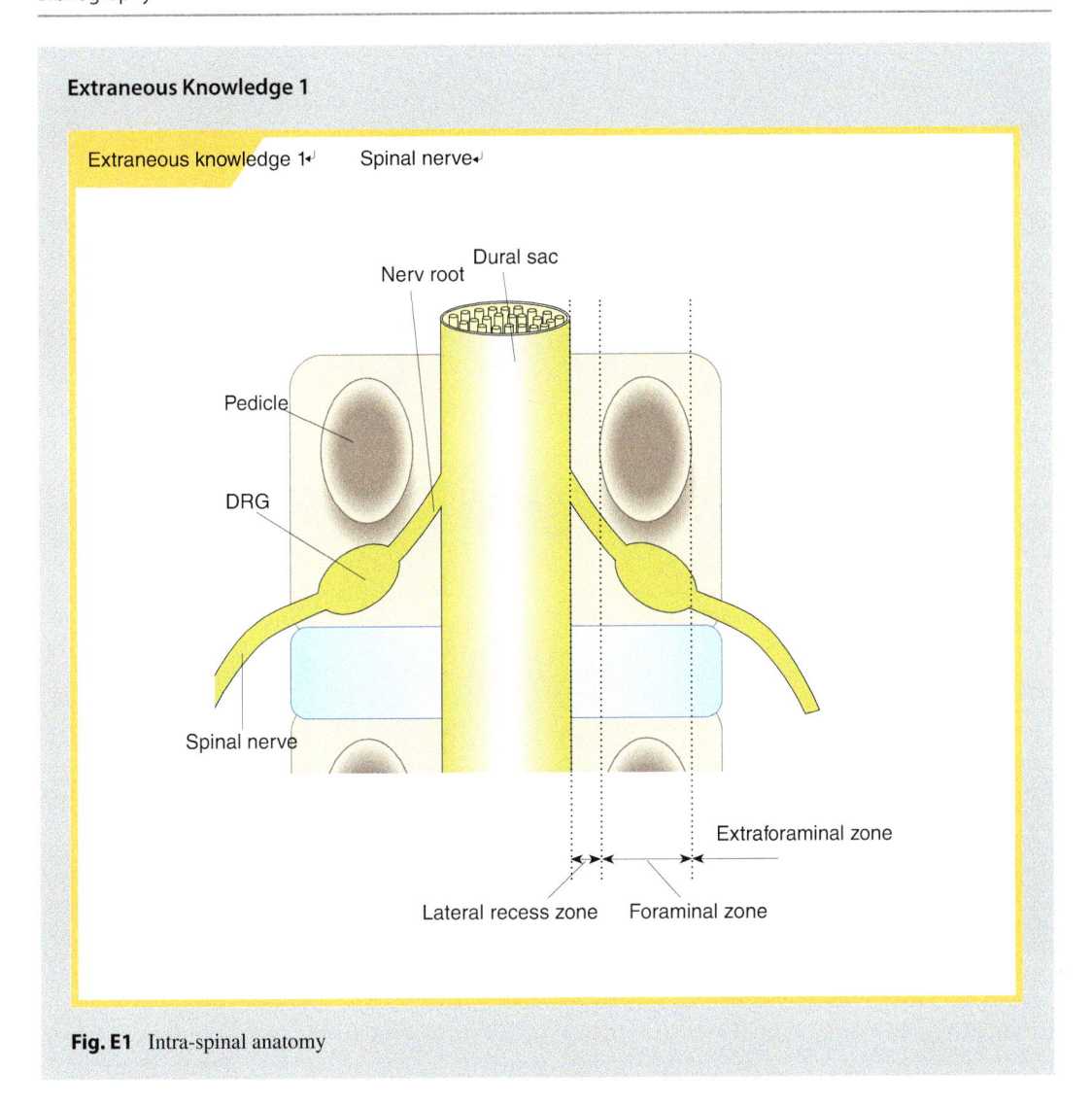

Bibliography

1. Basaran A, Topantan S. Spinal balloon nucleoplasty: a hypothetical minimally invasive treatment for herniated nucleus pulposus. Med Hypotheses. 2008;70:1201–6.
2. Bosscher HA, Heavner JE. Incidence and severity of epidural fibrosis after back surgery: an endoscopic study. Pain Pract. 2010;10(1):18–24.
3. Choi SS, Joo EY, Hwang BS, Lee JH, Lee G, Suh JH, Leem JG, Shin JW. A novel balloon-inflatable catheter for percutaneous epidural adhesiolysis and decompression. Korean J Pain. 2014;27(2):178–85.
4. Choi SS, Lee JH, Kim D, Kim HK, Lee S, Song KJ, Park JK, Shim JH. Effectiveness and factors associated with epidural decompression and adhesiolysis using a balloon-inflatable catheter in chronic lumbar spinal stenosis: 1-year follow-up. Pain Med. 2016;17(3):476–87.
5. Cooper RG, Freemont AJ, Hoyland JA, Jenkins JP, West CG, Illingworth KJ, et al. Herniated intervertebral disc-associated periradicular fibrosis and vascular abnormalities occur without inflammatory cell infiltration. Spine. 1995;20(5):591–8.
6. Erdine S, Talu GK. Precautions during epidural neuroplasty. Pain Pract. 2002;2:308–14.
7. Fritsch EW, Heisel J, Rupp S. The failed back surgery syndrome: reasons, intraoperative findings, and long-term results: a report of 182 operative treatments. Spine. 1996;21(5):626–33.
8. Schutze G. Epiduroscopy, spinal endoscopy. Berlin: Springer. p. 22–3.

9. Hammer M, Doleys DM, Chung OY. Transforaminal ventral epidural adhesiolysis. Pain Physician. 2001;4(3):273–9.
10. Harrington JF, Messier AA, Hoffman L, Yu E, Dykhuizen M, Barker K. Physiological and behavioral evidence for focal nociception induced by epidural glutamate infusion in rats. Spine. 2005;30(6):606–12.
11. Hong SJ, Kim DY, Kim H, Kim S, Shin KM, Kang SS. Resorption of massive lumbar disc herniation on MRI treated with epidural steroid injection: a retrospective study of 28 cases. Pain Physician. 2016;19(6):381–8.
12. Hoyland JA, Freemont AJ, Jayson MI. Intervertebral foramen venous obstruction. A cause of periradicular fibrosis? Spine. 1989;14(6):558–68.
13. Hwang BY, Ko HS, Suh JH, Shin JW, Leem JG, Lee JD. Clinical experiences of performing transforaminal balloon adhesiolysis in patients with failed back surgery syndrome: two cases report. Korean J Anesthesiol. 2014;66(2):169–72.
14. Joo EY, Koh WU, Choi SS, Choi JH, Ahn HS, Yun HJ, Shin JW. Efficacy of adjuvant 10% hypertonic saline in transforaminal epidural steroid injection: a retrospective analysis. Pain Physician. 2017;20(1):E107–14.
15. Kim KD, Wang JC, Robertson DP, Brodke DS, Olson EM, Duberg AC, et al. Reduction of radiculopathy and pain with Oxiplex/SP gel after laminectomy, laminotomy, and discectomy: a pilot clinical study. Spine. 2003;28(10):1080–7; discussion 7–8.
16. Kim DH, Cho SS, Moon YJ, Kwon K, Lee K, Leem JG, Shin JW, Park JH, Choi SS. Factors associated with successful responses to transforaminal balloon adhesiolysis for chronic lumbar foraminal stenosis: retrospective study. Pain Physician. 2017;20(6):E841–8.
17. King JS, Jewett DL, Sundberg HR. Differential blockade of cat dorsal root C fibers by various chloride solutions. J Neurosurg. 1972;36:569–83.
18. Kobayashi S, Shizu N, Suzuki Y, Asai T, Yoshizawa H. Changes in nerve root motion and intraradicular blood flow during an intraoperative straight-leg-raising test. Spine. 2003;28(13):1427–34.
19. Kuslich SD, Ulstrom CL, Michael CJ. The tissue origin of low back pain and sciatica: a report of pain response to tissue stimulation during operations on the lumbar spine using local anesthesia. Orthop Clin North Am. 1991;22(2):181–7.
20. Manchikanti L, Pampati V, Bakhit CE, Pakanati RR. Non-endoscopic and endoscopic Adhesiolysis in post-lumbar laminectomy syndrome. Pain Physician. 1999;2(3):52–8.
21. Massie JB, Huang B, Malkmus S, Yaksh TL, Kim CW, Garfin SR, et al. A preclinical post laminectomy rat model mimics the human post laminectomy syndrome. J Neurosci Methods. 2004;137(2):283–9.
22. Massie JB, Schimizzi AL, Huang B, Kim CW, Garfin SR, Akeson WH. Topical high molecular weight hyaluronan reduces radicular pain post laminectomy in a rat model. Spine J. 2005;5(5):494–502.
23. Matsuka Y, Spigelman I. Hyperosmolar solutions selectively block action potentials in rat myelinated sensory fibers: implications for diabetic neuropathy. J Neurophysiol. 2004;91:48–56.
24. McCarron RF, Wimpee MW, Hudkins PG, Laros GS. The inflammatory effect of nucleus pulposus. A possible element in the pathogenesis of low-back pain. Spine. 1987;12(8):760–4.
25. Parke WW, Watanabe R. Adhesions of the ventral lumbar dura. An adjunct source of discogenic pain? Spine. 1990;15(4):300–3.
26. Richardson J, McGurgan P, Cheema S, Prasad R, Gupta S. Spinal endoscopy in chronic low back pain with radiculopathy. A prospective case series. Anaesthesia. 2001;56(5):454–60.
27. Ross JS, Robertson JT, Frederickson RC, Petrie JL, Obuchowski N, Modic MT, et al. Association between peridural scar and recurrent radicular pain after lumbar discectomy: magnetic resonance evaluation. ADCON-L European Study Group. Neurosurgery. 1996;38(4):855–61; discussion 61-3.
28. Rydevik BL. The effects of compression on the physiology of nerve roots. J Manipulative Physiol Ther. 1992;15(1):62–6.
29. Shah RV, Ericksen JJ, Lacerte M. Interventions in chronic pain management. 2. New frontiers: invasive nonsurgical interventions. Arch Phys Med Rehabil. 2003;84(3 Suppl 1):S39–44.
30. Shah RV, Heavner JE. Recognition of the subarachnoid and subdural compartments during epiduroscopy: two cases. Pain Pract. 2003;3(4):321–5.
31. Songer MN, Ghosh L, Spencer DL. Effects of sodium hyaluronate on peridural fibrosis after lumbar laminotomy and discectomy. Spine. 1990;15(6):550–4.
32. Trescot AM, Chopra P, Abdi S, Datta S, Schultz DM. Systematic review of effectiveness and complications of adhesiolysis in the management of chronic spinal pain: an update. Pain Physician. 2007;10(1):129–46.

Types of ZiNeu Catheters and Their Features

2.1 ZiNeu Series

The ZiNeu series catheters generally feature similar structures.

The contrast dye port used for balloon inflation is situated in the middle section of the main body of the catheter. The size of the balloon can be adjusted by connecting the 1 cc Luer lock syringe filled with the contrast dye to the port and injecting the contrast dye amount as needed.

A guidewire or an endoscope can be inserted through the guidewire/drug injection port at the front of the catheter's main body. The contrast dye and therapeutic drugs can also be injected through this port.

Each side of the main body has a drain/irrigation port that can be used during an endoscopic procedure. There is a lock switch on the rear portion of the main body that is used to lock the movement of the catheter tip. There are many instances where the handle that was pulled from side to side at the lesion needs to be released for inflating the balloon or injecting the drug. In such instances, the catheter tip might slip out from the lesion. If the handle must be released, the lock switch could be pushed up to lock the tip; this measure allows the procedure to be performed safely (Fig. 2.1).

- Guidewire/drug injection port.
- Contrast dye injection port for balloon inflation.
- Lock.
- Drain/irrigation port.

Each catheter has the following features.

2.1.1 ZiNeu01

This catheter has an outer diameter of 2.3 mm. As the catheter lacks an articulated tip, it bends. This property renders adoption of a foraminal approach with this catheter more difficult than with other products with an articulated tip; however, this catheter offers greater strength, facilitating penetration into the intervertebral foramen and the detachment of adhesion. This catheter would be suitable for experienced operators who are highly competent in controlling the direction of the catheter (Fig. 2.2) (Video 2.1).

2.1.2 ZiNeuS

This catheter has an outer diameter of 2.3 mm and an articulated tip. It can be used together with a 0.9 mm endoscope. The articulated tip of the catheter facilitates the foraminal approach and induces less pain during the procedure. However, because this catheter is weaker than the ZiNeu01 catheter, which does not have an articulated tip, the force penetrating the intervertebral foramen may be relatively weak (Fig. 2.3).

Electronic Supplementary Material The online version of this chapter (https://doi.org/10.1007/978-981-15-7265-4_2) contains supplementary material, which is available to authorized users.

© Springer Nature Singapore Pte Ltd. 2021
J. W. Shin, *Spinal Epidural Balloon Decompression and Adhesiolysis*,
https://doi.org/10.1007/978-981-15-7265-4_2

Fig. 2.1 Description of the main body and structure of the ZiNeuS catheter

Guidewire/drug injection
Contrast dye injection port for balloon inflation
Lock
Drain/irrigation port

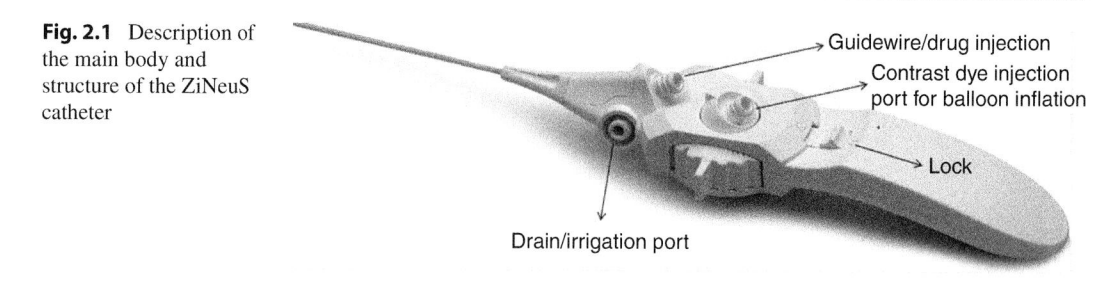

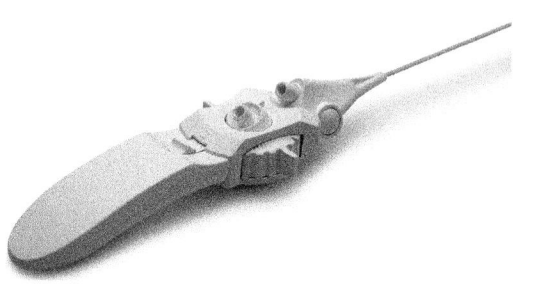

Fig. 2.2 An image of the main body of the ZiNeu01 catheter. The drain/irrigation port is blocked since it is not used for endoscopic procedures

2.1.3 ZiNeu02

This catheter has an outer diameter of 1.55 mm and an articulated tip. Since it is thinner than the others, it induces relatively less pain than its thicker counterparts during procedures. However, it is weaker than the 2.3-mm catheter. This catheter is suitable for young patients and when MRI findings indicate that the procedure will be simple (Video 2.2).

2.2 ZiNeuF Series

2.2.1 ZiNeuF

Although this is a thin 2F catheter, it is strengthened by a reinforcing wire. It is simple to operate and maneuver and is useful for approaching narrow spaces like the intervertebral foramen. Because it does not have a drug injection port, the drug must be injected with a needle after removing the catheter upon completion of the procedure. It

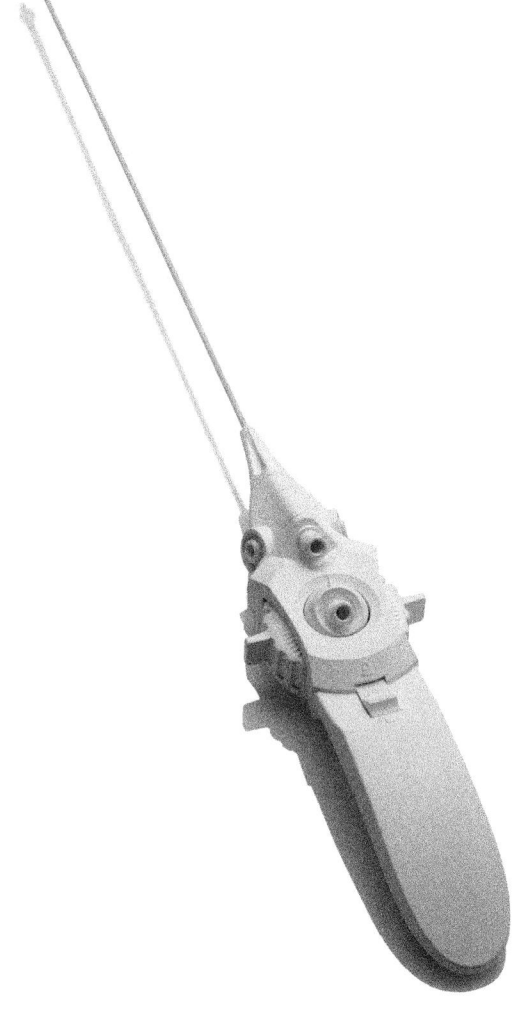

Fig. 2.3 The complete view of the ZiNeuS catheter with the balloon inflated

2.3 Differences Between Elastic and Inelastic Balloons

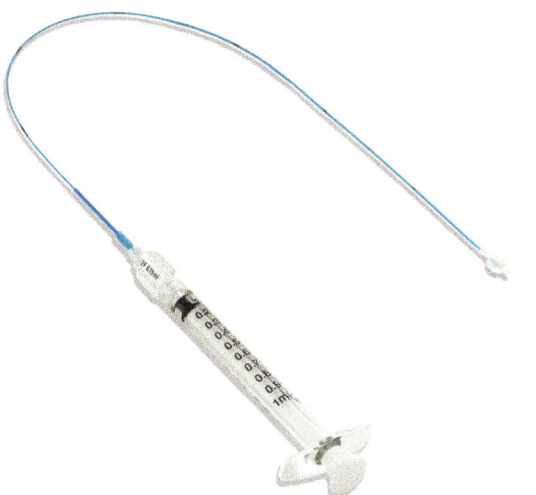

Fig. 2.4 An image of the ZiNeuF catheter with the balloon inflated

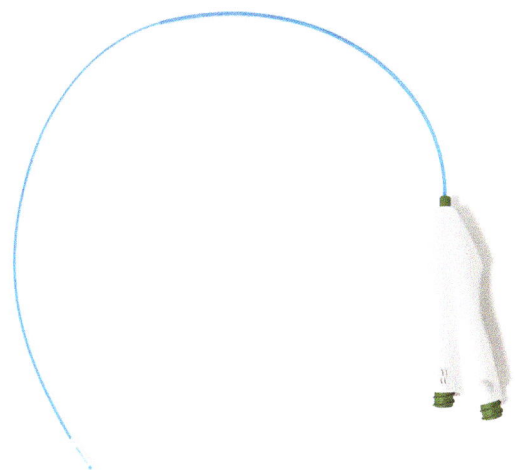

Fig. 2.5 An image of the ZiNeuF03 catheter

is suitable for use with transforaminal approach (Fig. 2.4).

2.2.2 ZiNeuF03

This slightly thicker 3F catheter features better strength and direction control relative to the ZiNeuF catheter. Because it has a drug injection port, drugs may be injected during the balloon procedure. The concept of adding the balloon dilation function to the Racz catheter informed the design of this catheter. It can be left in place for 2–3 days after the procedure to allow for additional performances of balloon dilation or drug injection. While it is used primarily for the caudal approach, it is also suitable for interlaminar (Fig. 2.5).

2.3 Differences Between Elastic and Inelastic Balloons

The materials for the balloon used in balloon catheters can be divided into two types: elastic and inelastic. The differences between the two include the following.

- When an inelastic balloon is deflated, its surface becomes wrinkled. Parts of the balloon may consequently come into contact with nerves when it is inserted; this can cause more nerve stimulation than when elastic balloons are used.
- Due to the nature of inelastic material, an inelastic balloon is limited in size, rendering it inappropriate for areas with varying degree of stenosis and adhesion. The objective of balloon decompression is to not only mitigate stenosis but also to reduce adhesion across the widest area possible. The effects expected from balloon decompression are more potent when areas with stenosis are alleviated to the greatest degree possible, and the areas with adhesion are expanded as far as possible. Using a small balloon with a fixed size offers no advantage over inserting a slightly thicker catheter.

2.3.1 Differences Between the Role of Elastic and Inelastic Balloons According to the Degree of Foraminal Stenosis or Adhesion

2.3.1.1 Cases of Mild-to-Moderate Stenosis or Adhesion

An elastic balloon can be inflated to its maximum size to achieve a relatively widespread alleviation of stenosis and adhesion, but an inelastic balloon cannot attenuate stenosis or adhesion in cases of

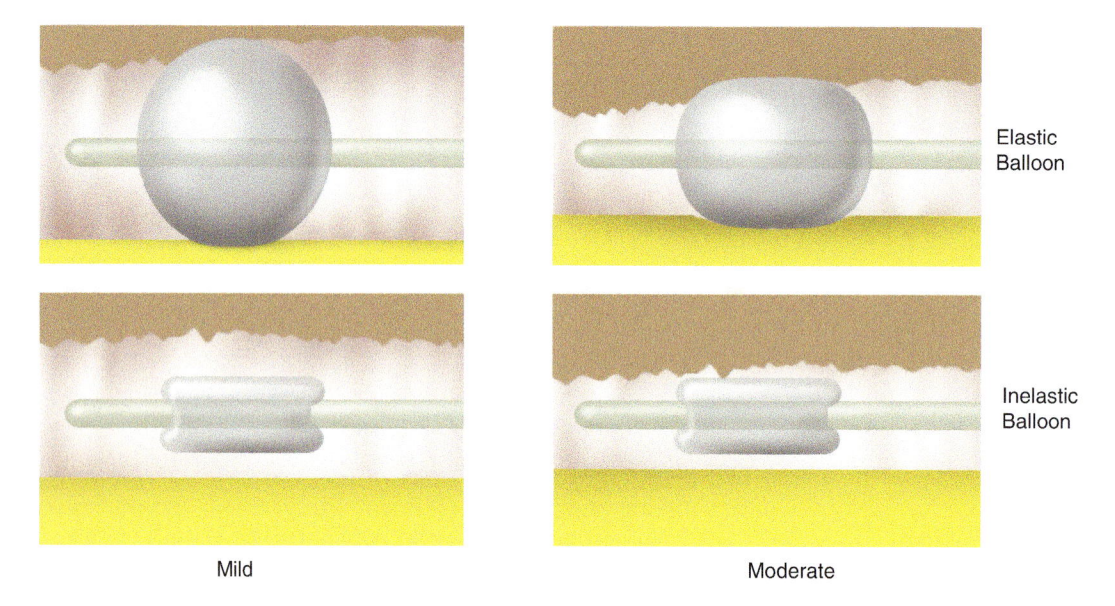

Fig. 2.6 Comparison between the elastic and inelastic balloons in cases of mild-to-moderate stenosis or adhesion. Because it is smaller, an inelastic balloon is less effective in alleviating mild-to-moderate stenosis

mild-to-moderate stenosis or adhesion due to its limited size. There is no difference as compared to inserting a slightly thicker catheter without a balloon and with an inelastic balloon (Fig. 2.6).

When using an elastic balloon, it is advisable to escalate the amount of injected contrast dye in a stepwise manner: from 0.05, through 0.1 and 0.2, to 0.3 cc. As long the patient does not complain of severe pain, inflate the balloon as far as possible when alleviating adhesion or stenosis; greater extents of inflation achieve greater levels of improvement. Balloon rupture is nonconsequential; hence, only the patient's pain need be considered during the procedure (Fig. 2.7). This method is impossible to perform with an inelastic balloon due to its size.

2.3.1.2 Cases Involving Severe Stenosis or Adhesion

An elastic balloon usually creates maximal space by expanding laterally in areas with severe stenosis. The application of excessive pressure applied to the balloon causes it to rupture, which precludes the exertion of excessive pressure onto the nerves. However, an inelastic balloon inflates only to a constant size without rupturing; as the pressure still rises in the balloon, however, the use of an inelastic balloon may induce nerve damage (Fig. 2.8).

The New Medical Technology Evaluation conducted by NECA recognized the safety of balloon decompression based on the fact that the balloon ruptures before the nerves are overly compressed. The confirmation of safety does not apply to an inelastic balloon. Because it does not rupture, a risk of severe nerve compression is present in cases with severe stenosis.

2.3.2 Differences Between the Role of Elastic and Inelastic Balloons in Cases Involving Central Stenosis or Adhesion

When performing spinal adhesiolysis with a conventional catheter lacking a balloon, the catheter tends to enter the same area following a previously made path. This prevents the detachment of adhesion from a wide area. Hence, using a balloon for detachment of adhesion from a wide area in a single round could be more effective and ultimately less time-consuming. In contrast with the use of a conventional catheter, the spinal canal must be widened as far as possible to achieve therapeutic effects when a balloon is used. However, a small and fixed balloon may not affect any differences relative to a moderately

2.3 Differences Between Elastic and Inelastic Balloons

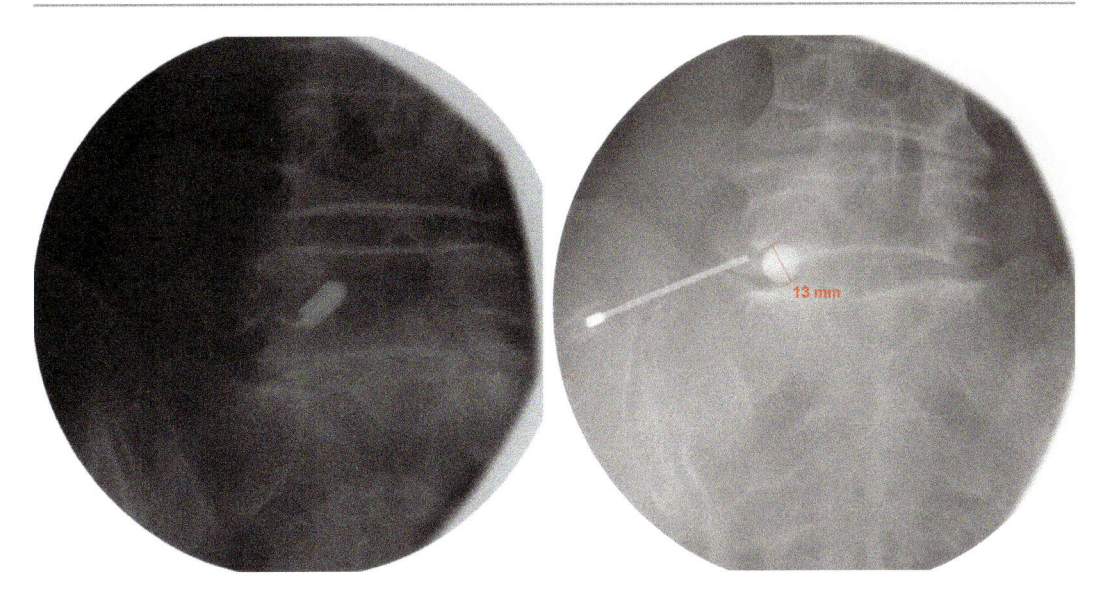

Fig. 2.7 An elastic balloon can provide widespread alleviation of an area with stenosis or adhesion by being inflated in all directions up to a diameter of ≥1 cm. It is impossible for an inelastic balloon to inflate to this extent

Fig. 2.8 Comparison between elastic and inelastic balloons in cases of severe stenosis or adhesion. Because an inelastic balloon does not rupture, pressure accumulates in the balloon. This may cause nerve damage in areas with severe stenosis

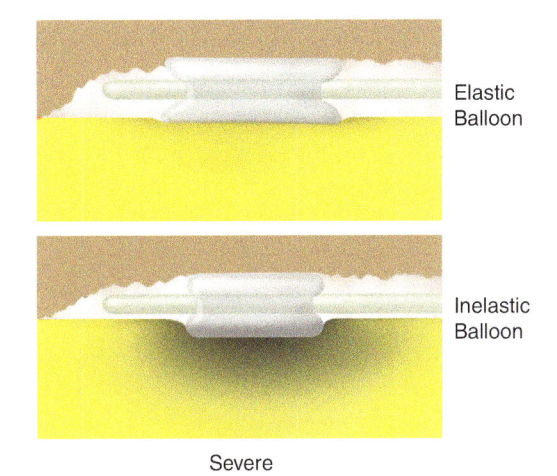

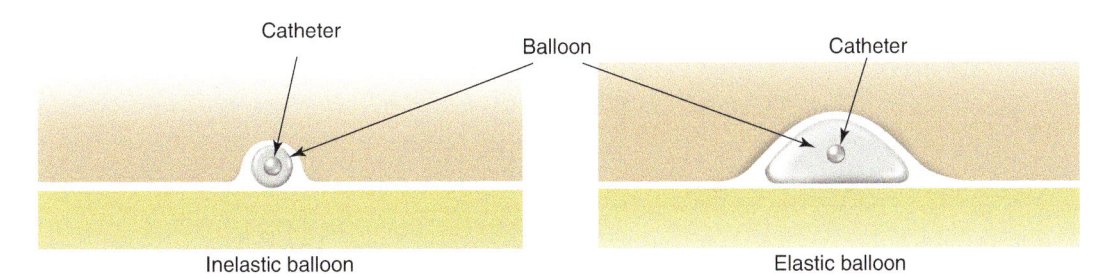

Fig. 2.9 Comparison of the width of the area treated by adhesiolysis between using inflated inelastic and elastic balloons. An elastic balloon is capable of removing adhesion from a much wider area

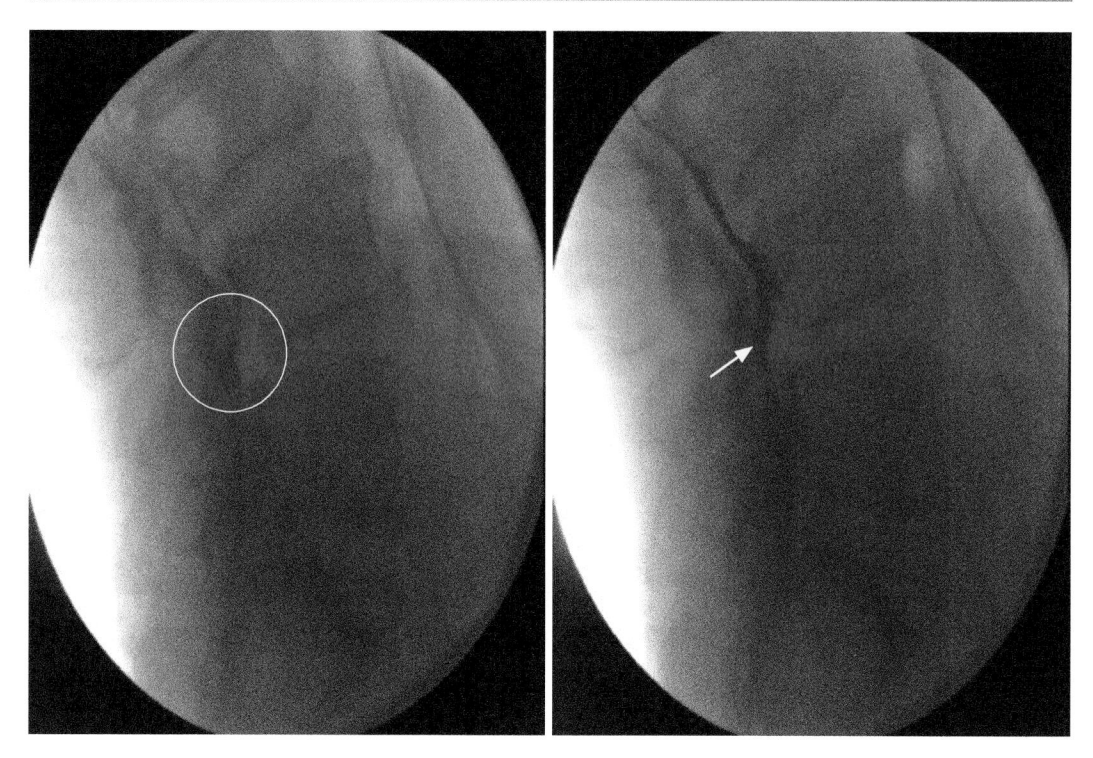

Fig. 2.10 Use of the ZiNeu catheter to perform the procedure on an area with spinal stenosis. Expansion of up to a diameter of 1.5 cm is possible. The expansion and removal of adhesion from a wide area are possible with just a single round of expansion. Circle: Inflated elastic balloon. Arrow: Contrast dye spreading after removal of adhesion

thick catheter that does not feature a balloon (Figs. 2.9 and 2.10).

Because of the large size of an elastic balloon, the height of dural lifting increases. When the drug is injected subsequently with the balloon extended in patients with severe disc extrusion, the drug can spread more efficiently due to the increase in space between the disc and dura (Fig. 2.11). This is another advantage of using an elastic balloon.

2.3 Differences Between Elastic and Inelastic Balloons

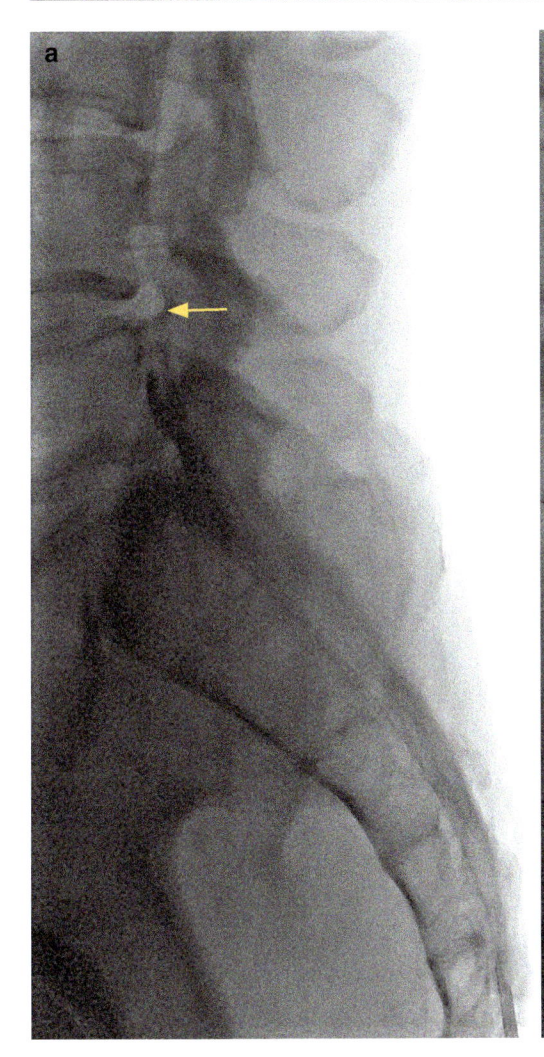

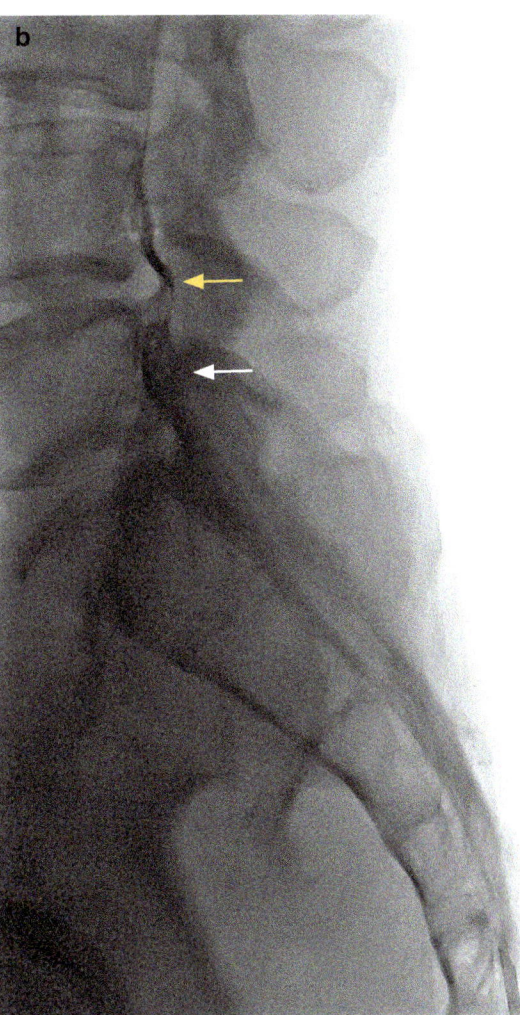

Fig. 2.11 (**a**) A case of the catheter being unable to gain entry and the contrast dye not spreading toward the head due to severe disc extrusion. (**b**) The drug injected with the increased space created between the disc and dura by balloon inflation. The contrast dye flows efficiently toward the head through the expanded space. Allowing for better drug spread is another advantage of using elastic balloons. Yellow arrow: Disc extrusion. White arrow: Inflated balloon

In Summary
1. In cases involving mild or moderate foraminal stenosis, central stenosis, or epidural adhesion, there is very little difference between using a catheter with an inelastic balloon and no balloon.
2. In cases of severe stenosis, an inelastic balloon could actually cause nerve damage due to excessive nerve compression. In the new medical technology certification process, a balloon that does not rupture presents a safety-related issue.
3. Rupturable, adjustable elastic balloons are appropriate balloons for balloon decompression.

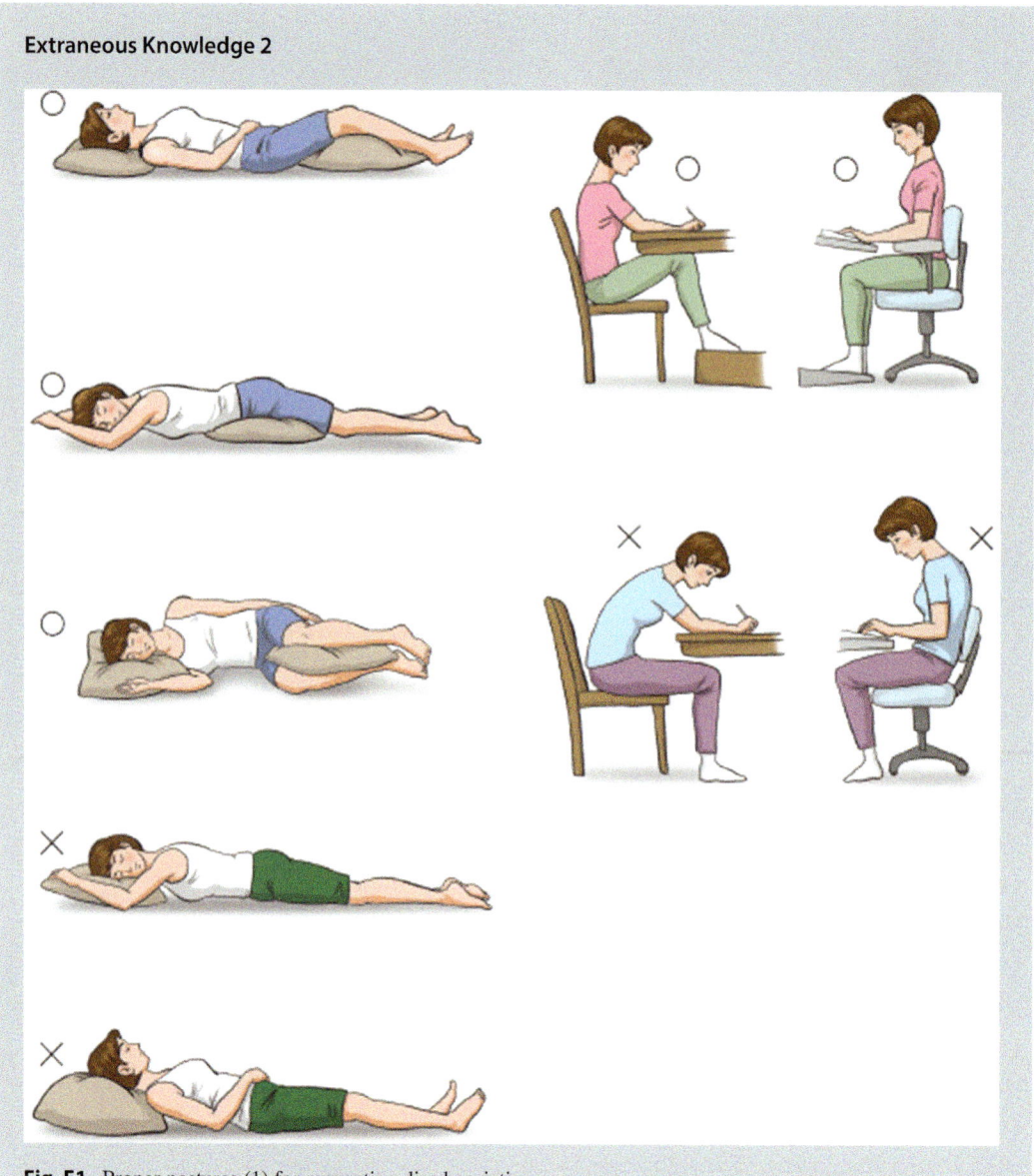

40 2 Types of ZiNeu Catheters and Their Features

Extraneous Knowledge 2

Fig. E1 Proper postures (1) for preventing disc herniation

2.3 Differences Between Elastic and Inelastic Balloons

Extraneous Knowledge 2

Important to maintain adequate lumbar lordosis

1. When standing
2. When sitting (chair)
3. When sitting (couch)
4. When lifting on object
5. When working while kneeling

Fig. E2 Proper postures (2) for preventing disc herniation

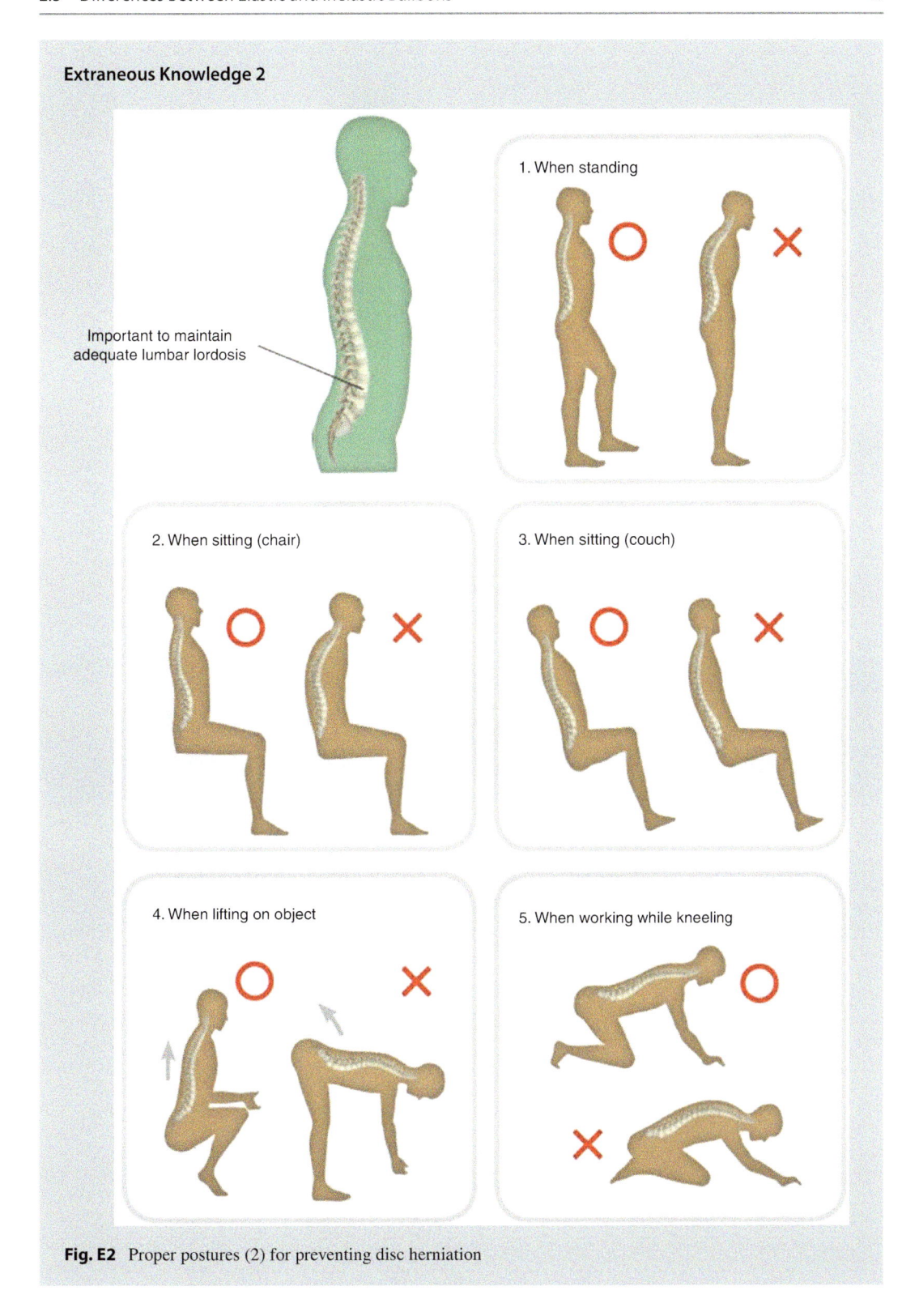

Pre-Procedural Preparation and Precautions

3.1 Before the Procedure

The preparation for the balloon procedure is the same as those employed for other invasive spinal interventional treatments.

1. The procedure for transforaminal or interlaminar balloon decompression using the ZiNeuF catheter is similar that of an epidural block and does not require the administration of antibiotics, but caudal balloon decompression requires the intravenous administration of antibiotics prior and subsequent to the procedure to prevent infection. The oral administration of antibiotics and analgesics for 3 days following the procedures is required.
2. Any medication for hypertension or diabetes taken prior to the procedure should not be discontinued.
3. Although the procedure does not involve general anesthesia, fasting for at least 6 h prior to the procedure is recommended in case of emergency.
4. The extensive vascularization of the epidural space increases the risk of bleeding during the procedure. While this is nonproblematic in most cases, the use of antiplatelets or anticoagulants should be discontinued according to the following guidelines before proceeding with the procedure because epidural hematoma may occur in rare cases. Balloon decompression falls under the category of "high-risk patients" (Table 3.1). When patients cannot discontinue their medication, it is recommended not to perform the procedure in the interest of their safety. The primary physician who prescribed the drug(s) should be consulted on whether it is safe to discontinue taking the drug(s) according to the criteria outlined above.

3.2 Drugs Used

While there are no differences in the drugs used during the balloon procedure and those used during neuroplasty or adhesiolysis, the selection of drugs varies between operators. In this section, the drugs usually employed by the author are introduced.

3.2.1 Dexamethasone

The effects of steroids within the epidural space are explained by various mechanisms, including the reduction of perineural inflammation, stabilization of neural cell membrane, inhibition of C-fiber activation, and reduction of edema. However, their efficacy and safety remain controversial. The pathophysiology of degenerative changes in the spine includes persistent compression or irritation of the spinal nerves that may impair microcirculation, restrict nutrient supply, and cause edema and inflammation. These

Table 3.1 Recommendations for the discontinuation of drugs according to the risk of procedure

Stratification of risk According to procedures		
Low Risk	Intermediate Risk	High Risk
- Peripheral nerve blocks - Joint injections - Sacroiliac joint block	- Neuraxial injections - Facet procedures - Viceral sympathetic blocks	- Spinal Cord Stimulator trial and implantation - Intrathecal Drug Delivery System implantation - Vertebroplasty - Epiduroscopic procedures - Epidural balloon procedures

Drugs	Low risk	Intermediate risk	High risk
	When to stop		
Aspirin	X	6days	6days
NSAIDs	X	1day - Ibuprofen 4days - Naproxen 10 days - Piroxicam	1days - Ibuprofen 4days - Naproxen 10 days - Piroxicam
Warfarin (Coumadin)	5days	5days	5days
Heparin	IV - 6h SC - 24h	IV - 6h SC - 24h	IV - 6h SC - 24h
LMWH	Prophylaxis - 12h Treatment - 24h	Prophylaxis - 12h Treatment - 24h	Prophylaxis - 12h Treatment - 24h
Fondaparinux (Arixtra)	42h(4days)	42h(4days)	42h(4days)

Drugs	Low risk	Intermediate risk	High risk
	When to stop		
Dabigatran (Pradaxa)	4days		
Rivaroxavan (Xarelto)	26h(3days)		
Apixavan (Eliquis)	30h		
Edoxaban (Lixiana)	Minimum 24h to 72h		
Clopidogrel (Plavix)	X	7days	7days
Prasugrel (Effient)	X	7-10days	7-10days
Ticagrelor (Brilinta)	X	5days	5days

consequences could induce a vicious cycle and adhesion/fibrosis. For example, while it is easy to think that disc herniation and the consequent compression of nerves would induce severe pain, muscle weakness or paralysis mainly would develop from the decline in nerve conduction. Familiar symptoms, such as pain or radiculopathy, occur when stimulation is applied to nerves that have been sensitized by perineural inflammation. Therefore, while steroids can effectively reduce inflammation in the epidural space, their employment in cases of chronic spinal stenosis without inflammation is inadvisable. In the past, triamcinolone was primarily used in the epidural space. While triamcinolone had reportedly achieved greater therapeutic effect in the epidural space than did dexamethasone, particulated steroids with large sized particle were later found to increase the risk of arterial embolization; hence, the use of non-particulated steroids with smaller particle size and less cohesion, such as dexamethasone, is now recommended.

As a reference, the injection of steroids into the epidural space could promote or exacerbate adhesion. Further of note, triamcinolone may promote adhesion to a greater degree than can dexamethasone.

It is recommended that therapeutic drugs be added to the injected steroid due to the extensive application of irritation during the procedure: 5 mg of dexamethasone is mixed with 1% lidocaine and 3 cc is injected into the intervertebral foramen and 4 cc is injected into the spinal canal. For patients with diabetes, the amount of steroid used should be reduced.

3.2.2 Lidocaine and Contrast Dye

When obtaining an epidurogram prior to the procedure, a 10 cc mixture of 1% lidocaine and contrast dye is injected into the epidural space. Lidocaine can help to reduce pain during the procedure and exerts what is believed to be a preemptive analgesic effect by diminishing pain for 2–5 days afterward. The operator should take care to prevent the local anesthetic from spreading to a blood vessel or the intrathecal area, as it could result in dangerous consequences. Therefore, approximately 3–5 cc of 100% contrast dye alone should always be administered to confirm the site of the epidural space. The epidurogram can be subsequently performed with the contrast dye/local anesthetic mixture.

As aforementioned, the 10 cc mixture of 5 mg of dexamethasone and 1% lidocaine should be divided into smaller portions to administer to the affected areas for therapeutic purposes after the epidural space is confirmed with 100% contrast dye.

While lidocaine tends to be regarded only as a local anesthetic, it is primarily used in the field of pain medicine as a neurotherapeutic drug. Local anesthetics not only inhibit pain transmission but also act as a potent blocker of sodium channels that modulate the pain pathway, promote muscle relaxation, and improve blood circulation by blocking sympathetic nerves in the epidural space. Therefore, if used properly, local anesthetics can achieve excellent pain reduction and therapeutic effects. In particular, they exhibit excellent efficacy in reducing hyperexcitability and nerve sensitivity. However, improper administration could lead to fatal complications in patients, including total spinal anesthesia, a drop in blood pressure, cardiac arrest, and loss of consciousness. Therefore, injecting the contrast dye to confirm the epidural space must be performed prior to administering the drug.

3.2.3 Hyaluronidase

Hyaluronidase is an enzyme that degrades hyaluronic acid and can thus be used to dissolve adhesion areas and enhance the effects of steroids. However, a review of various reports has shown that this drug may induce potential adverse effects and may not be cost-effective.

The author uses this hyaluronidase when performing an epidurogram at the beginning of the procedure or when adhesion is severe during the procedure; adhesion is attenuated 3–5 min subsequent to the injection of the drug, rendering previously impeded entry and the administration of the catheter possible. Accordingly, the selective use of hyaluronidase is recommended when it is difficult to proceed with the procedure due to severe adhesion.

3.2.4 Normal Saline

Irrigation with normal saline is often used in endoscopic adhesiolysis procedures to secure the field of view (FOV), alleviate adhesion with hydraulic pressure, and remove pain-related substances. The amount of irrigation is reportedly proportional to the level of improvement in patients. However, the operator should be cautious: excessive amounts of normal saline could cause various complications, such as increased intracranial pressure and intraocular hemorrhage.

The evidence for the ability of saline irrigation to remove pain-related substance is lacking. While irrigation with normal saline can indeed attenuate adhesion with hydraulic pressure, the effect may not be that significant. Moreover, if the balloon decompression procedure can directly alleviate stenosis or adhesion, the importance of effect of adhesiolysis by hydraulic pressure may not be low. Hence, the author does not perform aggressive saline irrigation. It is recommended that irrigation be applied to areas adjacent to the site of balloon adhesiolysis at which sufficient adhesion was not achieved. The author usually irrigates the intervertebral foramen with 5 cc of saline and the spinal canal with 10 cc of saline after balloon adhesiolysis. Consequently, there are very few cases in which ≥ 100 cc is used for irrigation. Even when an epiduroscope is used, the amount of saline necessary for securing an optimal FOV can be reduced with balloon dilation. In other words, balloon dilation can help to reduce the amount of normal saline irrigation, regardless of whether the saline is used for obtaining the FOV or therapeutic purposes.

3.2.5 Hypertonic Saline

Hypertonic saline
NaCl 1 mEq = 58.44 mg/mmol
5% NaCl: NaCl 50 mg/mL —>Na 0.855 mEq/mL
10% NaCl: NaCl 100 mg/mL —> Na 1.71 mEq/mL

The following method is used at Asan Medical Center for preparing hypertonic saline
NaCl 40 mEq/20 cc = 2 mEq/cc
NaCl content per 1 mL: 0.117 g/mL (11.7%)
Na content per 1 mL: Na—2.002 mEq/mL

 # 5% hypertonic saline 4 mL
⇒ (0.855 mEq/mL × 4 mL)/2 mEq/mL = 1.71 mL
1.7 mL (NaCl 40 mEq sol) + distilled water
2.3 mL = 4 mL

 # 10% hypertonic saline 4 mL
⇒ (1.71 mEq/mL × 4 mL)/2 mEq/mL = 3.42 mL
3.4 mL (NaCl 40 mEq sol) + distilled water
0.6 mL = 4 mL

: Instead of distilled water, local anesthetic and steroid can be used for dilution

The injection of hypertonic saline may cause severe pain. Anesthesia should therefore be performed first with 1% lidocaine at a slightly higher dose than that used for the hypertonic saline, which is to be administered after confirming the site of the epidural space with the contrast dye. Approximately 2–4 cc of the hypertonic saline should then be injected into each area. The author administers hypertonic saline with steroids during the final round of drug administration: The hypertonic saline is diluted to the desired concentration by mixing it with the steroid according to the aforementioned method, and the injection is then administered. If hypertonic saline is injected after the steroid has been administered, the steroid may be washed away; hence, the steroid is typically used only in the final injection.

Hypertonic saline is the primary therapeutic agent used during neuroplasty. Leaving the drug-injection epidural catheter in place after the balloon procedure and administering hypertonic saline through the catheter for 2–3 days would be equivalent to performing neuroplasty together with balloon decompression and adhesiolysis; both maximize the effect of the pharmacotherapy. This option should be considered, especially in patients who show a tendency to develop neuropathic pain or complain of severe pain.

While various reports of the attenuation of spinal stenosis or post-spinal surgery pain with hypertonic saline have engendered the belief that hypertonic saline reduces adhesion and pain, no reports indicate hypertonic saline itself actually reduces adhesion. On the other hand, numerous articles have reported that hypertonic saline can reduce pain by various mechanisms; specifically, it can inhibit C-fiber conduction and reduce neuronal excitability by inducing hyperosmolarity and highly concentrated chloride content. It has further been demonstrated that hypertonic saline can reduce cell swelling and inflammation.

Even without neuroplasty, pain could be reduced by injecting hypertonic saline in the perineural area. Reports of the effects of administering hypertonic saline to patients with foraminal stenosis are described below.

Pain Physician 2013; 16:197-211 • ISSN 1533-3159

Randomized Trial

Transforaminal Hypertonic Saline for the Treatment of Lumbar Lateral Canal Stenosis: A Double-Blinded, Randomized, Active-Control Trial

Won Uk Koh, MD[1], Seong Soo Choi, MD, PhD[1], Seung Yong Park, MD[1], Eun Young Joo, MD[1], Sung Hoon Kim, MD[1], Jae Do Lee, MD[2], Jae Young Shin[3], Jeong Hun Suh, MD, PhD[1], Jeong Gil Leem, MD, PhD[1], and Jin-Woo Shin, MD, PhD[1]

3.2 Drugs Used

Fig. 3.1 Changes in numerical rating scale over time in the two groups. 0 = base line, *$P < 0.05$ vs. *baseline*, †$P < 0.05$ vs. *baseline*

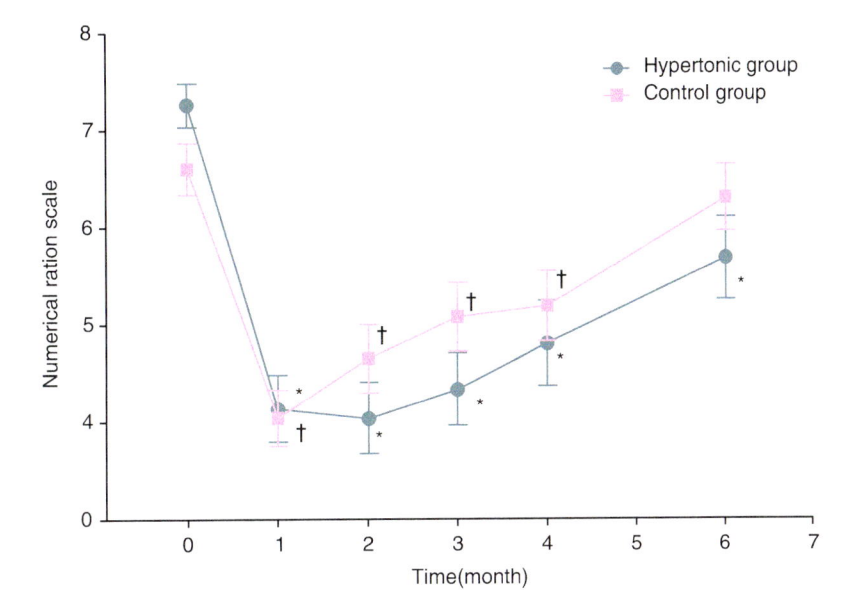

Fig. 3.2 Changes in Oswestry Disability Index over time in the two groups. 0 = baseline *$P < 0.05$ vs. *baseline*, †$P < 0.05$ vs. *baseline*

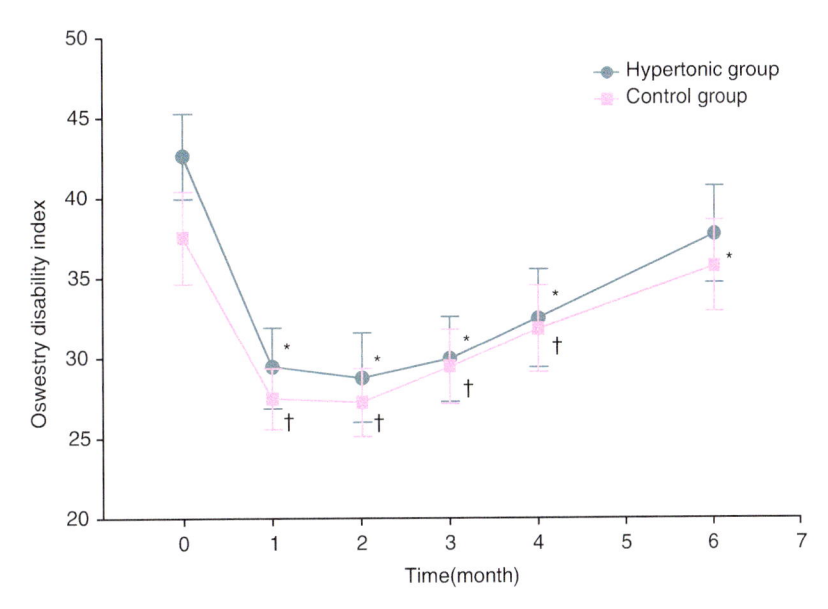

Among 53 patients with intractable lumbar lateral canal stenosis, 27 received 2 cc of 1% lidocaine via transforaminal epidural block followed by 2 cc of 10% hypertonic saline mixed with 20 mg of triamcinolone; 26 patients in the control group received normal saline instead of hypertonic saline.

Follow-up observations showed that pain attenuation was maintained for 4 months in the control group and 6 months in the hypertonic saline group, while improvement in the Oswestry Disability Index was maintained for 4 months in both groups. Comparison between the two groups revealed that the responder rate, the level of pain attenuation, and the Oswestry Disability Index were superior in the hypertonic saline group (Figs. 3.1, 3.2 and 3.3).

These results indicate that hypertonic saline itself could have a beneficial effect on pain, even if it is not used for adhesiolysis.

The intraneural injection of hypertonic saline could cause pain, tremor, and partial weakness,

Fig. 3.3 Comparison of the responder rate over time between the two groups. *P = 0.007, hypertonic* vs. *control. The data are presented as percentage (%)*

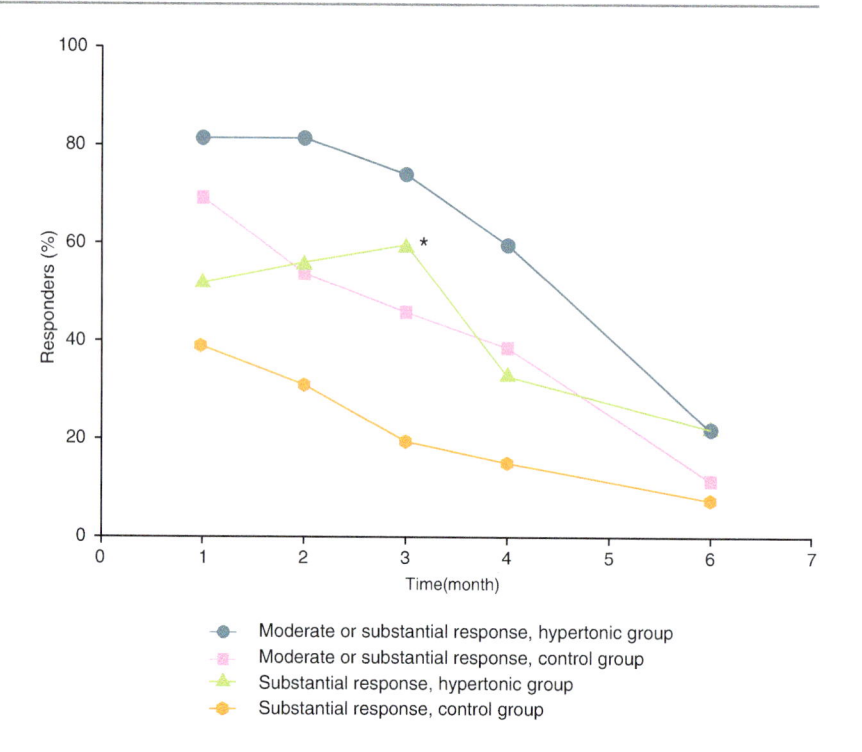

- Moderate or substantial response, hypertonic group
- Moderate or substantial response, control group
- Substantial response, hypertonic group
- Substantial response, control group

while an intrathecal injection of a large volume of hypertonic saline could cause serious adverse events, including arachnoiditis, hypertension, tachycardia, and pulmonary edema. Hence, confirmation of the correct site of administration using contrast dye is absolutely necessary before the drug is injected.

Moreover, only small volumes should be used.

Recently published articles have reported that 5% saline achieves a similar effect as does 10% while being safer. Dr. S.S. Choi from Asan Medical Center checked pain reduction in rats after different concentrations of saline were injected into their intrathecal spaces. The results showed that the injections of 5%, 10%, and 20% hypertonic saline produced excellent mechanical allodynia reduction and the extents of such effects did not differ significantly according to the concentration of saline. Accordingly, the use of 5% hypertonic saline is advisable: it is safer and causes less pain than using ≥10% hypertonic saline (Fig. 3.4).

3.3 Procedure-Related Precautions

3.3.1 Method for Preventing Balloon Rupture

Using a balloon that does not rupture could be dangerous, as it can exert excessive pressure on surrounding nerves. Therefore, the capacity of a balloon to rupture under excessive pressure is very important for the safety of the patient. Nevertheless, balloon rupture prior to the completion of the procedure could be frustrating. Accordingly, a method to safely inflate the balloon and prevent balloon rupture during the procedure is outlined below:

1. Whenever possible, using a sheath instead of a guide needle. Although inserting a guide needle may be simpler, microdamage to the balloon occurs often when the needle tip passes through it, which could increase the

3.3 Procedure-Related Precautions

Fig. 3.4 Injection of 5%, 10%, and 20% NaCl showed excellent mechanical allodynia reduction effect in rats. The extents of the effects did not differ significantly according to the concentrations used

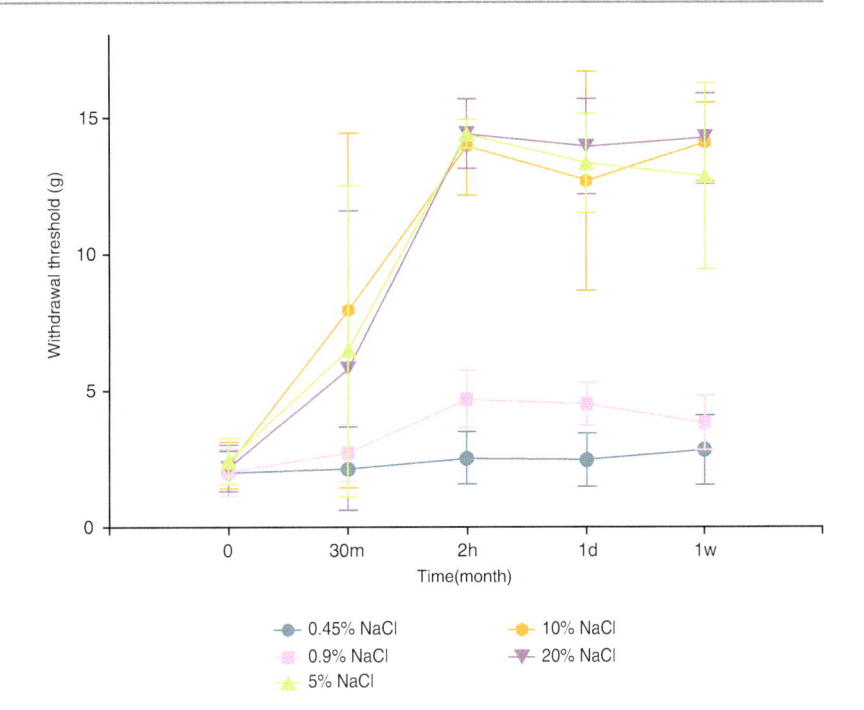

likelihood of rupture during the procedure. In particular, the balloon is often damaged by the needle tip when the catheter is withdrawn from the guide needle. If the use of a guide needle is unavoidable, then caution should be taken when passing the needle tip through the balloon portion of the catheter.

2. The author recommends the method of performing the procedure on the entire affected area by inserting the catheter into the affected area and slowly withdrawing it while repeating the process of inflating and deflating the balloon. If possible, reinsert the catheter to perform the procedure once more time in the affected area. It is important to increase the size of the balloon by inflating it in a stepwise manner: inflate the balloon slowly by injecting only 0.05 cc of contrast dye for the initial procedure and 0.1 cc of contrast dye for the second procedure. This allows the elasticity of the balloon to increase, and the widened area by the small balloon can reduce the pressure in the larger balloon of the next step, resulting in less bursting and less patient pain. If the balloon did not rupture and the patient's pain was not severe when the procedure was performed on the target area when 0.1 cc of contrast dye was used, then the size of the balloon could be increased by inflating it with 0.2–0.3 cc as long as the patient's pain is not too severe. Beyond this point, it does not matter whether the balloon ruptures or not. By increasing the size of the balloon in such a stepwise manner, the therapeutic effect could be maximized without balloon rupturing prematurely or inducing severe pain. When a balloon is inflated, it could rupture at any point. Balloon rupturing is not problematic since medical balloons do not leave any debris when they rupture.

3. When inflating the balloon, the contrast dye should be injected slowly to minimize the risk of rupture. Injecting the contrast dye rapidly could excessively increase the pressure in the balloon and rupture it, causing severe pain. Accordingly, it is recommended that the contrast dye should be injected slowly while the level of the patient's pain is monitored. If the level of pain is too severe, the injection should be terminated, even if all 0.1 cc has not been injected, and the balloon should be deflated after 2–3 s.

3.3.2 Method for Preventing Catheter Damage During the Procedure

Although rare, using a guide needle instead of a sheath could scratch or damage the catheter. In particular, there is a greater likelihood of damaging the catheter when it is withdrawn than when it is inserted due to the snagging by the needle tip. However, if a needle is used instead of a sheath, adopting the following method can help to prevent damage:

1. If possible, the guide needle should be inserted at an angle parallel to the epidural space. When employing a caudal approach, the guide needle should be inserted parallel to the caudal epidural space to minimize damage to the catheter during the procedure. When adopting a transforaminal approach, the needle should be inserted as flat as possible when gaining entry in the intervertebral foramen; this helps minimize resistance of the catheter during insertion and reduce the likelihood of damage to the catheter.
2. When the catheter is withdrawn, it should be pulled slowly. If any resistance is felt, the bevel of the needle should be turned little by little to find the specific angle at which it can be withdrawn without resistance. If there is appreciable resistance despite various maneuvers, the needle should be withdrawn slightly to decrease snagging, or the needle and catheter should be removed together. If the catheter is withdrawn forcibly despite obvious resistance, the catheter may be scratched or may break, and a broken piece may be left inside the body. Caution should thus be taken when the catheter is withdrawn, especially when a guide needle is used.

3.3.3 Method for Preventing Injection into the Intrathecal Space

Extreme caution should be taken to prevent serious complications that may occur if the dura is punctured preceding or during the administration of local anesthetic or steroid. Dural puncture can be identified by referencing contrast findings.

Therefore, before injecting the drug into the affected area, the possible presence of dural puncture must be checked every time by injecting 2–3 cc of 100% contrast dye.

For further details, please refer to the section dedicated to dural puncture in Chap. 7.

3.3.4 Method for Reducing Pain During the Procedure

If the patient experiences a significant amount of pain during the procedure, pain unrelated to the lesion may persist for 3–10 days. Therefore, pain should be minimized as much as possible during the procedure. This can be achieved as follows:

3.3.4.1 Caudal Approach

1. Apply sufficient local anesthesia before inserting the guide needle. If pain is severe during needle insertion despite anesthesia, remove the stylet of the needle and inject an additional 2–3 cc of local anesthetic through the needle.
2. During pre-procedure epidurogram, mix lidocaine with the contrast dye to dilute the lidocaine to a concentration below 1% and perform epidural anesthesia. This level of anesthesia can reduce pain while maintaining the functions of motor and sensory nerves. Accordingly, it enables a provocation test—asking the patient whether the stimulation applied to the site of the procedure is the same area where the patient felt pain—and provides comfort to both the patient and operator.
3. When inserting the catheter into the caudal epidural space, the advancement of the catheter must be adjusted within the medial boarders of the bilateral sacral foramen. This approach helps to ensure that less pain is inflicted by avoiding the sacral nerve. Avoid excessively tilting the catheter laterally when inserting to prevent touching the sacral nerve that runs toward the sacral foramen, as this can cause unnecessary pain.
4. The catheter must be moved slowly and cautiously. Rough movement can irritate nerves and exacerbate pain.

5. Slight pain during the procedure is unavoidable, but if abnormally severe pain occurs, the procedure must be stopped, and the cause of such pain must be identified. Pain may be severe when an area with neurogenic inflammation is contacted, when tissue is damaged, or when the catheter irritate cauda equina fibers after dura puncture. Whatever its cause, abnormally severe pain can also cause postoperative pain; hence, the procedure should not be performed hastily or forcibly.

3.3.4.2 Transforaminal Approach

1. Apply sufficient local anesthesia before inserting the guide needle. If the patient's pain is severe during needle insertion despite the administration of anesthesia, remove the stylet of the needle and inject an additional 2–3 cc of local anesthetic through the needle. However, if the guide needle is inserted near the intervertebral foramen, this method should not be used. If the nerves are anesthetized from the local anesthetic being injected into the intervertebral foramen, nerve damage caused by the guide needle may not be recognized. Hence, caution is required when adopting the transforaminal approach.
2. If possible, the guide needle or sheath should be laid flat in the intervertebral foramen when gaining entry. This will help to prevent pain induced by nerve irritation when the catheter is inserted.

Extraneous Knowledge 3

Differences in contrast findings according to the position of the needle tip during transforaminal epidural block

The insertion of the needle into the intervertebral foramen often indicates a successful transforaminal block. However, because many cases often involve perineural adhesion inside the intervertebral foramen, positioning the catheter or needle closer to the spinal nerves could be important for allowing the drug to spread better to the affected area.

Figure **a** represents a case in which the contrast dye was injected with the needle having entered through the inferior aspect of the intervertebral foramen, rendering the filling defect near the spinal nerve visible. In Figure **b**, when the drug was injected in the same patient after the needle was inserted just below the pedicle—i.e., close to the perineural area—the drug spread well with no sign of filling defect. The drug spread more efficiently into the affected area in the case represented by Figure **b**.

When the needle is inserted through a safe triangle, the approach should be made as close as possible to the superior aspect of the intervertebral foramen—i.e., the area just below pedicle—to ensure that the drug spreads accurately into the perineural area.

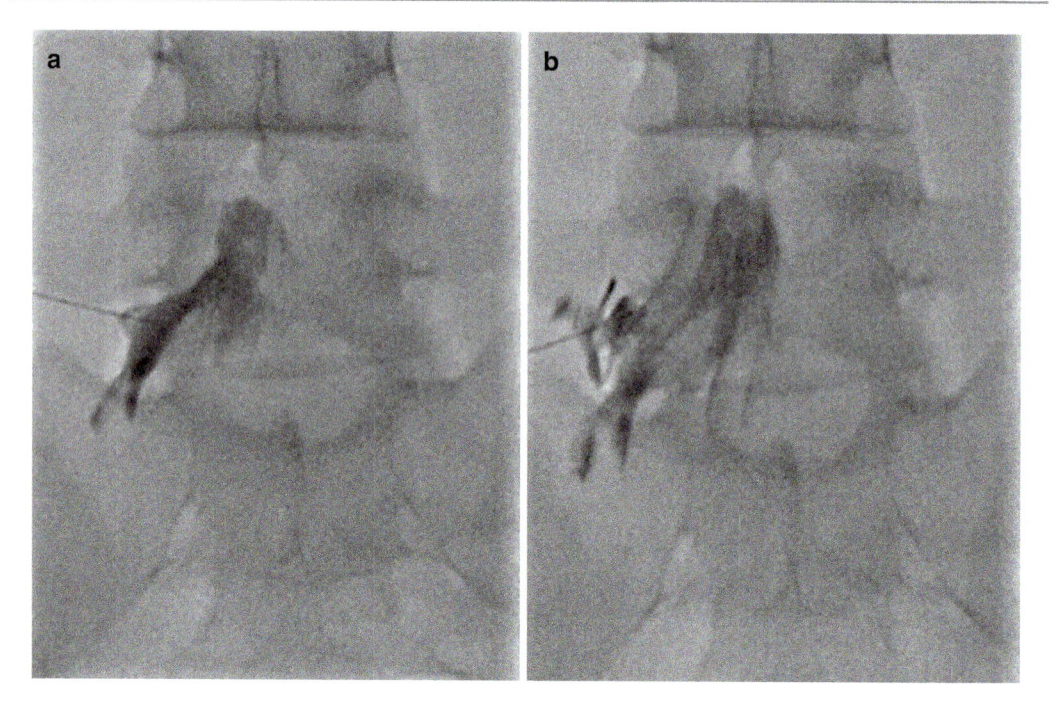

Fig. E1 Differences in contrast findings according to the position of the needle tip. (**a**) The needle inserted into the inferior aspect of the intervertebral foramen. (**b**) The needle inserted into the superior aspect of the intervertebral foramen

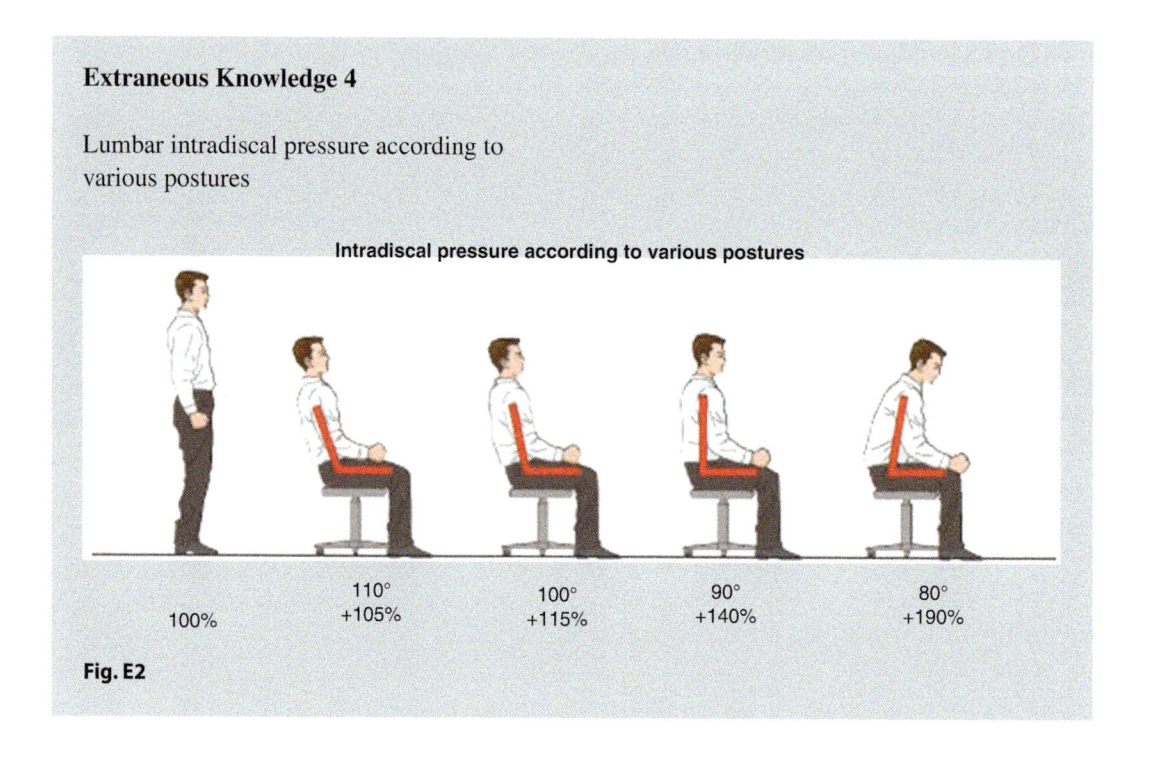

Extraneous Knowledge 4

Lumbar intradiscal pressure according to various postures

Intradiscal pressure according to various postures

100%	110° +105%	100° +115%	90° +140%	80° +190%

Fig. E2

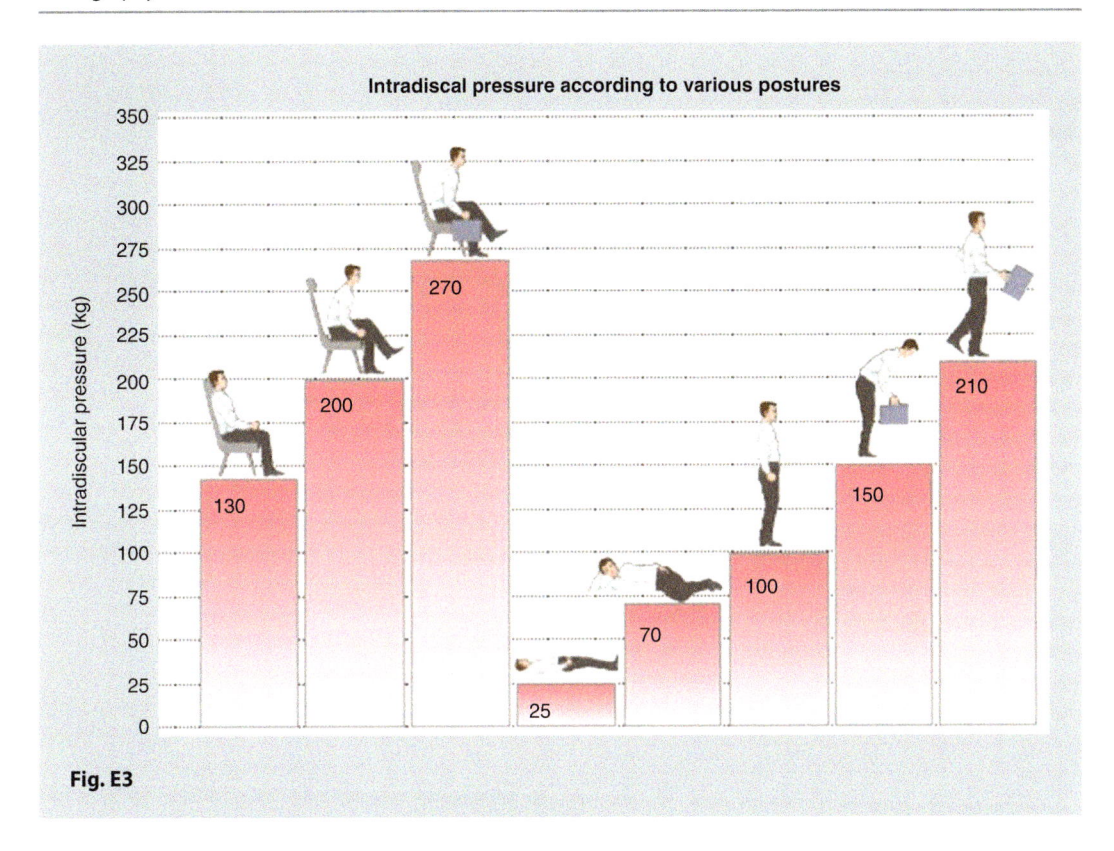

Intradiscal pressure according to various postures

Fig. E3

Bibliography

1. Pain medicine. 4th ed. p. 585.
2. Joo EY, Koh WU, Choi SS, Choi JH, Ahn HS, Yun HJ, Shin JW. Efficacy of adjuvant 10% hypertonic saline in transforaminal epidural steroid injection: a retrospective analysis. Pain Physician. 2017;20(1):E107–14.
3. Koh WU, Choi SS, Park SY, Joo EY, Kim SH, Lee JD, Shin JY, Suh JH, Leem JG, Shin JW. Transforaminal hypertonic saline for the treatment of lumbar lateral canal stenosis: a double-blinded, randomized, active-control trial. Pain Physician. 2013;16(3):197–211.
4. King JS, Jewett DL, Sundberg HR. Differential blockade of cat dorsal root C fibers by various chloride solutions. J Neurosurg. 1972;36:569–83.
5. Matsuka Y, Spigelman I. Hyperosmolar solutions selectively block action potentials in rat myelinated sensory fibers: implications for diabetic neuropathy. J Neurophysiol. 2004;91:48–56.
6. Narouze S, Benzon HT, Provenzano DA, Buvanendran A, De Andres J, Deer TR, Rauck R, Huntoon MA. Interventional spine and pain procedures in patients on antiplatelet and anticoagulant medications: guidelines from the American Society of Regional Anesthesia and Pain Medicine, the European Society of Regional Anaesthesia and Pain Therapy, the American Academy of Pain Medicine, the International Neuromodulation Society, the North American Neuromodulation Society, and the World Institute of Pain. Reg Anesth Pain Med. 2015;40(3):182–212.

Methods for Executing the ZiNeu Series Catheter Procedure

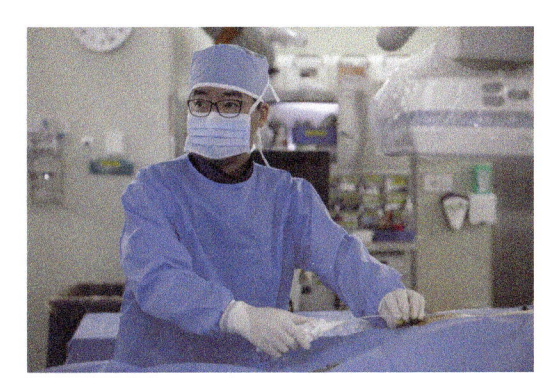

4

Image of balloon decompression being according to the caudal approach

4.1 Target Diseases

Low back and leg pain caused by spinal stenosis
Low back and leg pain caused by chronic intervertebral disc herniation
Low back and leg pain caused by epidural adhesion
Postspinal surgery pain syndrome

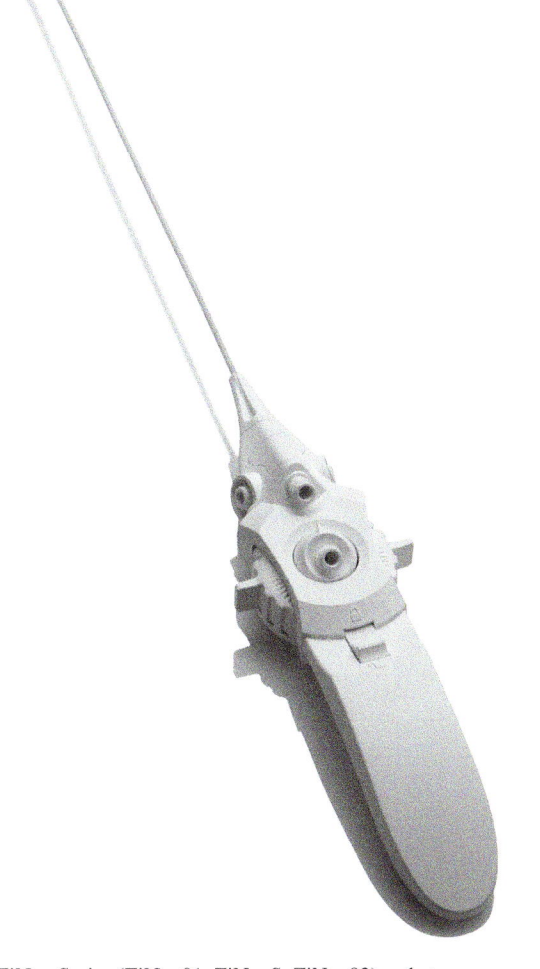

ZiNeu Series (ZiNeu01, ZiNeuS, ZiNeu02) catheter

Electronic Supplementary Material The online version of this chapter (https://doi.org/10.1007/978-981-15-7265-4_4) contains supplementary material, which is available to authorized users. The videos can be accessed by scanning the related images with the SN More Media App.

© Springer Nature Singapore Pte Ltd. 2021
J. W. Shin, *Spinal Epidural Balloon Decompression and Adhesiolysis*,
https://doi.org/10.1007/978-981-15-7265-4_4

4.1.1 Best Indication

Patients for whom conventional epidural block or neuroplasty achieved short-lived effects. Patients wanting to improve claudication caused by spinal stenosis.

4.2 Pre-Procedure Preparations

4.2.1 Posture and Disinfection

While the patient is lying in a prone position, a slightly high pillow is placed underneath the patient's abdomen to reduce lumbar lordosis. The spinal canal becomes relatively straighter when lordosis is reduced. This can lower resistance when the catheter is inserted. Hence, it is helpful to use the lateral view in C-arm lateral while the patient is in a prone position and adjust the height of the pillow accordingly.

Before disinfecting the site of operation, gauze should be placed in the area between the coccygeal vertebra and anus to prevent Betadine from flowing into the anus. Disinfection and preparation should be performed as shown in (Fig. 4.1).

To reduce pain during the procedure, 100 μg of Fentanyl is injected portion-wise before and during the procedure. General anesthesia is not recommended since the patient's pain and systemic condition must be monitored continuously through conversation with the patient. Moreover, a provocation test must be performed during the procedure.

When epidurography is performed at the beginning of the procedure, pain is not severe since epidural anesthesia is performed simultaneously. Light sedation is possible for sensitive patients.

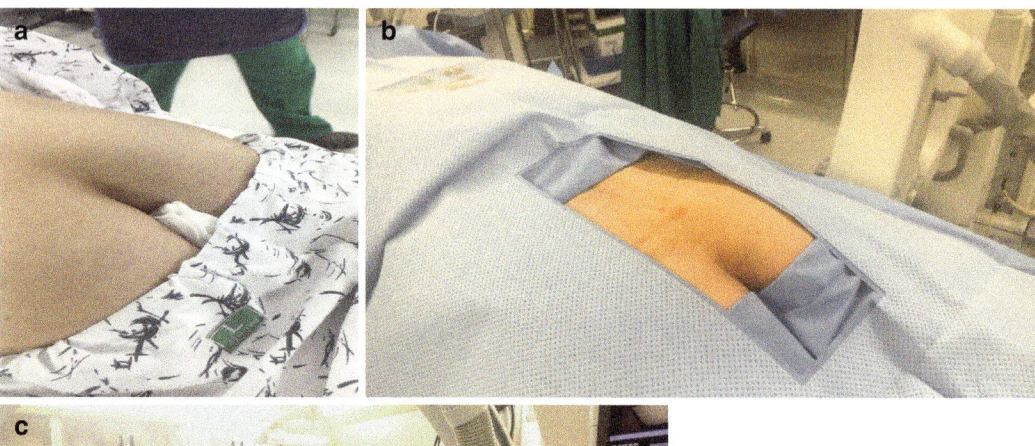

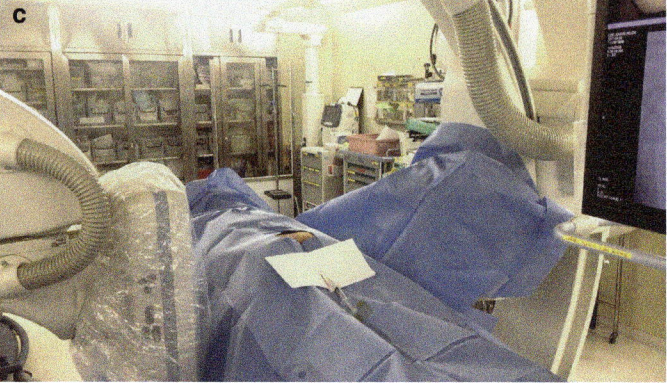

Fig. 4.1 (**a**) A gauze is placed in between the buttocks. (**b**) A surgical drape is placed up to the area above the gauze, and the area is disinfected. (**c**) Preparation for the procedure has been completed

4.2 Pre-Procedure Preparations

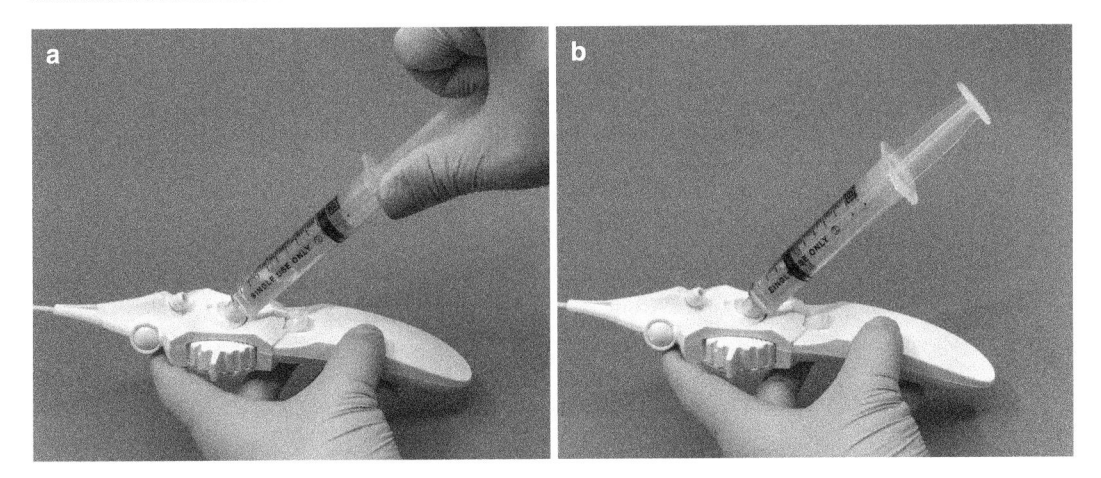

Fig. 4.2 (**a**) The pulling of the syringe plunger to remove the air inside the catheter. (**b**) The release of the plunger and then its subsequent filling with contrast dye

4.2.2 Removal of Air Inside the Catheter and Contrast-Dye Filling

A 10 cc syringe filled with approximately 3–4 cc of contrast dye is connected to the contrast dye inlet component of the ZiNeu catheter. The syringe plunger is pulled sufficiently to maintain strong negative pressure for 2–3 s. The plunger is then released. This alone can remove the air inside the catheter and fill the space with the contrast dye (Fig. 4.2).

If strong negative pressure is not applied while the plunger is pulled, the air inside the catheter may not be completely removed. This can cause air to appear during balloon inflation. The air remaining in the balloon may present complicate the identification of the degree of balloon inflation in the C-arm images—in severe cases, the degree of inflation could be mistaken for a ruptured balloon. It is therefore important to apply strong negative pressure when removing the air (Fig. 4.3).

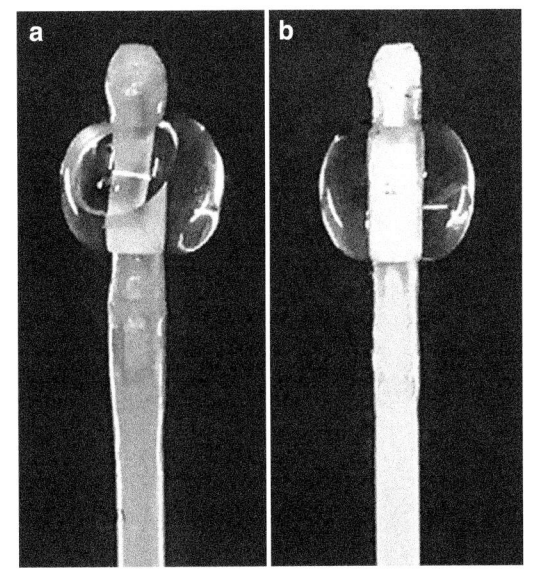

Fig. 4.3 (**a**) Inflated balloon contains air because the air inside the catheter had not been removed completely. (**b**) Inflated balloon when the air inside the catheter has been completely removed

4.2.3 Connecting the Syringe for Balloon Decompression

A 1 cc Luer lock syringe filled with 0.1 cc of contrast dye is connected to the contrast dye inlet for balloon decompression. If the procedure is performed when the syringe is filled with more than 0.1 cc of contrast dye, the operator may unknowingly over-inflate the balloon. It is therefore recommended that the syringe should not be filled past 0.1 cc to prevent this possibility. Injecting 0.1 cc of contrast dye could inflate the balloon to a diameter of approximately 10 mm. Of course, the balloon size could be re-adjusted by modifying the amount of contrast dye as needed during the procedure (Fig. 4.4).

The Luer lock syringe attached to the catheter should be twisted to the left or right to be loaded together with the drug-injection syringe (Fig. 4.5).

It is advisable for a right-handed person to twist the Luer lock syringe to the left (Fig. 4.5b, c).

4.2.4 Balloon Expansion

Injecting 0.1 cc of contrast dye with a 1 cc Luer lock syringe can be completed quickly and with very little resistance. However, the pressure applied to the balloon at the tip of the catheter is unexpectedly strong (Fig. 4.6).

If the degree of stenosis on the lesion is severe, the pressure inside the balloon increases even more. However, a quick injection with 0.1 cc of contrast dye can be completed without feeling such a pressure difference. In other words, pressure in the balloon and nearby nerves may be higher than what is felt by the operator.

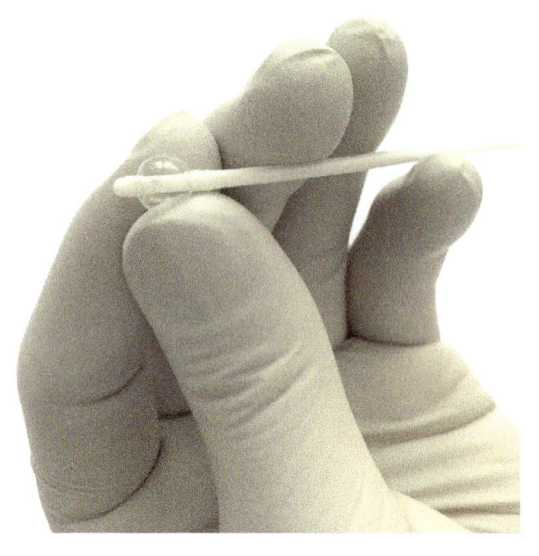

Fig. 4.4 A balloon that has been fully inflated with an injection of 0.1 cc of contrast dye

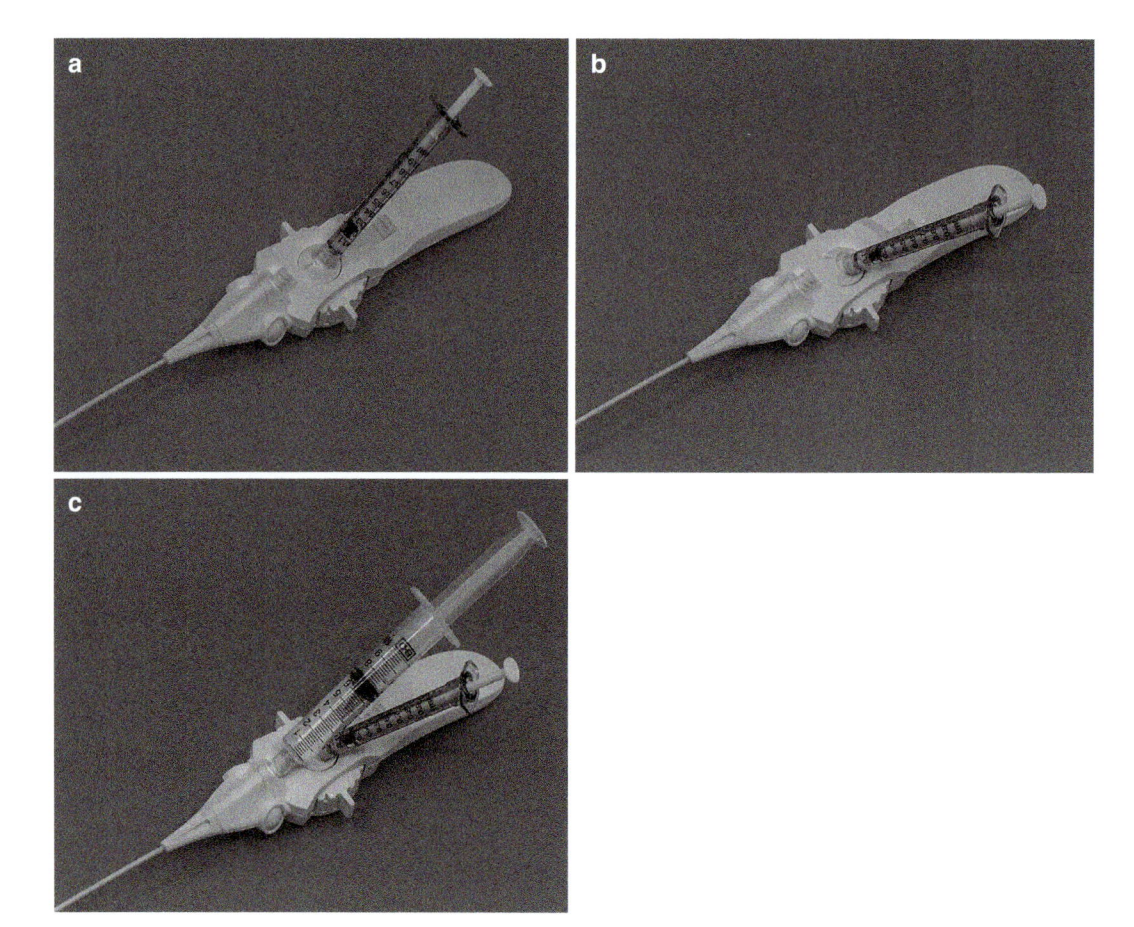

Fig. 4.5 (**a**) A 1 cc Luer lock syringe is connected to the contrast-dye inlet. (**b**) The syringe is rotated by 45°. Connection of the drug-injection syringe is possible only in this manner. (**c**) The drug-injection and balloon decompression syringes are connected together

4.3 Recommended Procedure

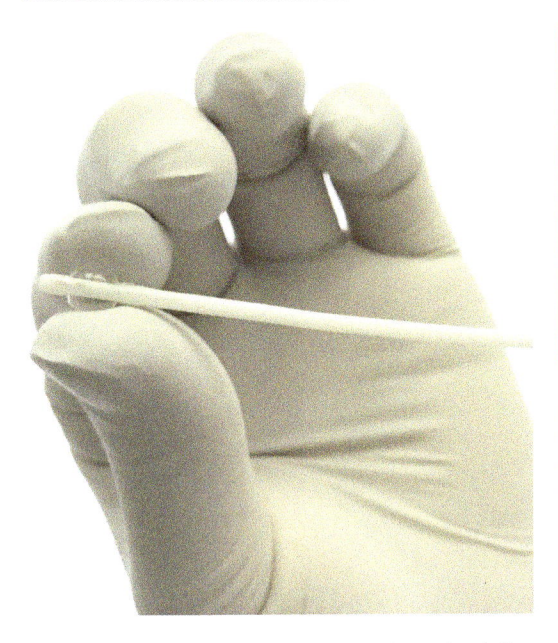

Fig. 4.6 Feeling the pressure on the balloon after inflating the balloon with 0.1 cc of contrast dye. Unexpectedly strong pressure can be felt in the balloon

Excessive, rapid balloon inflation may cause severe pain and balloon rupture. Balloon expansion should therefore be performed slowly with gradual, step-by-step increases in balloon size.

> **Rules to abide by during balloon decompression:**
> 1. Inject the dye slowly.
> 2. If the patient complains of severe pain during balloon expansion, do not inflate further. Stop for 2–3 s and deflate the balloon.
> 3. A single inflation should not exceed 5 s.
> 4. The procedure should be performed by repeatedly inflating and deflating the balloon while moving gradually.
> 5. Catheter must move inside the intervertebral foramen in deflated state (for prevention of nerve stretching injury).
> 6. The balloon should be increased in size in stepwise manner. Do not inflate the balloon to its fullest size from the beginning.

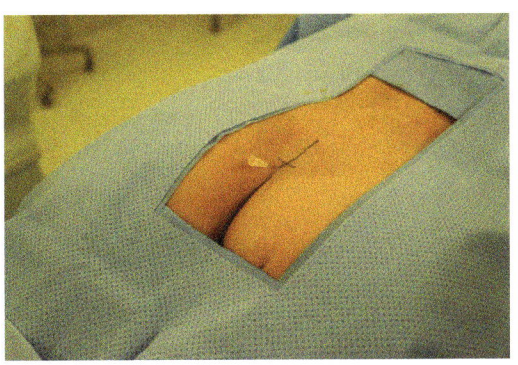

Fig. 4.7 The entry point is slightly below the point where the line connecting the middle of the spine and the line connecting the left and right cornua meet. The exact location is decided with C-arm lateral view

4.3 Recommended Procedure

4.3.1 Guide Needle Insertion

Accurately position the guide needle at the midline to allow the catheter tip to move freely from side to side and to facilitate its approach to the target site.

Draw a line connecting the middle of the spine and another line connecting the left and right cornua. A point slightly below where the two lines meet and a point where the needle can be inserted parallel to the caudal epidural space in the lateral view is set as the entry point (Fig. 4.7).

While performing local anesthesia, it is advisable to estimate the position and angle of the guide needle under the C-arm lateral view using the anesthetic needle. If the guide needle insertion position and angle were approximated while the patient was under local anesthesia, insert the guide needle at the calculated angle. Subsequently insert the guide needle along the previously marked midline. Alternatively, with his or her free hand, the operating clinician can feel and check for the lumbar spinous process, along which the guide needle can be inserted. (Both methods prescribe inserting the guide needle into the midline.) (Fig. 4.8).

The needle should be inserted in such a manner that it forms a straight line with the caudal

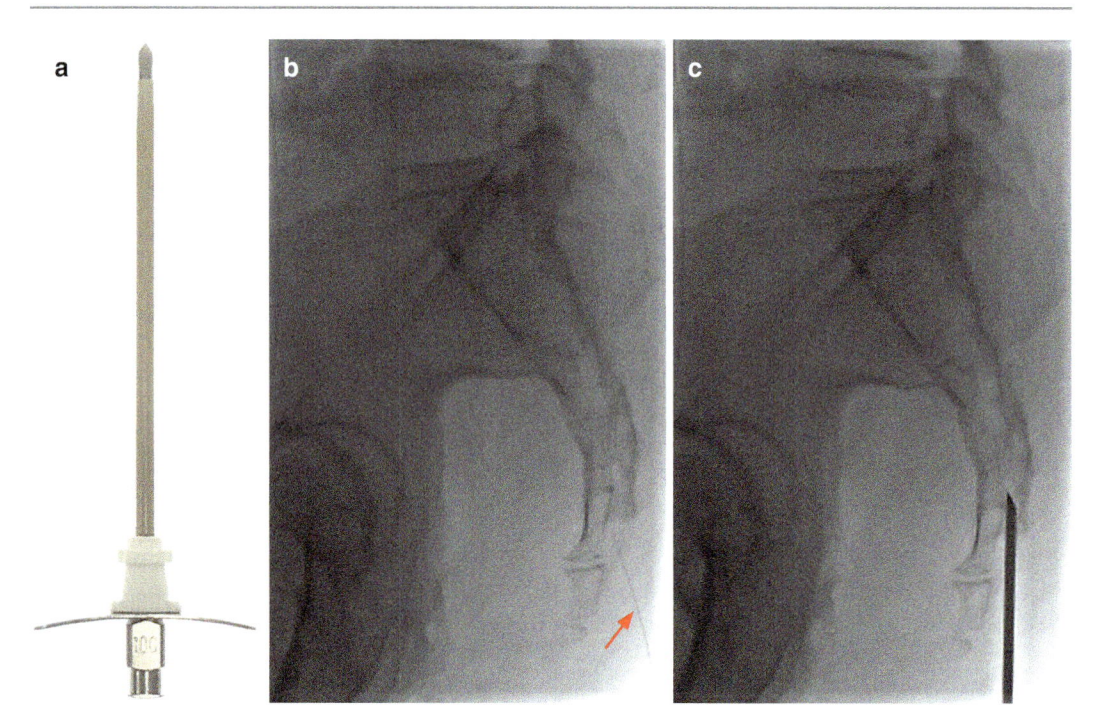

Fig. 4.8 (**a**) 10 G guide needle, including the sheath. (**b**) During local anesthesia, an anesthetic needle was inserted into the sacral hiatus to confirm the approach angle and path in advance. Arrow: Local anesthetic needle. (**c**) A guide needle is inserted and placed at a similar angle

epidural space to minimize any damage or resistance when the catheter is maneuvered during the procedure (Fig. 4.9).

When the needle tip passes through the sacrococcygeal ligament, immediately rotate the needle by 180° so that the bevel faces downward (ventral) to minimize damage to the bone from the needle. Subsequently advance the needle further by 1–3 cm. Determine the direction of the bevel that facilitates catheter insertion based on lateral view in that state. If rotating the bevel to face upward (dorsal) would facilitate the insertion of the catheter, rotate it accordingly. If not, keep the bevel facing downwards. When using the sheath, the final position of the bevel does not matter; however, even in this case, the sheath should be advanced by only 2–3 cm after passing through the sacrococcygeal ligament. Inserting it too deeply can complicate the manipulation of the catheter (Fig. 4.10).

When using the guide needle alone, place it with its bevel facing upward, as shown in Fig. 4.10d. In most cases, this reduces the resistance generated by the movement of the catheter. However, it may be preferable to have the bevel face downward, as shown in Fig. 4.11. The selection of the bevel's orientation depends on the angle that the guide needle forms with the caudal epidural space as well as the optimal approach to the anterior epidural space.

4.3.1.1 Reference: When Guide Needle Entry Is Difficult

1. Although rare, the caudal epidural space can be congenitally narrow. The width of the caudal epidural space can be measured in advance by MRI. In patients with a caudal epidural space width of <2.3 mm, catheters with a thickness of 2.3 mm cannot be used. Instead, the ZiNeu02 catheter with a thickness of 1.55 mm should be employed (Fig. 4.12).
2. In the case that only the initial entry point to the caudal epidural space is narrow, the guide needle should be tapped with a hammer to allow for its passage through the narrow entry

4.3 Recommended Procedure

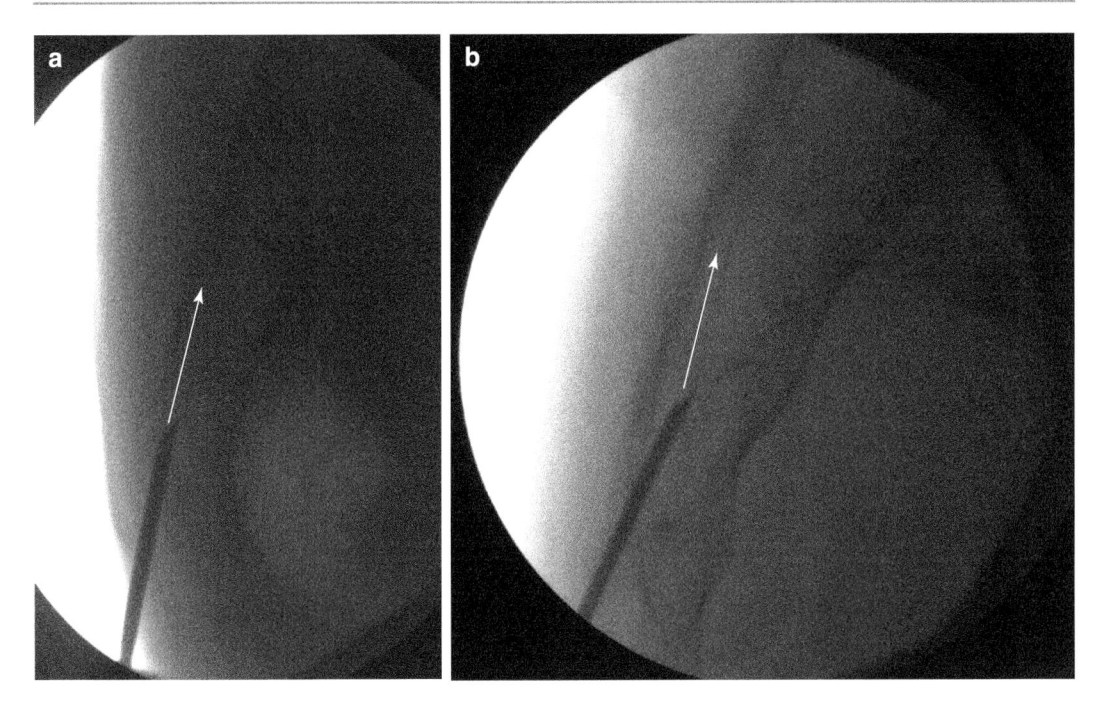

Fig. 4.9 During its insertion, the guide needle should form a straight line with the caudal epidural space, as shown by the arrow

point and the tip of the guide needle to enter the wide caudal epidural space (Fig. 4.13).

Other reasons that prevent the guide needle from being inserted into the causal epidural space usually involve the sacral hiatus: it is either not situated in the normal position or otherwise prevents entry into the midline of the sacral hiatus. Many cases that rely solely on the lateral view for guide needle insertion could prevent the operator from noticing deviations in the guide needle's trajectory from the midline. If the entry into the epidural space cannot be performed—despite the entry angle appearing correct in the lateral view—the operator should reference the AP view to determine whether the needle is deviating from the midline. As aforementioned, such possibility can be reduced if the midline is located before and the skin is marked accordingly, and then the entry is made in that direction (Fig. 4.14).

If entry cannot be made despite the maintenance of needle's course along the midline, the caudal epidural space should be localized first using a different, thinner epidural needle; when a thick guide needle is used, it may be difficult to locate the sacral hiatus, and the patient may feel severe pain after several attempts to localize the sacral hiatus with the thicker needle. Hence, the guide needle should be inserted only after the optimal angle has been found with the thin needle.

Blood vessels may occasionally appear contrast-enhanced after the needle is inserted and the contrast dye is injected. This is due to the penetration of the needle through the sacral bone and the consequent leakage of the contrast into the bone marrow. In such cases, the damaged bone area should be bypassed by repositioning the needle should into the epidural space. Otherwise, the ZiNeu catheter should be inserted and the contrast dye injected after placing the ZiNeu catheter to the epidural space at the L5–S1 level (Figs. 4.15 and 4.16).

4.3.2 Epidurogram and Regional Anesthesia

Before starting the procedure, an epidurogram should be performed to confirm the pathologic lesion. At this time, mixing 2% Lidocaine with

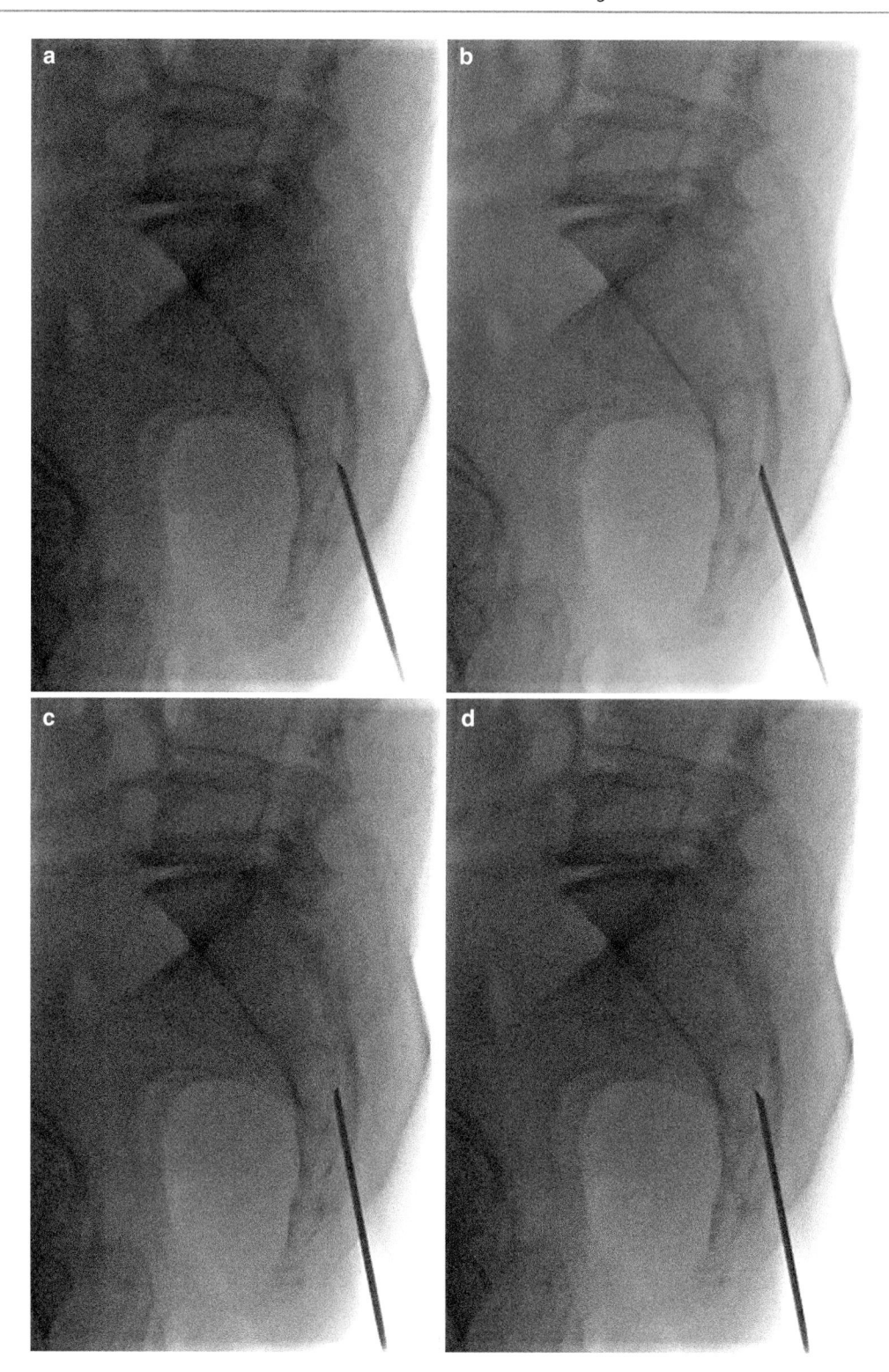

Fig. 4.10 (**a**) Insert the guide needle parallel to the epidural space as much as possible with bevel of the guide needle facing upward (dorsal). Stop when the needle tip passes through the sacrococcygeal ligament. (**b**) Rotate the bevel of the guide needle by 180° so that it faces downward (ventral). (**c**) Advance the guide needle further by approximately 1–3 cm. (**d**) If advantageous for catheter insertion, rotate the guide needle again by 180°

4.3 Recommended Procedure

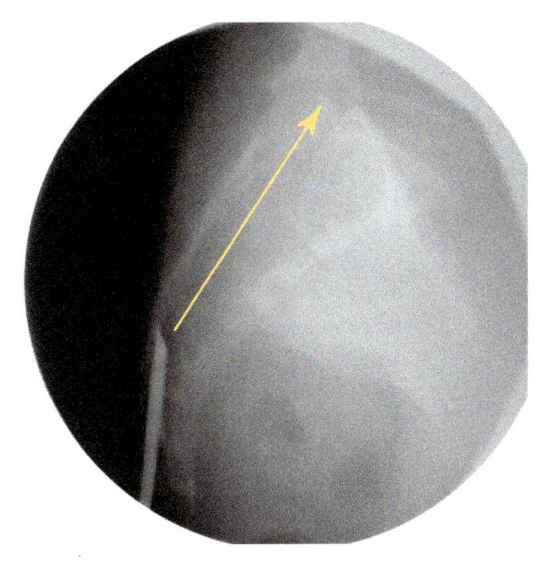

Fig. 4.11 In this patient's case, having the bevel of the guide needle facing downward (ventral) allowed for smoother catheter insertion into the anterior epidural space. Arrow: The direction of catheter entry into the anterior epidural space

the contrast dye to prepare 1% Lidocaine mixture and injecting this mixture into the epidural space is very useful to achieve adequate regional anesthesia at the site of the procedure. Regional anesthesia administered to the epidural space can increase the success rate of the procedure by reducing pain, while also temporarily reducing pain. However, when a mixture of regional anesthetic and contrast dye is injected epidurally, caution should be exercised to prevent the injection of the into the intrathecal space: even small amounts can induce total spinal anesthesia and cause unconsciousness, low blood pressure, and cardiac arrest.

4.3.2.1 Recommended Method

After placing the guide needle, inject 3–5 cc of 100% contrast dye to check whether it was injected into a blood vessel or the intrathecal space. If the injection of the dye into the epidural

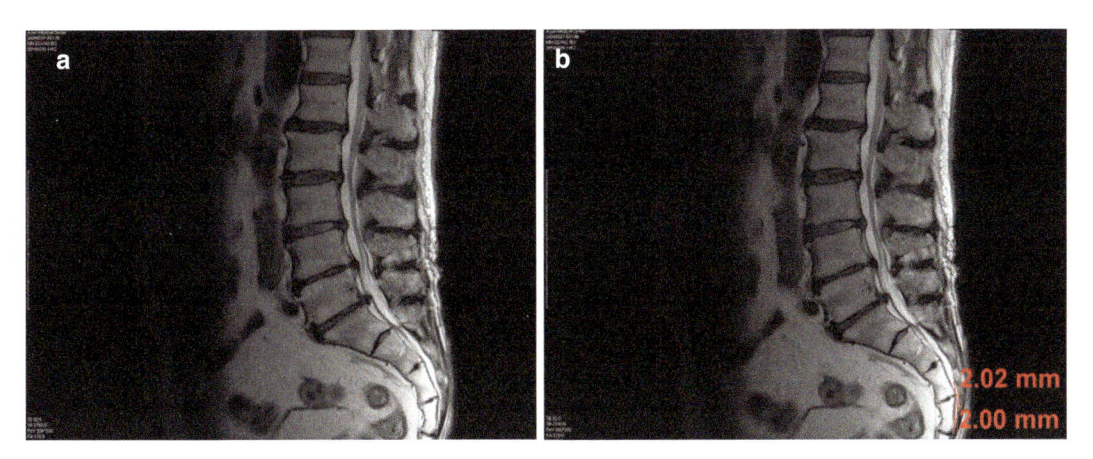

Fig. 4.12 Patient with a caudal epidural space width of <2.3 mm

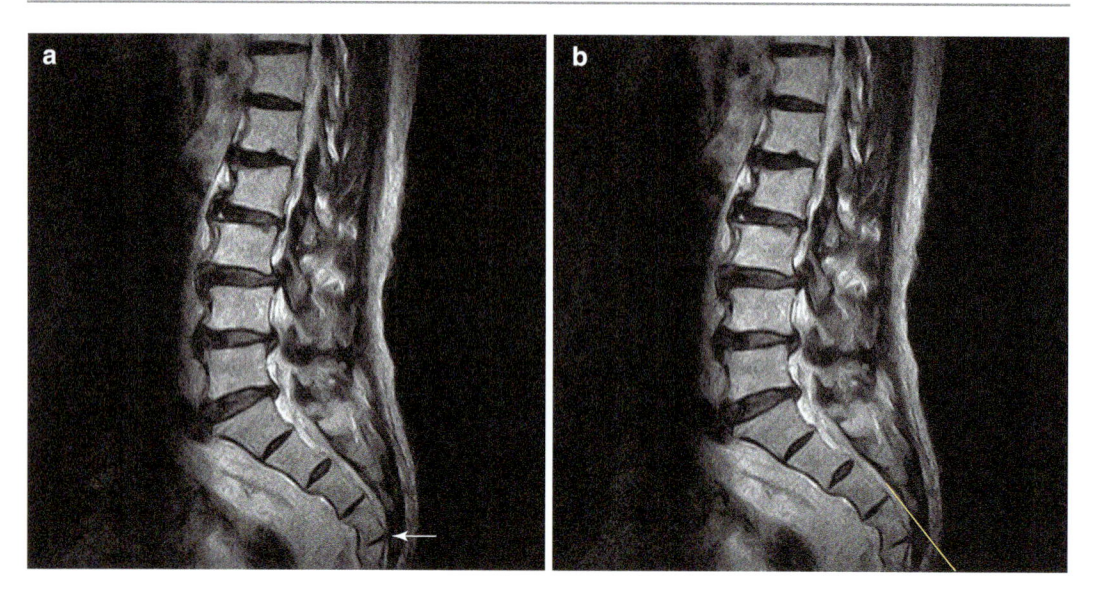

Fig. 4.13 Case of a narrow initial entry point to the caudal epidural space. Arrow: Narrow initial entry point. Yellow line: The passage of a virtual needle through the narrow area

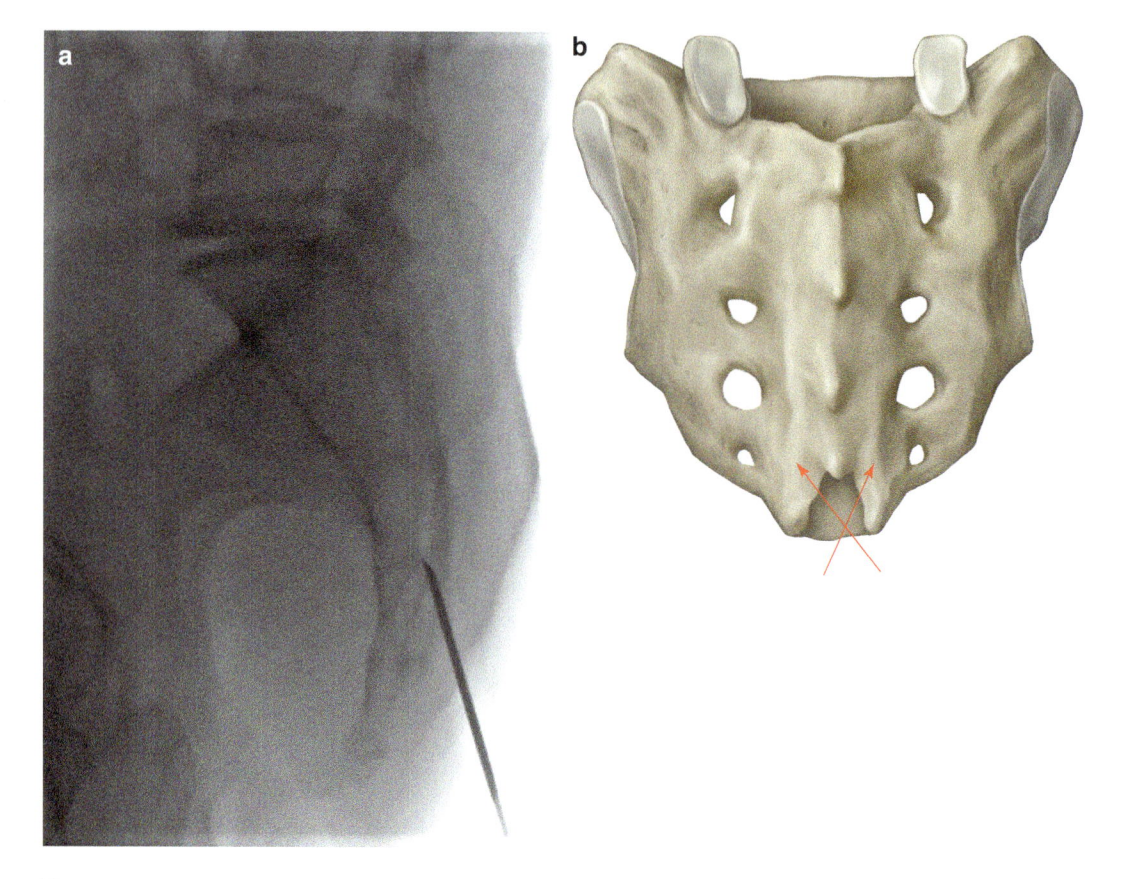

Fig. 4.14 (**a**) Entry under the lateral view. (**b**) A schematic diagram of the inability to enter the sacral hiatus due to deviation from the midline as indicated by the arrow. (**c**) An AP view of the correct placement of the guide needle on the midline. Yellow line: midline

4.3 Recommended Procedure

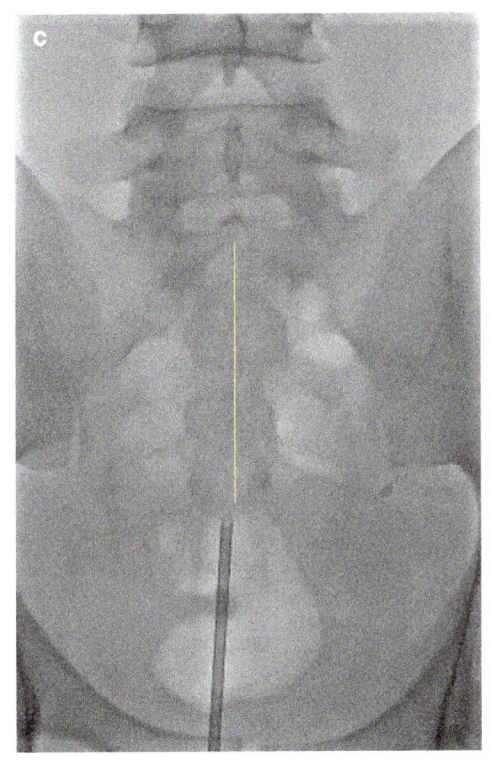

Fig. 4.14 (continued)

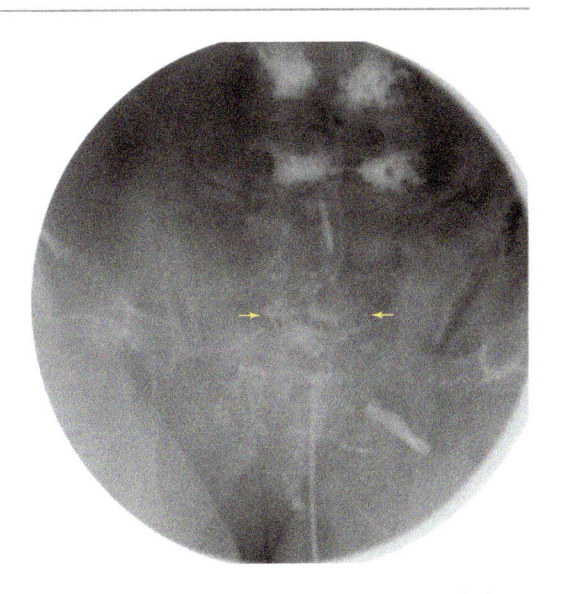

Fig. 4.15 The leakage of the contrast dye into the bone marrow due to the needle-induced damage of the sacral bone. Arrow: The contrast dye spread to the vessels

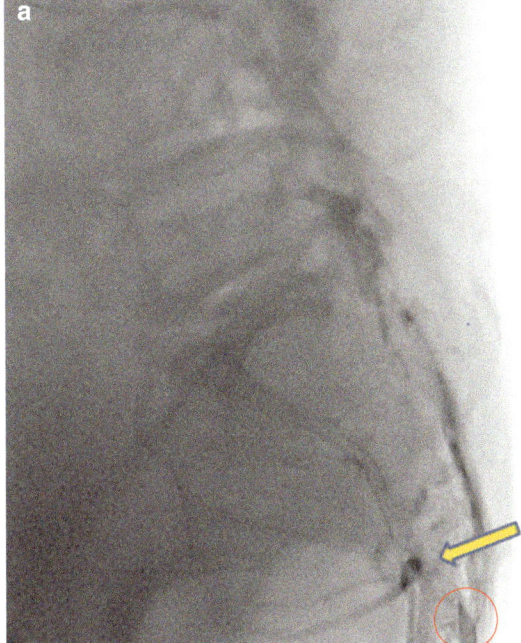

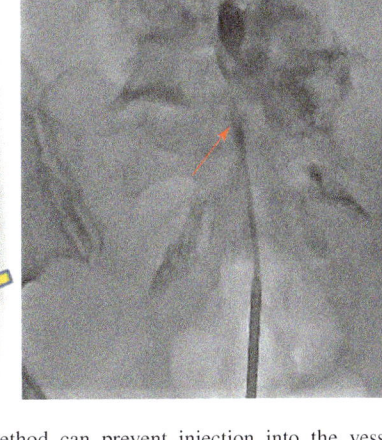

Fig. 4.16 (a) The leakage of a portion of the contrast dye into the vessels due to the needle-induced damage of the sacral bone. (b) The injection of the contrast dye at L5–S1 level following the insertion of the ZiNeu catheter. This method can prevent injection into the vessels. Yellow arrow: The contrast dye inside the blood vessel. Red arrow: The position of the catheter tip. Circle: The tip of the guide needle

space is confirmed, the following should be considered:

1. If the 3–5 cc of 100% contrast dye has spread up to the target site of procedure, inject 10 cc of contrast dye mixed with local anesthetic and perform the epidurogram.
2. If the 100% contrast dye has not spread well to the target site due to adhesion in the caudal epidural space, carefully raise the ZiNeu catheter along the midline to the vicinity of the L5–S1 and reinject 3 cc of 100% contrast dye. (If the catheter has deviated from the midline, contact between the catheter and the sacral root may cause pain during entry.) Upon localization of the epidural space, administer 7 cc of the contrast dye with local anesthetic to the site to confirm adhesion of the target lesion and anesthetize the site of procedure (Fig. 4.17).
   - 100% contrast dye must be used to check the epidural space. The drug containing the local anesthetic should be injected only if the epidural space has been confirmed.
   - Concentration of diluted local anesthetic used for epidurogram:
     - 1% Lidocaine for patients aged <70 years
     - 0.7% Lidocaine for patients aged ≥70 years.
   - It is helpful to inject hyaluronidase prior to the procedure since it can effectively loosen adhesion. It could be injected as a mixture during epidurogram or injected separately as a mixture with 10 cc of normal saline.

4.3.3 ZiNeu Series Catheter Insertion

The epidural space can be divided into the anterior and posterior epidural spaces (Fig. 4.18). Stenosis or adhesion alleviation in the anterior epidural space should be prioritized because the sinuvertebral nerve, which is associated with low back pain, innervates most of the structures in the anterior epidural space and most degenerative spinal diseases, including disc herniation, involve lesions in the anterior epidural space. Moreover, confirming that the drug spreads into the anterior epidural space prior to treatment is essential to

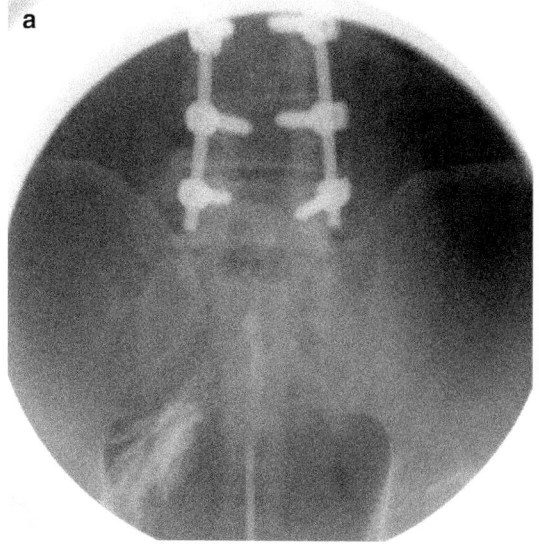

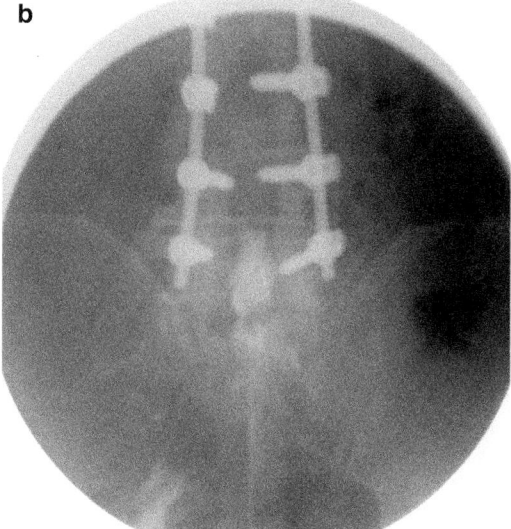

Fig. 4.17 (a) The 3–5 cc of injected 100% contrast dye, did not spread to the L5–S1 level. In such cases, even a 10 cc dose of contrast dye with local anesthetic will not anesthetize the target site of procedure. (b) In the same patient, a catheter was inserted along the midline up to the L5–S1 level, and 3 cc of 100% contrast dye is reinjected. Upon localization of the epidural space, 7 cc of the contrast dye with local anesthetic is injected

4.3 Recommended Procedure

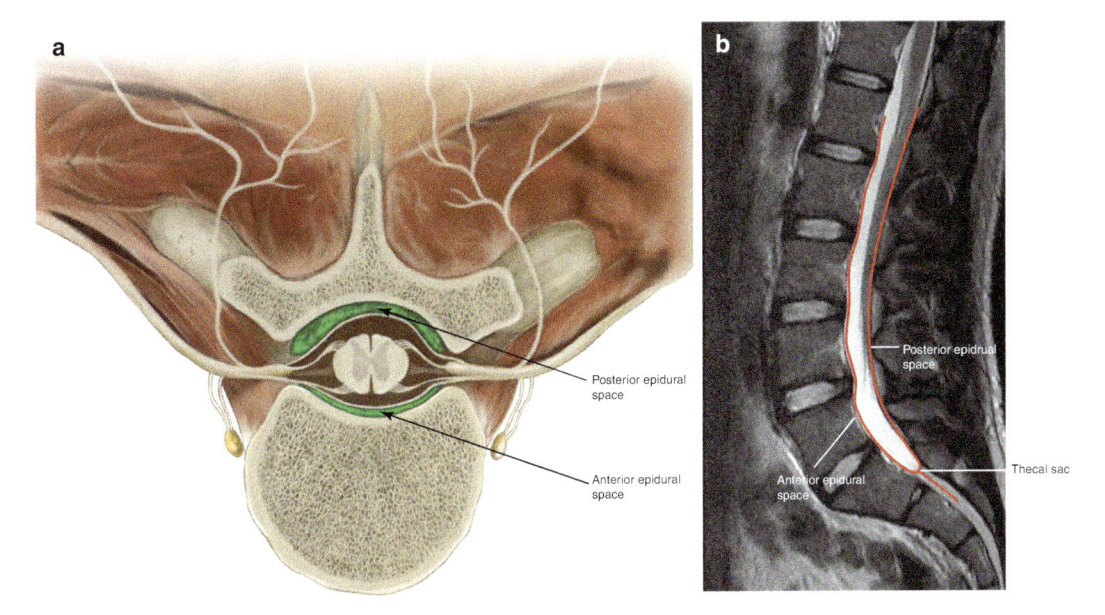

Fig. 4.18 (a) Anterior and posterior epidural spaces. The posterior epidural space is wider than the anterior epidural space. (b) Division of the anterior and posterior epidural spaces along the thecal sac area, with the dura in between

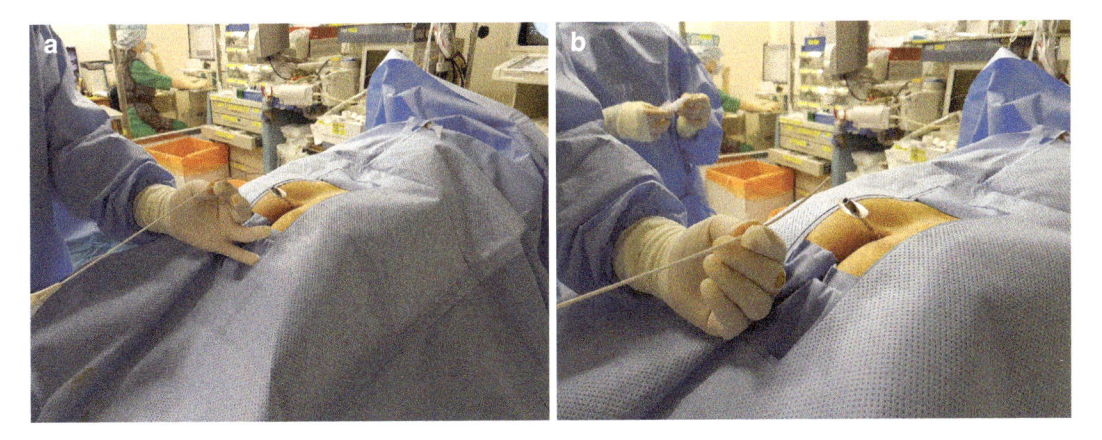

Fig. 4.19 (a) Insertion into the anterior epidural space. The catheter tip is slightly bent toward the front of the patient. (b) For insertion into the posterior epidural space, the catheter tip is slightly bent toward the back of the patient

successful outcomes. It is thus paramount that the catheter be inserted into the anterior epidural space during balloon decompression. However, because adhesion in the posterior epidural space is also associated with movement-induced low back pain caused, the procedure should also be performed in the posterior epidural space.

To insert the catheter into the anterior epidural space, the ZiNeu catheter body is turned to one side and the handle is pulled gently so that the catheter tip is pointing toward the front of the patient (Fig. 4.19a). (When inserting the catheter into the posterior epidural space, the insertion is performed in an opposite fashion like that presented in Fig. 4.19b.)

Entry into the anterior epidural space should be attempted while viewing radiological images by adjusting the handle of the ZiNeu catheter in real time in the lateral view or by turning the catheter's body so that the catheter tip enters along the anterior epidural space. When the handle is pulled too much, the catheter tip might not be able to enter the midline; it may slip to one of the sides of the foramen. Hence, the catheter tip should be inserted while it is adjusting carefully according to the lateral view (Fig. 4.20).

Once the entry has been made close to the L5–S1 level, whether the catheter has been placed on the midline should be checked with the AP view. If the lateral view shows that the catheter was inserted along the anterior epidural space while the AP view shows that it has been placed near the midline, the catheter may have been inserted along the anterior epidural space (Figs. 4.21 and 4.22).

If the catheter tip appears to be placed within the anterior epidural space in lateral view but is tilted to one side of the spine in the AP view, there is a high likelihood that the catheter has been placed within the posterior epidural space while its tip has slipped laterally towards the foramen. Hence, the tip area in this case is situated at one side of the anterior epidural space. While the location of the catheter tip is not important, there are cases where the entire catheter needs to be inside the anterior epidural space. When the procedure must be performed in the anterior epidural space of the center of the L5–S1 level, the catheter should be withdrawn and re-inserted (Fig. 4.23).

Another method that can be used to gain entry into the anterior epidural space is to adjust the catheter tip so that it is placed within the anterior epidural space at the S1–2 level in the lateral view like Fig. 4.20b and changing the C-arm to the AP view: if the catheter tip is tilted laterally in the AP view, it can be adjusted toward the midline in that state and advanced toward the head (Figs. 4.24a and 4.25a). By doing so, the catheter tip in the posterior epidural space could be slipped through the anterior epidural space and be advanced into the anterior epidural space toward the head. Ultimately, whether the catheter tip has entered the anterior epidural space or not can be checked in lateral view (Figs. 4.24b and 4.25b). While this method is easier than the previous method, it tends to tilt the catheter tip to one side at the L5–S1 level; hence, the previous method is better when the procedure must be performed on the entire anterior epidural space at the center of the L5–S1 level.

A comparison is made between the first and second methods in Fig. 4.26 through the lateral view.

The relative narrowness of the anterior epidural space may lead to the feeling of slightly more resistance to entry than when entering the posterior epidural space. However, this transition in resistance becomes clear with experience.

At the initial stage of catheter insertion, the direction of entry must be adjusted upon reaching the middle area—i.e., the medial aspect of the sacral foramen—to avoid contact with the sacral nerve. This step requires caution, especially when the catheter is inserted into the anterior epidural space: advancing the catheter into the sacral foramen while it is excessively tilted to one side could bring the catheter into contact with the sacral nerve and induce severe pain (Fig. 4.27).

4.3.4 Method for Adjusting the Direction of the Catheter

Two methods allow for changing the direction or angle of entry. One method involves pulling the handle to bend the tip of the catheter, while the other involves rotating the catheter body with the tip slightly bent to change the angle of the tip. When modifying the direction of entry, more delicate direction control is possible by slightly

Fig. 4.20 (**a**) In MRI images, the thecal sac is located at the S2 level; this is where the anterior and posterior epidural spaces split. (**b**) An attempt to enter the anterior epidural space by bending the catheter tip toward the front of the patient. If it is bent too much, it may slip laterally. Hence, the catheter should be advanced while the bent portion is straightened slightly if the catheter tip has been crossed over the anterior epidural space line. (**c**) The catheter has been well-placed within the anterior epidural space. Arrow: Catheter

4.3 Recommended Procedure

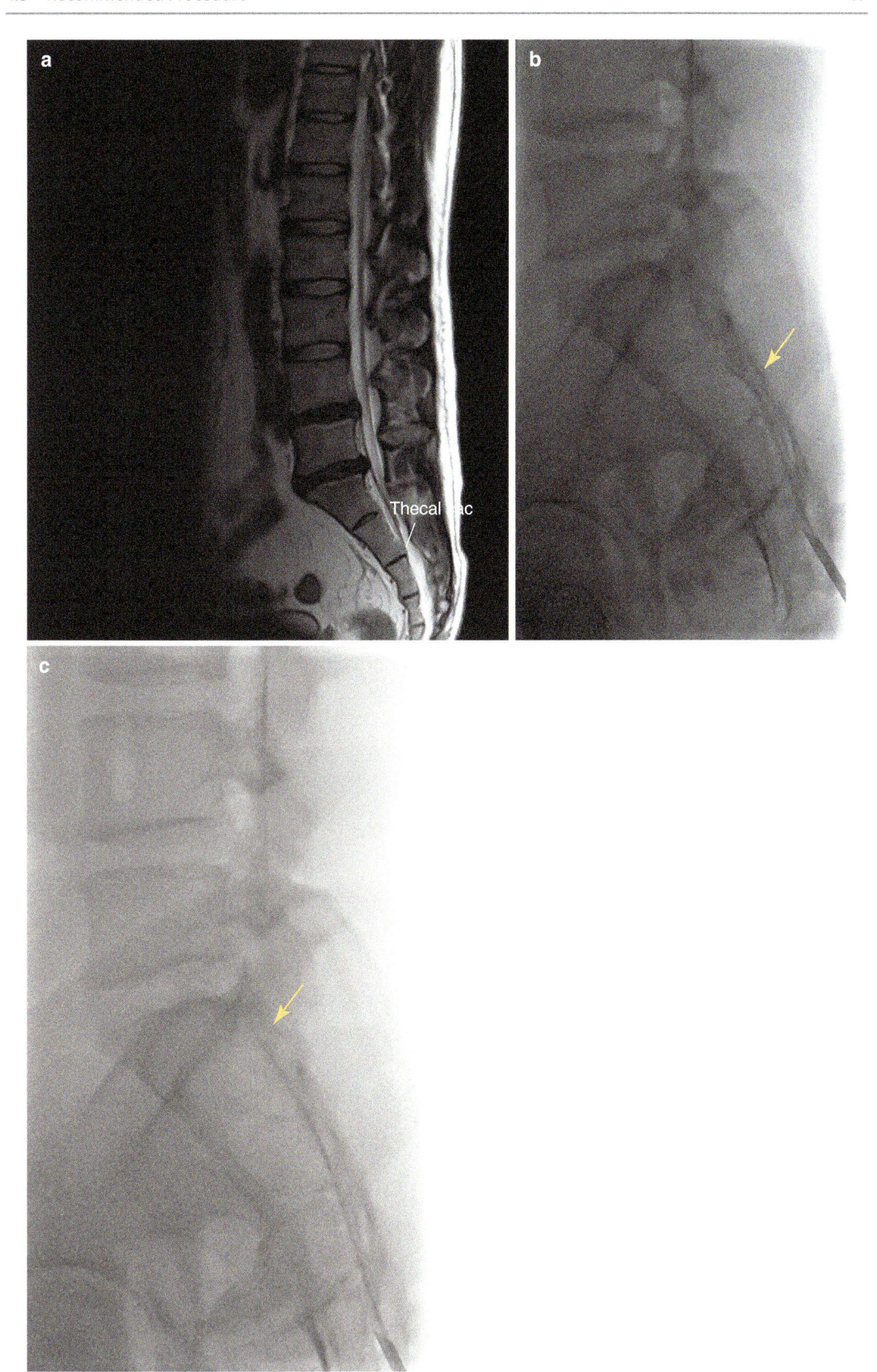

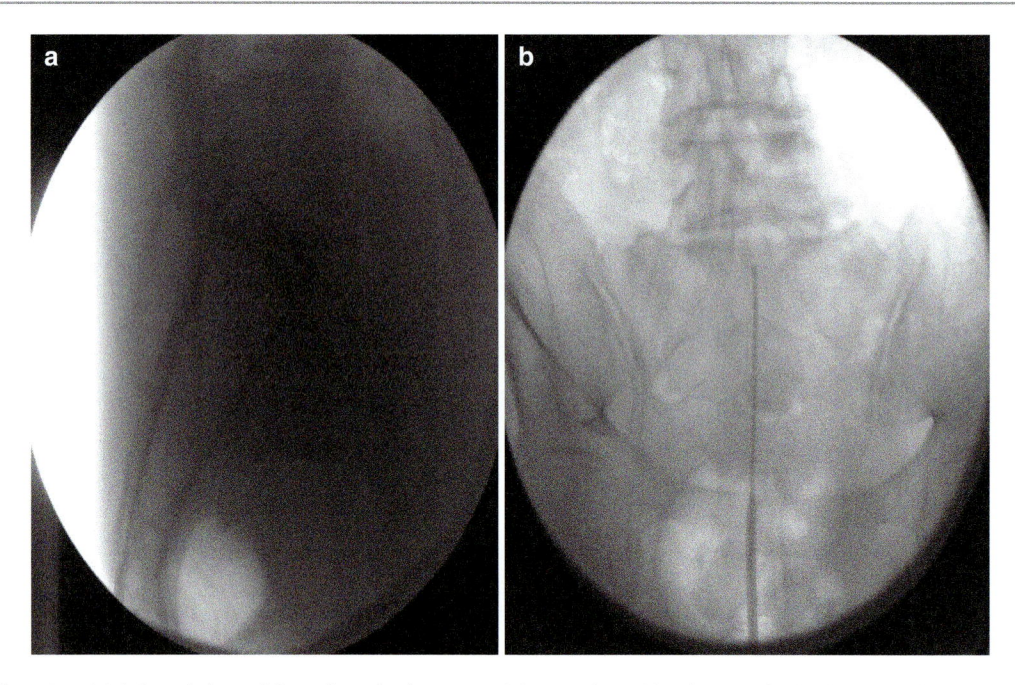

Fig. 4.21 (**a**) A lateral view of the catheter having entered the anterior epidural space. (**b**) An AP view of the catheter having been placed on the midline. As shown here, both AP and lateral views should be checked

Fig. 4.22 (**a**) The catheter within the anterior epidural space and the balloon inflated. Circle: Inflated balloon. (**b**) The catheter has been placed within the posterior epidural space

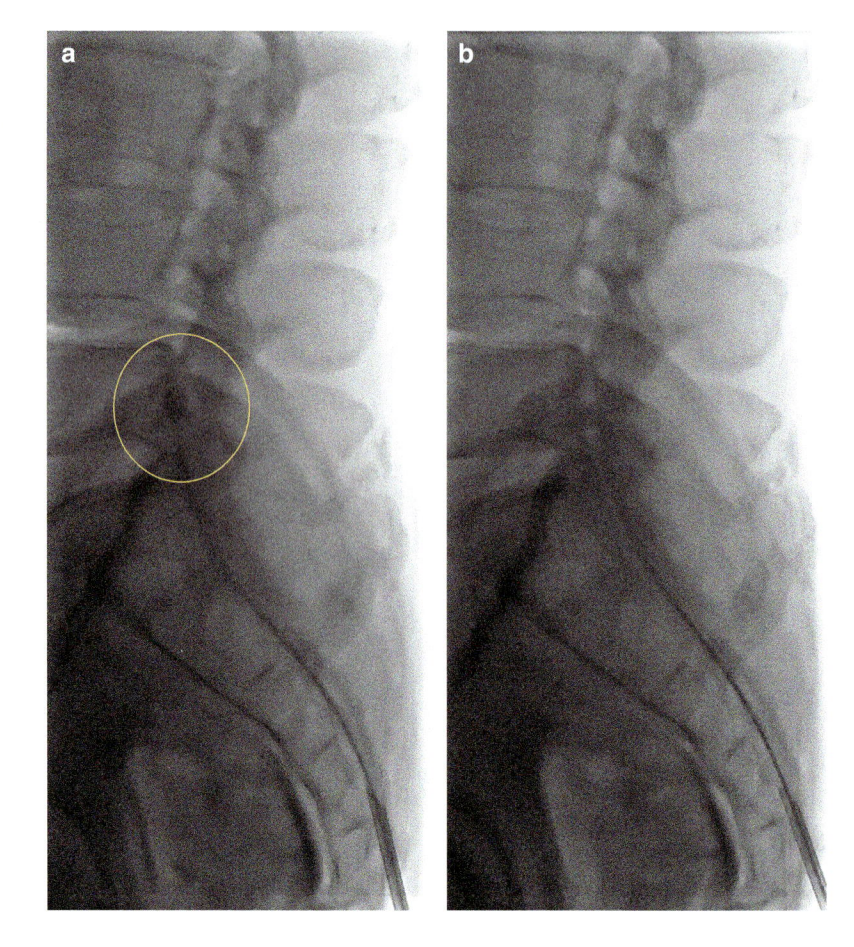

4.3 Recommended Procedure

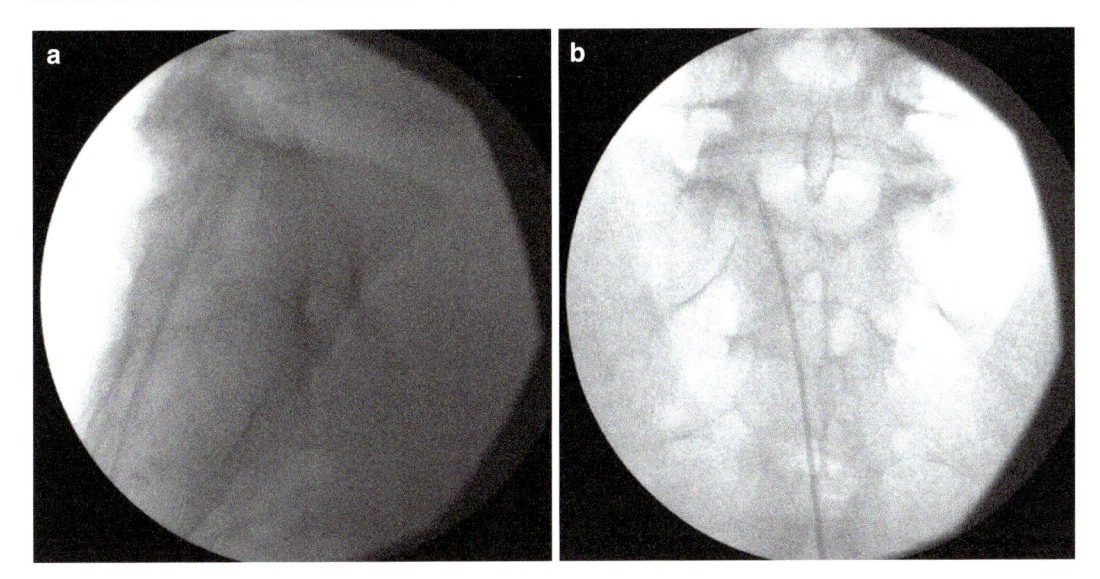

Fig. 4.23 (**a**) A lateral view showing that the tip area is situated within the anterior epidural space. (**b**) An AP view showing that the catheter tip has slipped to one side. Based on the findings in (**a**) and (**b**), it was determined that the catheter was placed within the posterior epidural space, but the catheter tip only had slipped out toward one side of the anterior epidural space

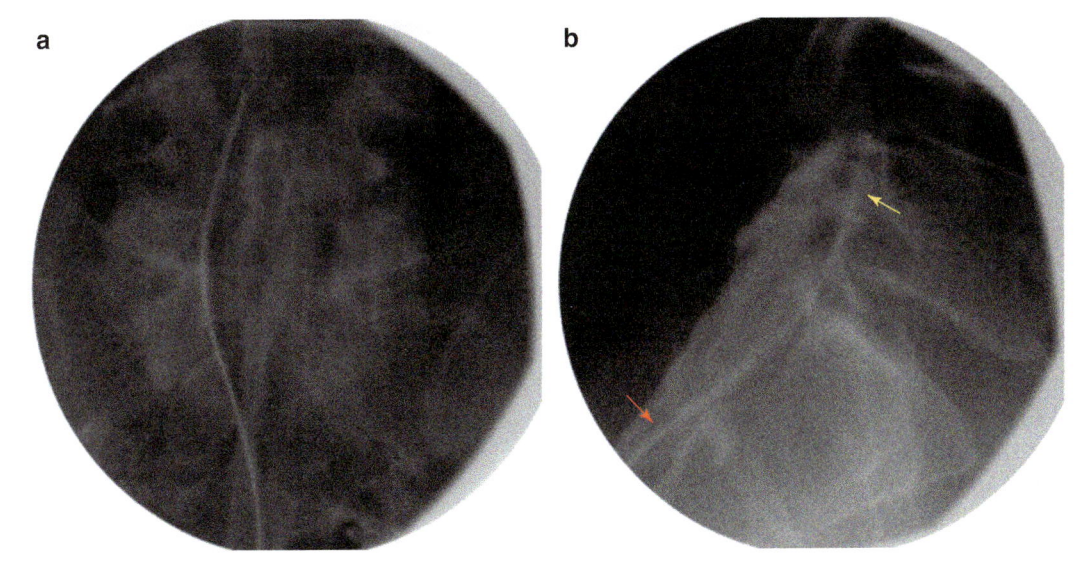

Fig. 4.24 (**a**) After inserting the catheter by tilting it to one side, the tip is adjusted toward the middle and is advanced toward the head. (**b**) When gaining entry according to the method shown in **a**, the catheter being inserted into the posterior epidural space may often rotate halfway around the dura and slip through the anterior epidural space and be advanced toward the head. Red arrow: Catheter placed inside the posterior epidural space. Yellow arrow: Catheter tip slipped through the anterior epidural space

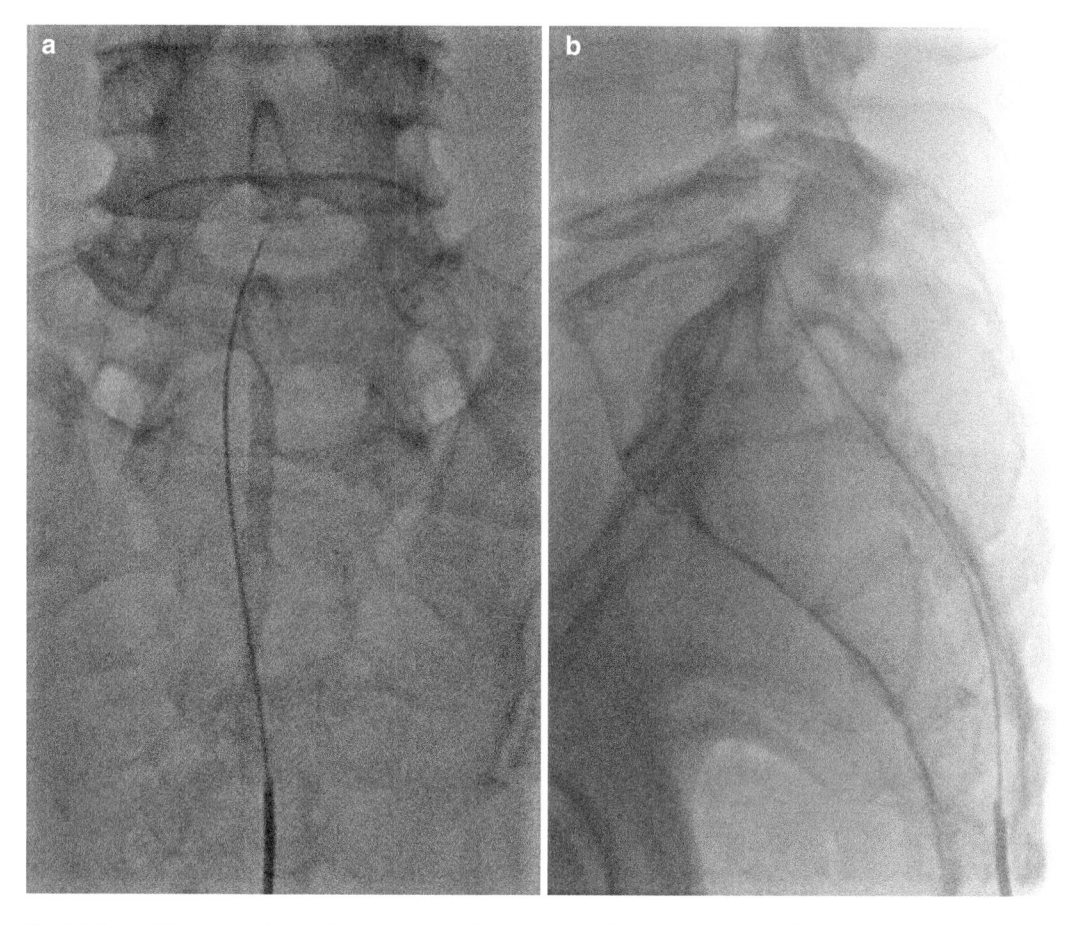

Fig. 4.25 A different case in which the catheter is inserted according to the method referred to in Fig. 4.24

rotating the main body of the catheter instead of simply moving its handle from side to side.

The sides of the epidural space are not flat; rather, its left and right sides are short and convoluted (Fig. 4.28). Accordingly, shifting the catheter to the left or right does not accurately change the direction of the tip to either the left or the right: when pulled excessively to one side, the tip may even bend toward the opposite direction because of the lack of available space to allow the catheter to bend. Hence, changing the direction by pulling on the catheter handle is primarily employed when entering the intervertebral foramen. To gain directional control within the spinal canal, rotating the main body can allow more delicate adjustments.

The method of rotating the catheter itself—i.e., its main body—when it is slightly bent to one side is similar to the method used to bend the tip of the Racz catheter to adjust its direction. When inserting the Racz catheter into the epidural space, the tip of the catheter should first be bent slightly to rotate the catheter itself, set its direction and advance it to the target point. Similarly, when controlling the direction of ZiNeu catheter, its tip is slightly bent, while its body is slightly rotated (Fig. 4.29).

In other words, the handle is pulled gently to bend the tip area while the main body is rotated to delicately guide the direction of the tip (Fig. 4.30).

The target area can be reached easily and accurately with the delicate control of the extent of bending of the catheter tip by using either method: pulling the handle to from side to side or rotating the catheter's main body while it is slightly bent.

4.3 Recommended Procedure

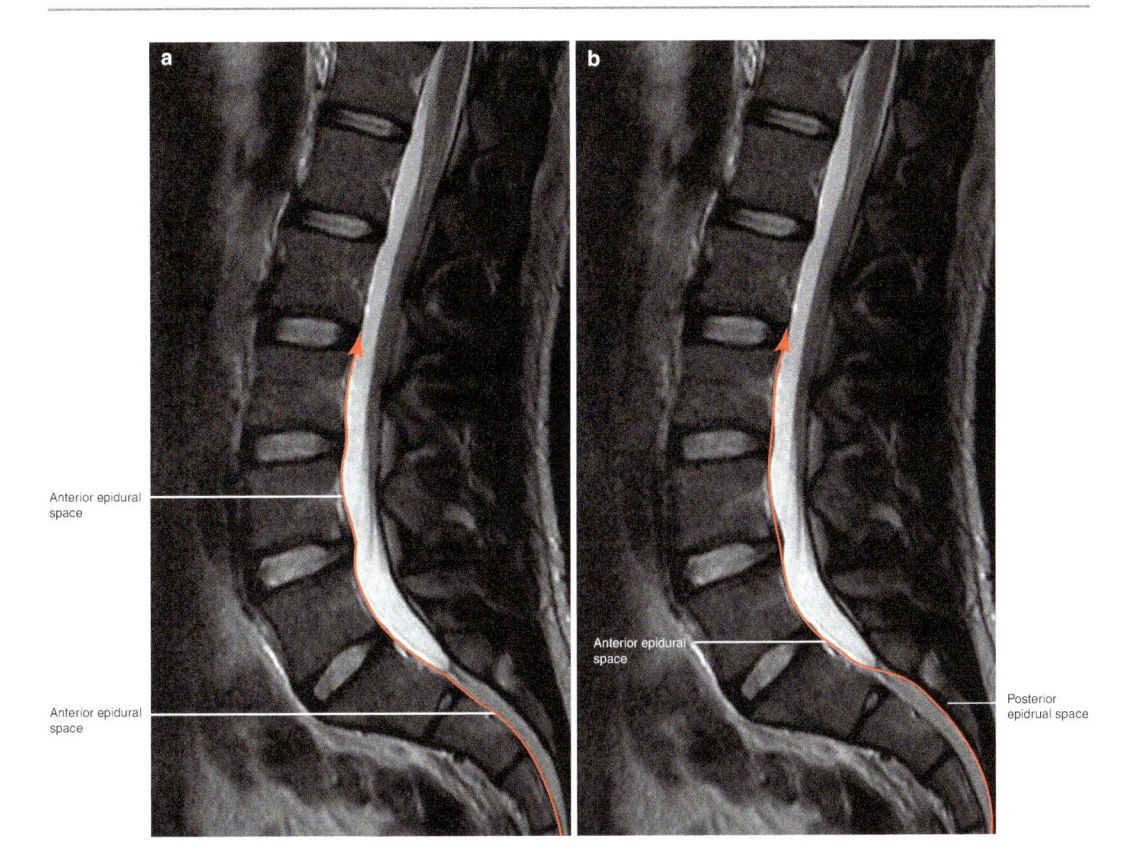

Fig. 4.26 Two methods of entering the anterior epidural space. (**a**) Entry into the midline of the anterior epidural space from the initial opening. (**b**) Entry by rotating to the anterior epidural space after crossing through the posterior epidural space

4.3.5 Entry into the Intervertebral Foramen

The likelihood of dural puncture during the procedure is higher in the central area than in the intervertebral foramen area. Therefore, it is advisable to perform the procedure in the central area subsequent to its completion in the targeted intervertebral foramen area.

In many cases, balloon expansion in the intervertebral foraminal area decisively influences the prognosis of the patient. Whenever possible, balloon decompression should be performed up to the extraforaminal area.

The performance of balloon expansion in narrow areas may create excessive pressure on and around the balloon, which could cause severe pain or balloon rupture. Hence, the balloon should be inflated gradually while the C-arm images are referenced in real-time. If the patient complains of severe pain during balloon decompression, inflation of the balloon should be ceased—even if the balloon has not been fully inflated. After 2–3 s, the balloon should then be deflated. The site of the procedure should be divided into two to three zones, and the inflation/deflation of the balloon should be repeated twice or thrice for each zone as the catheter is gradually moved between zones.

Drug administration after the procedure may differ depending on the patient and physician; typically, however, a local anesthetic/steroid mixture is administered after confirmation with the 100% contrast dye.

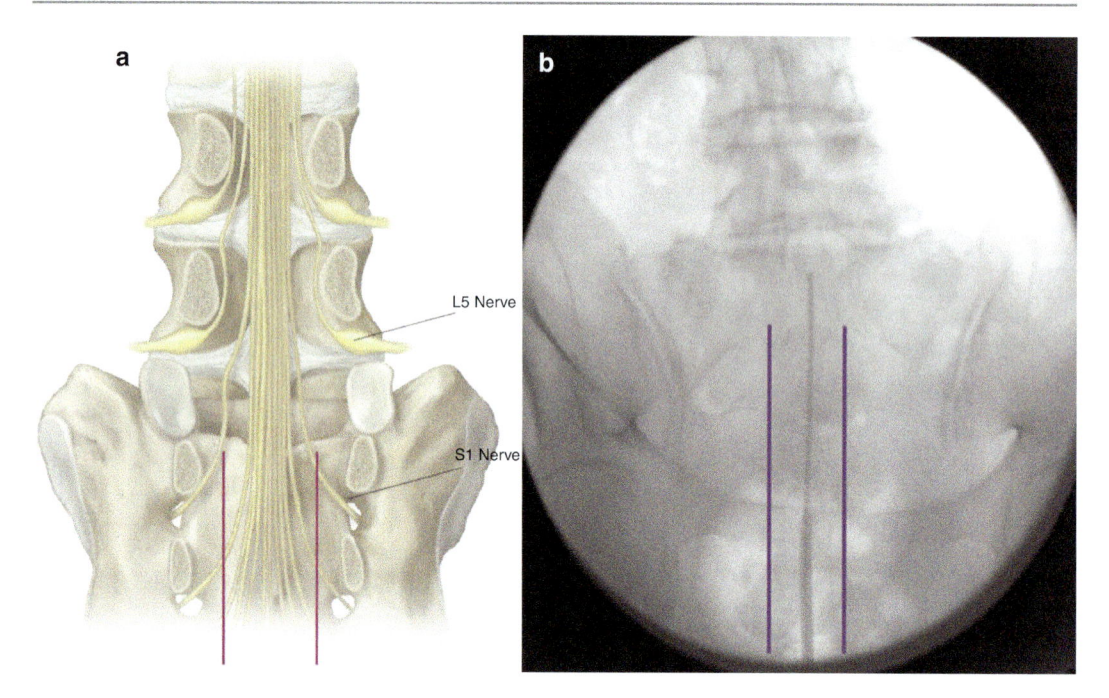

Fig. 4.27 (**a**) To prevent nerve-irritation symptoms, the catheter must be inserted within the purple lines to prevent its contact with the sacral nerve that runs through the sacral foramen. (**b**) Image of the catheter being inserted within the purple lines. There is virtually no pain under this state. The purple lines connect the medial sides of the sacral foramina

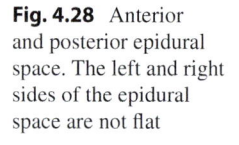

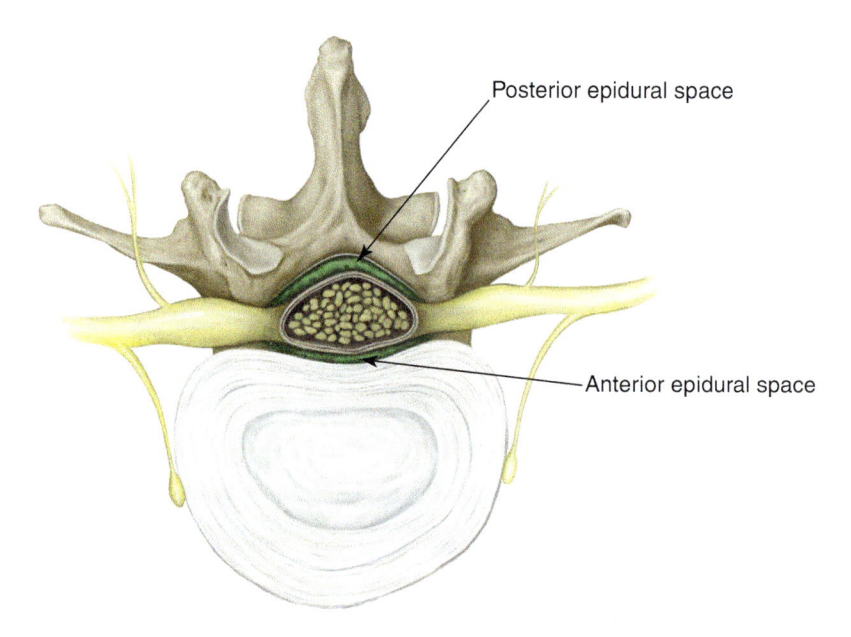

Fig. 4.28 Anterior and posterior epidural space. The left and right sides of the epidural space are not flat

Methods for entry into the intervertebral foramen include entry into the superior and inferior aspect of the intervertebral foramen. The former refers to the area just below the upper pedicle where the spinal nerves run; the latter, to the area right above the lower pedicle often referred to as Kambin's triangle (Fig. 4.31).

4.3 Recommended Procedure

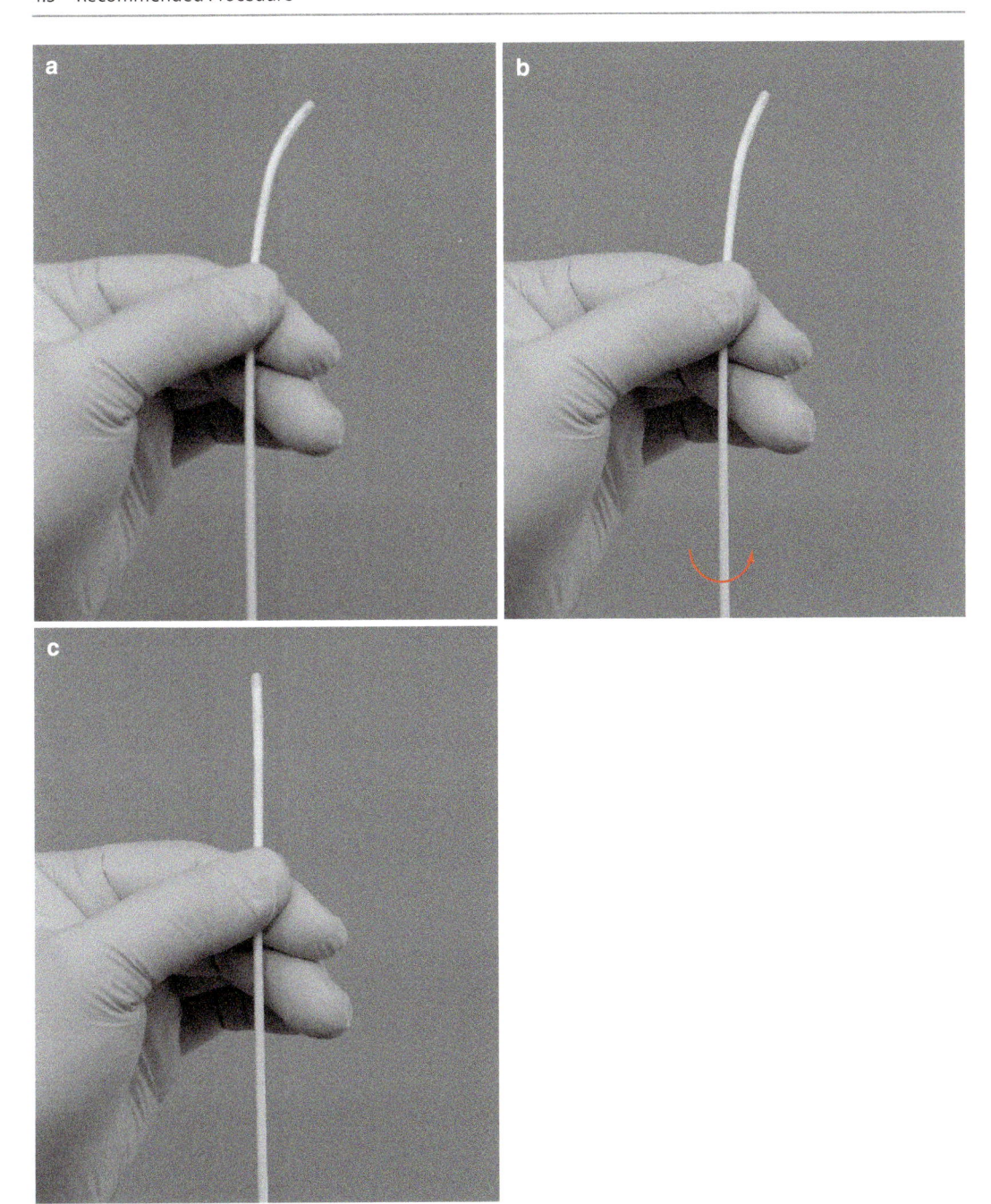

Fig. 4.29 (a) Catheter bent to the right. (b) The catheter in A is rotated by 45 degrees. (c) The catheter in **a** is rotated by 90°. **c** appears close to a straight line because the effect of bending diminishes smaller as position **a** is rotated to position **c**. (**a**, **b**) The catheter is advanced to the right within the epidural space as far as the catheter tip can bend to the right. (**c**) The catheter is advanced in a straight line inside the epidural space, as the tip is not tilted to either side

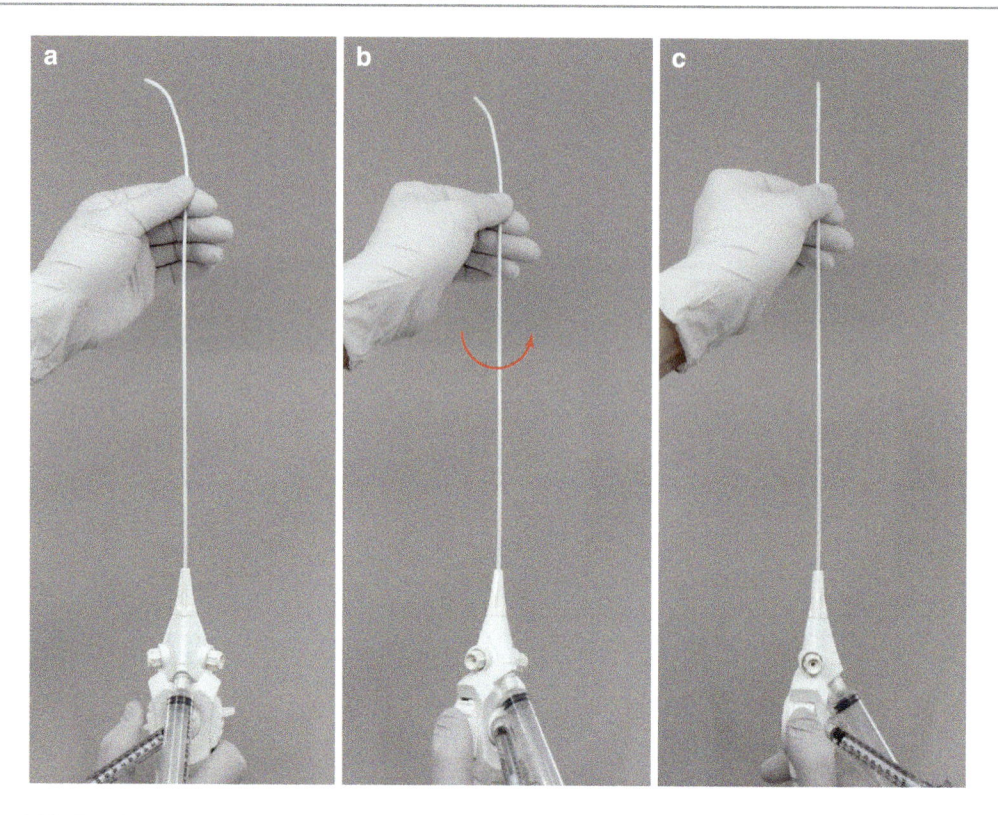

Fig. 4.30 Rotating the main body of the catheter as the tip is bent slightly to the left. (**a**) The catheter tip is slightly bent. (**b**) The catheter body is rotated by 45° from state **a**. The extent of bending becomes smaller with rotation. (**c**) The catheter body is rotated by 90° from state **a** and appears as a straight line without any bending. By slowly rotating the main body of the catheter as the bending of the tip transitions from position **a** to **c**, the effect of the bending of the tip diminishes

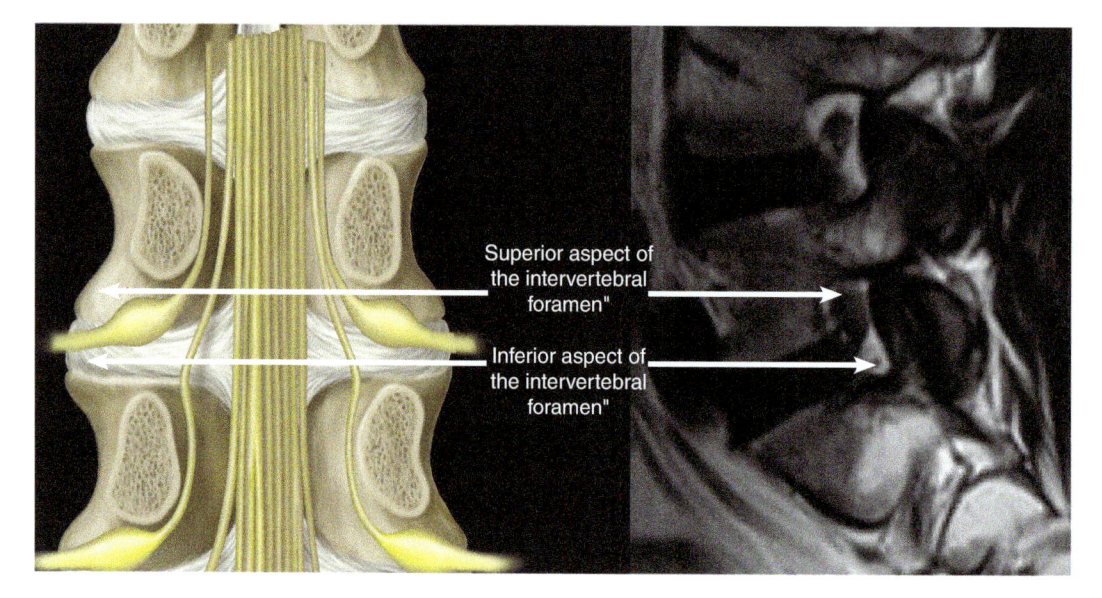

Fig. 4.31 Location of the superior and inferior aspects of the intervertebral foramen

4.3 Recommended Procedure

The method of entry should be decided according to the location of the lesion. If adhesion or stenosis is suspected near the spinal nerves, the balloon should be inflated after the entry is made into the superior aspect of the intervertebral foramen. However, if there is a lesion in the inferior aspect of the intervertebral foramen or impingement of the traversing nerve due to the pathology of retrodiscal area, the entry should be made into the inferior aspect of the intervertebral foramen.

The angles of entry through the superior and inferior aspects of the intervertebral foramen differ. The former requires entry along the upper pedicle; the latter, close to the upper part of the lower pedicle (Fig. 4.32).

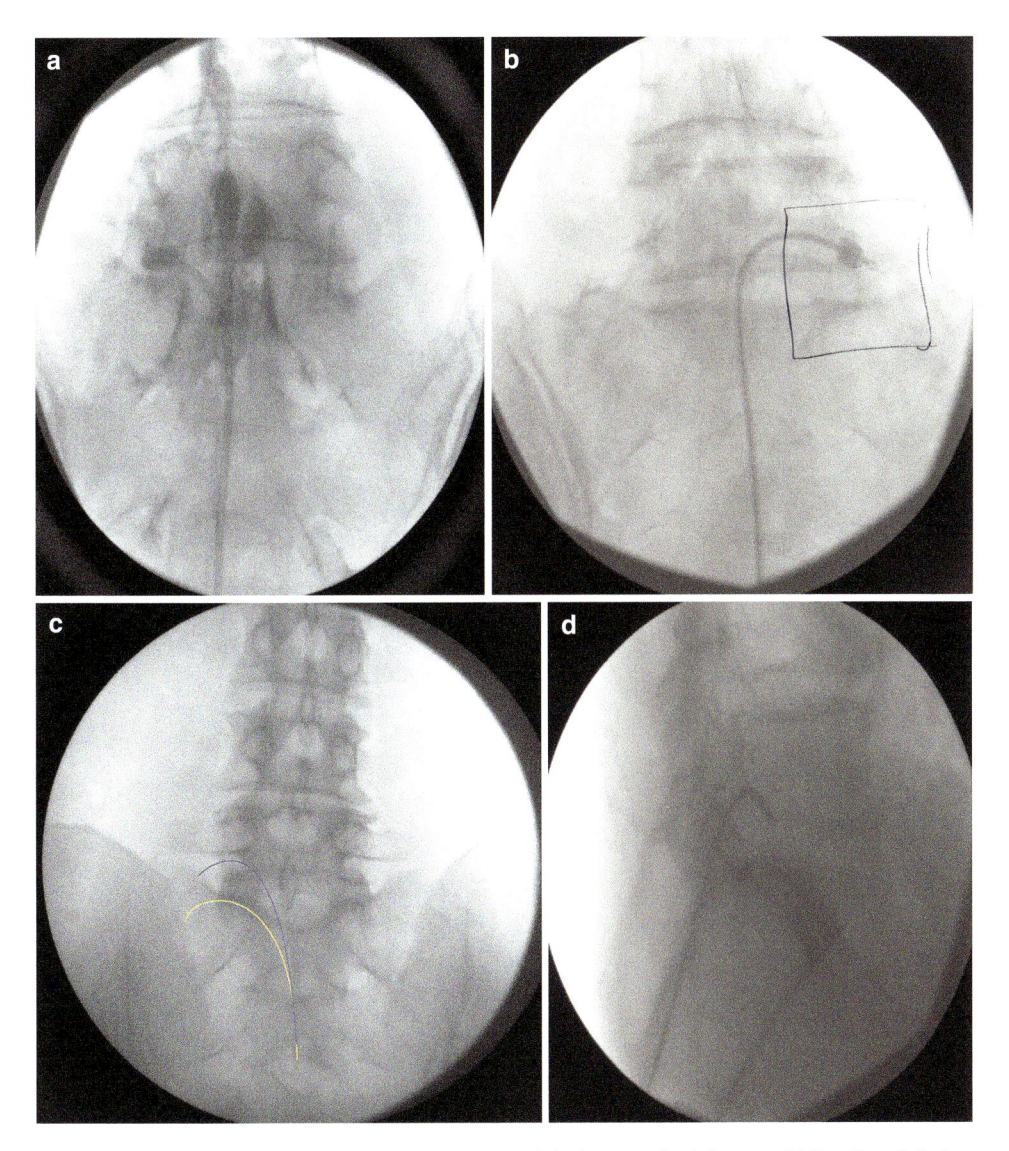

Fig. 4.32 (**a**) Entry into the inferior aspect of the intervertebral foramen. (**b**) Entry into the superior aspect of the intervertebral foramen. (**c**) Schematic diagram of the entry into the superior and inferior aspects of the intervertebral foramen. Purple line: Entry into the superior aspect of the intervertebral foramen. Yellow line: Inferior aspect of the intervertebral foramen. (**d**) Lateral view of the entry into the superior aspect of the intervertebral foramen. The catheter passes through the anterior epidural space to reach the intervertebral foramen

Below are two cases that required the procedure to be performed in the superior aspect of the intervertebral foramen:

Case 1 A 73-year-old man visited the pain clinic at our hospital for Rt. L5 radiculopathy and 200 m claudication. MRI findings showed multilevel central stenosis with Rt. L4 foraminal stenosis but no Rt. L5 foraminal stenosis (Fig. 4.33). Informed by the supposition that the patient's main symptoms were caused by adhesion along the Rt. L5 root, ZiNeu catheter-mediated balloon decompression in the Rt. L5 foramen and Rt. L4–5 retrodiscal area was planned.

During the procedure, an attempt was made to insert the catheter into the superior aspect of the Rt. L5–S1 intervertebral foramen; however, insertion into the inferior aspect alone was possible. Injection of the contrast dye showed a filling defect in the superior aspect of the intervertebral foramen, but the defect could not be resolved. The balloon decompression of the patient's L4–5 retrodiscal and preganglionic areas was successful (Fig. 4.34).

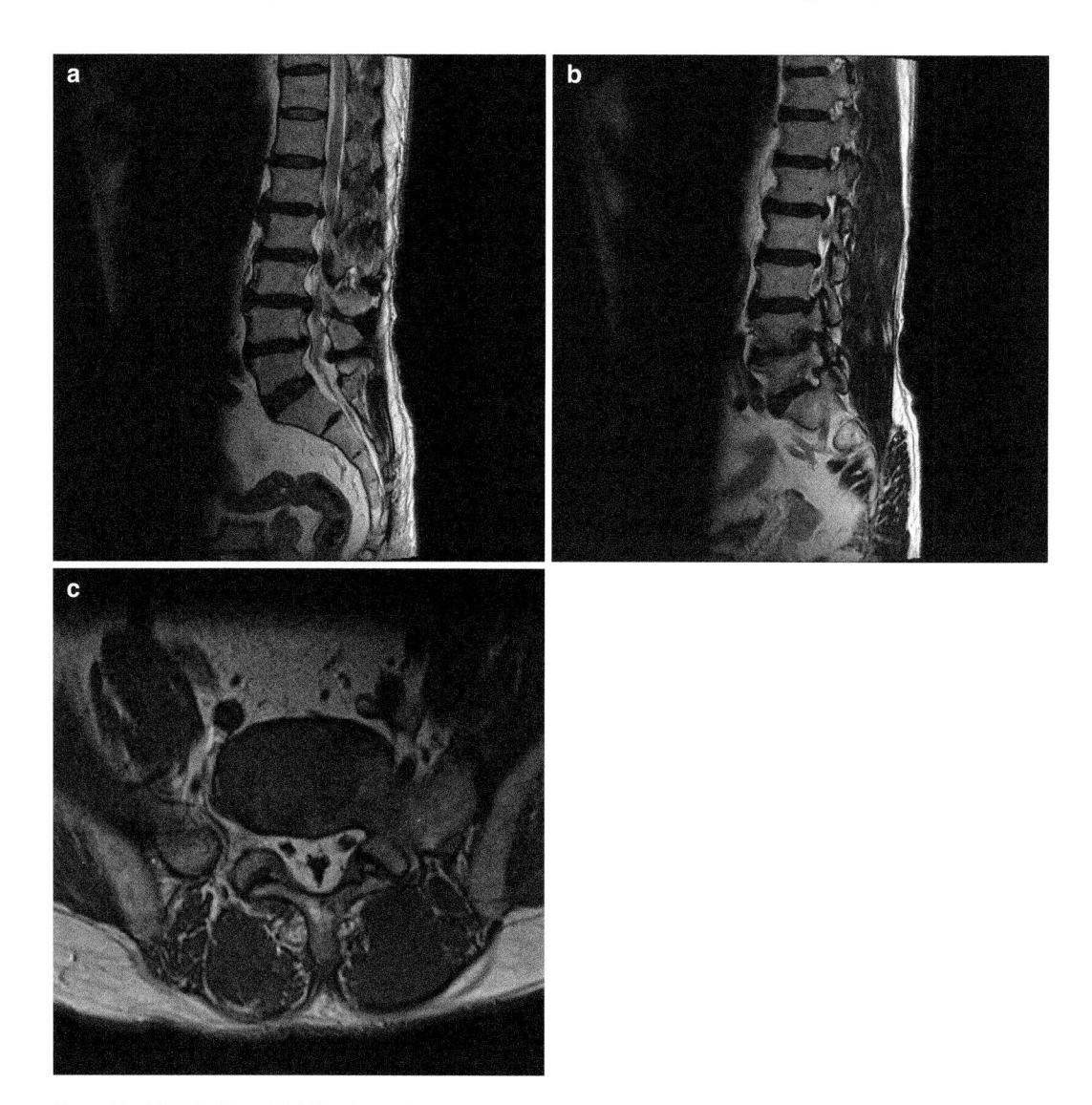

Fig. 4.33 MRI findings. Multilevel central stenosis with Rt. L4 foraminal stenosis Rt. L5 foraminal stenosis was not found

4.3 Recommended Procedure

As the patient's symptoms showed no improvements within 1 month of the procedure, the previously observed filling defect was suspected as the primary site of the lesion. Accordingly, balloon decompression using the ZiNeuF catheter was performed at the superior aspect of the intervertebral foramen, and the filling defect was resolved (Fig. 4.35).

The patient reported that his symptoms improved significantly following the procedure. This case confirms the importance of balloon decompression along the superior aspect of the intervertebral foramen—i.e., along the spinal nerve—when adhesion near the spinal nerve is suspected.

Case 2 A 78-year-old man presented with symptoms similar to those of the patient described in Case 1. An attempt was made to insert the ZiNeu02 catheter through the superior aspect of Rt. L5–S1 intervertebral foramen; however, insertion into the inferior aspect alone was possible. The filling defect near the Rt. L5 nerve in the superior aspect of the intervertebral foramen could not be resolved. As the patient's symptoms did not improve, the procedure was performed once more a month later. Entry into the superior aspect of the intervertebral foramen was successful, and the filling defect near the Rt. L5 nerve was resolved. The patient showed significant improvement since the procedure (Fig. 4.36).

If only the success rate of entry into the superior or inferior aspects of the intervertebral foramen entry is considered, the ZiNeuF catheter is superior to the ZiNeu catheter. In Case 2, the use of the ZiNeuF catheter during the second procedure increased the likelihood of success, just as in Case 1. However, this patient had undergone the procedure before the ZiNeuF catheter was released, and thus, the second procedure was performed using the ZiNeu02 catheter.

These two cases suggest that, when addressing lesions in the intervertebral foramen, the success of the procedure depends on accurately approaching the lesion.

While several novel procedural methods for foraminal decompression have been recently developed, most of these techniques attempt entry into the inferior aspect of the intervertebral foramen to avert the risk of spinal nerve damage. These techniques cannot directly remove perineural adhesion or stenosis in the superior aspect of the interverte-

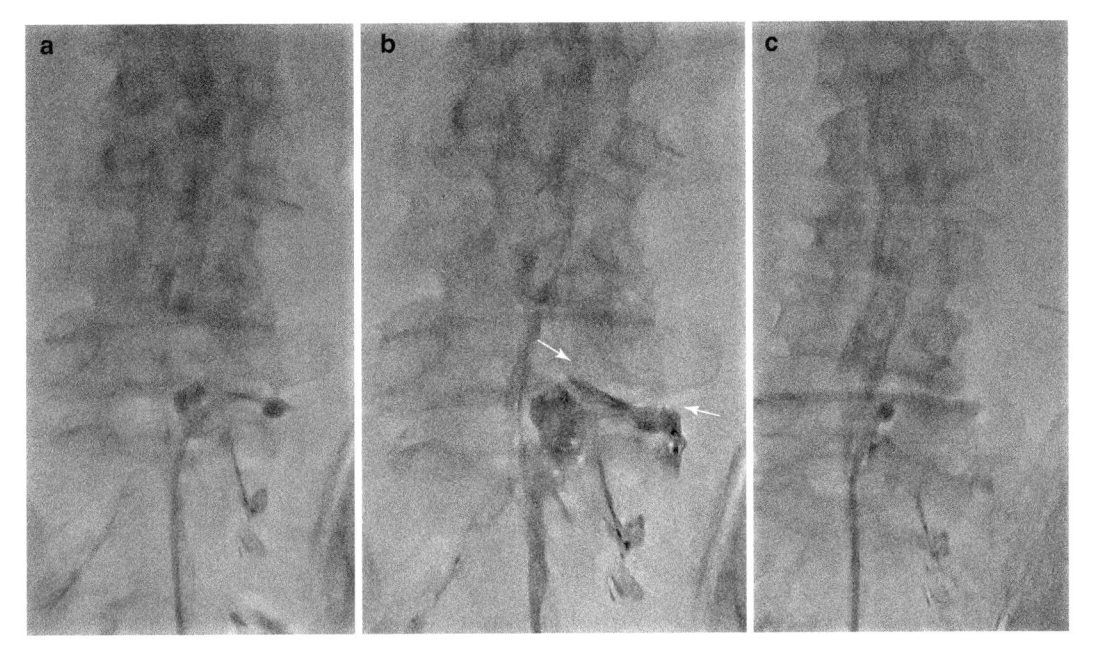

Fig. 4.34 (**a**) An attempt was made to insert the catheter into the superior aspect of the Rt. L5 foramen, but only insertion into the inferior aspect was possible. (**b**) Filling defect in the superior aspect of the intervertebral foramen. Arrow: filling defect. (**c**) Balloon being inflated in the preganglionic area

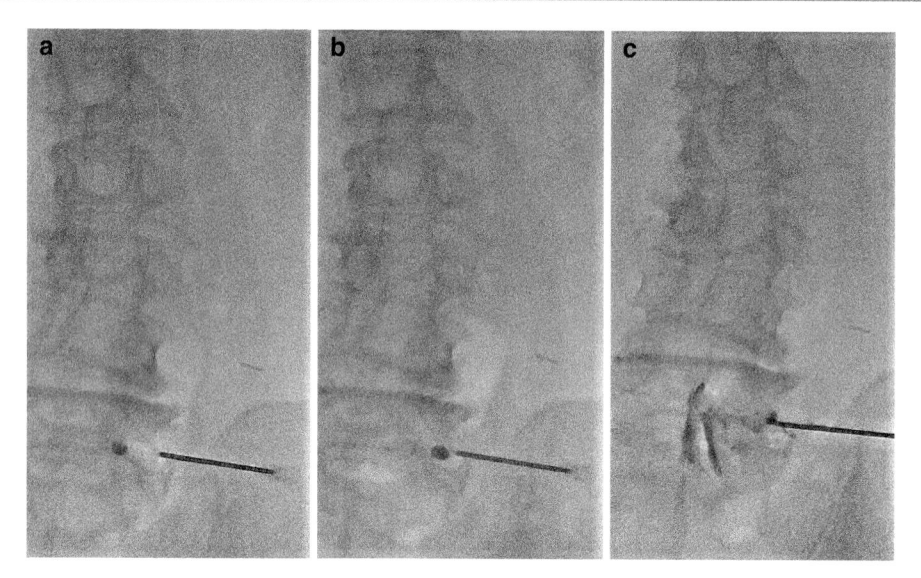

Fig. 4.35 Performance of balloon decompression with the ZiNeuF catheter at the superior aspect of the intervertebral foramen in the patient shown in (Fig. 4.34). (**a**, **b**) The inflation of the balloon following the entry into the superior aspect of the intervertebral foramen. (**c**) The filling defect in the superior aspect of the intervertebral foramen was resolved after the procedure

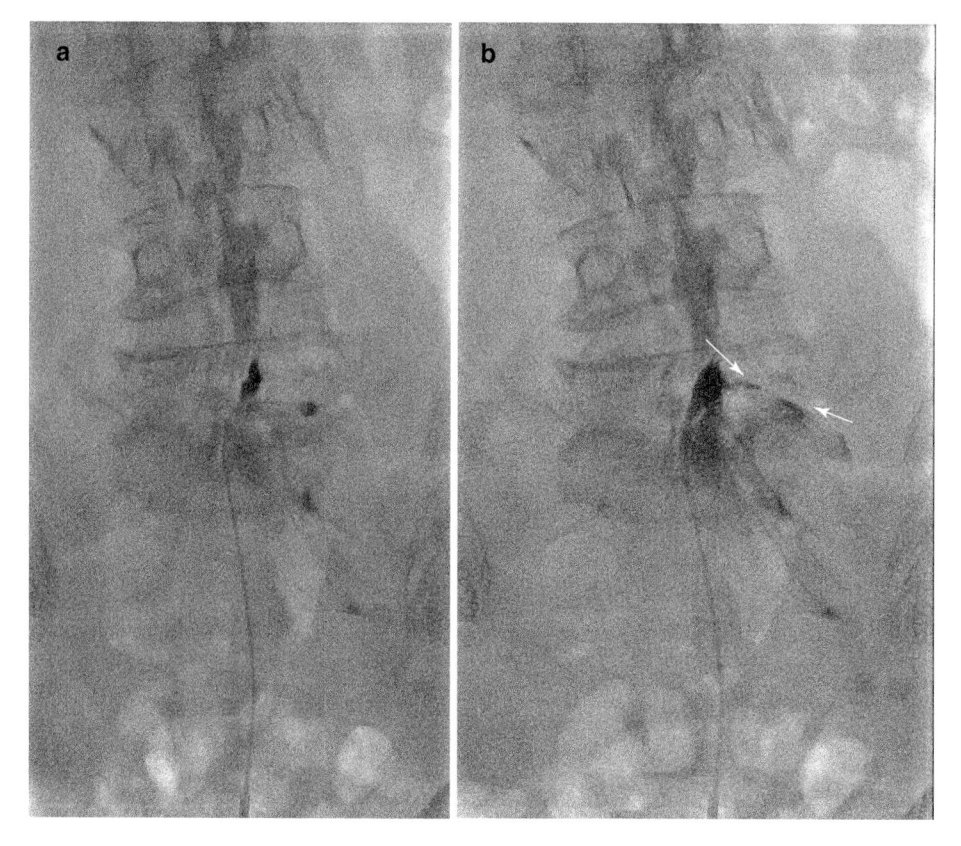

Fig. 4.36 (**a**, **b**) The filling defect in the superior aspect of the intervertebral foramen could not be resolved because the ZiNeu02 catheter could only be inserted into the inferior aspect of the Rt. L5 intervertebral foramen. Arrow: filling defect. (**c**) The successful entry into the superior aspect of the intervertebral foramen when the procedure was performed again. (**d**) The filling defect in the superior aspect of the intervertebral foramen was resolved after the procedure

4.3 Recommended Procedure

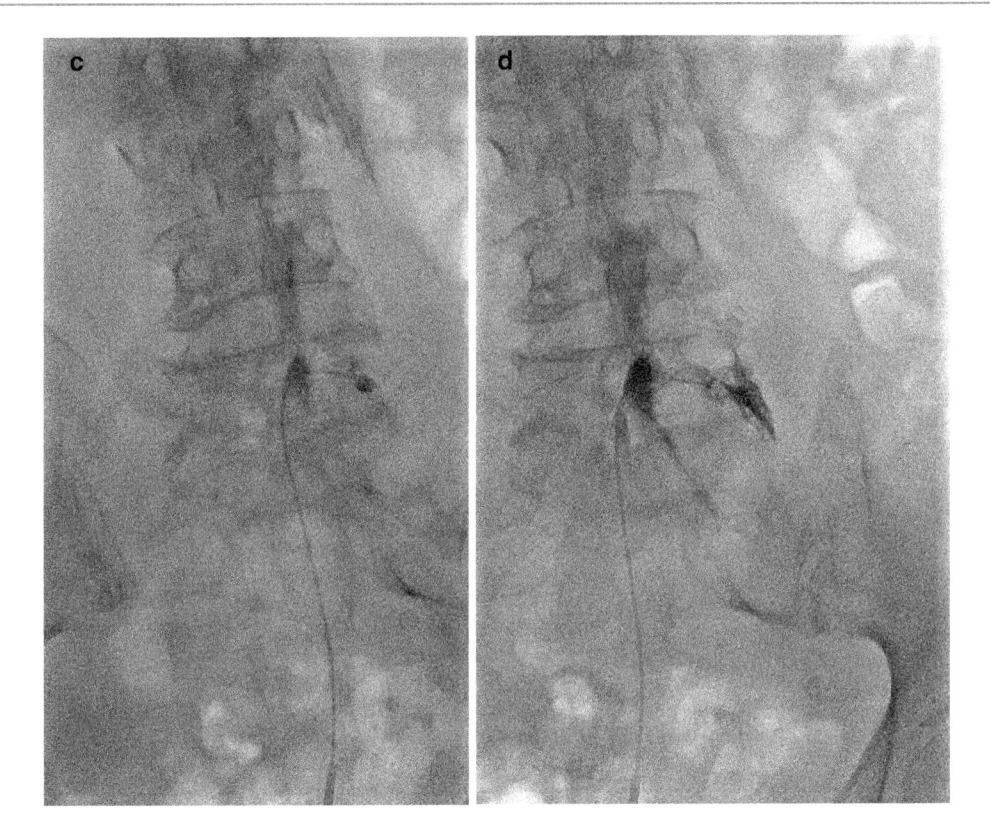

Fig. 4.36 (continued)

bral foramen and may expand only the inferior aspect. As the cases described above illustrate, this area may be unrelated to the symptoms, and the procedure may therefore be ineffectual. Balloon decompression is a safe procedure with almost no possibility of nerve damage; thus, it features the major advantage of allowing the catheter to approach the nerves closely during the procedure.

For cases that require entry into the inferior aspect of the intervertebral foramen and retrodiscal area, please refer to the detailed explanation presented on pages 43–45 as well as Chap. 9.

L5 radiculopathy could be caused by lesions in the L5 intervertebral foramen, but also by the irritation of the L5 nerve, which traverses lower levels, by L4–5 retrodiscal lesions. Furthermore, S1 radiculopathy may occur due to L5–S1 retrodiscal lesions (Fig. 4.37).

Following the foraminal procedure, it is therefore important to perform balloon decompression and adhesiolysis by inserting the ZiNeu catheter up to the retrodiscal area of the upper level, close to the preganglion. As aforementioned, this is on account of the difficulty in localizing the primary cause of L5 radiculopathy to the intervertebral foramen, preganglion, or retrodiscal area of the upper level (Fig. 4.38).

As explained in the Introduction, balloon decompression in patients with Rt. L5 radiculopathy may require the insertion of the catheter into the inferior aspect of the Rt. L4–5 intervertebral foramen, in addition to the retrodiscal area.

MRI findings should be referenced to find the optimal location for the alleviation of adhesion and traversing nerve compression prior to the adoption of this approach.

In cases involving degenerative spinal diseases, common lesion sites include the left and right L4, L5 foramen and L4–5 retrodiscal area, and L5–S1 retrodiscal area. Accordingly, these areas become the main target for balloon decompression; however, which of these areas require the procedure must be accurately determined prior to its performance (Fig. 4.39).

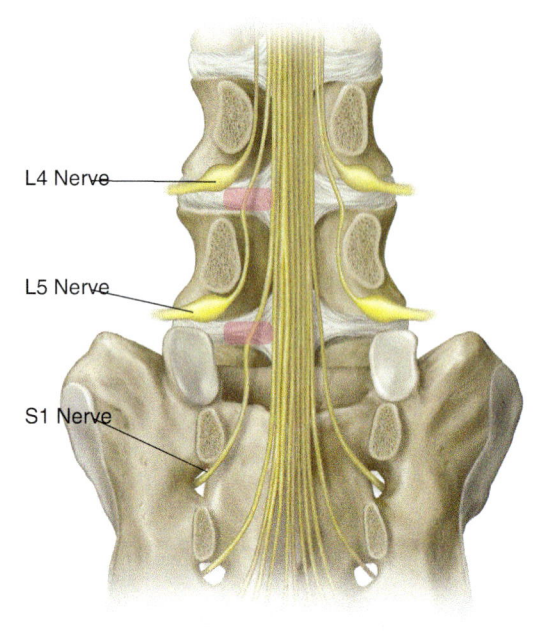

Fig. 4.37 Schematic diagram showing that L5 radiculopathy may be caused by the irritation of the L5 traversing nerve by the L4–5 retrodiscal lesion. S1 radiculopathy may be caused by L5–S1 retrodiscal lesions. Red mark: retrodiscal lesion

When S1 radiculopathy is present, catheter insertion into the S1 foramen is often attempted. However, stenosis does not occur in the S1 foramen; S1 radiculopathy is usually caused by lesions in the retrodiscal area of the L5–S1 level. Hence, because lesions in the retrodiscal area must be resolved, inserting the catheter directly into the S1 foramen is ineffective (Fig. 4.40).

Pain or nerve-irritation symptoms may present during the inflation of the balloon or contact between the catheter and a nerve. In such cases, it is important to ask the patient if the site of stimulation corresponds to the site of pain (provocation test): if the sites correspond, it is highly likely that the stimulated site is causing the pain.

Useful tip for performing the intervertebral foraminal procedure

1. When entering into the caudal space, advancing the catheter between the midline and medial border of the S1 pedicle on the affected side is more advantageous for adjusting the angle of entry into the intervertebral foramen and applied strong force during inserting the catheter into the intervertebral foramen to allow it to penetrate to the extraforaminal area—i.e., the catheter should ideally pass through the blue mark presented in Fig. 4.41. Entry into the midline weakens the force penetrating into the intervertebral foramen, which can lower the success rate. In contrast, if the catheter is advanced upward while being tilted too much to the affected side, it may touch the sacral nerve or be blocked by the S1 pedicle, preventing entry into the intervertebral foramen. Therefore, the catheter should be directed to pass through the blue mark in Fig. 4.41 (Figs. 4.41, 4.42 and 4.43).

2. Sometimes, entry into the intervertebral foramen can be facilitated by approaching it from the opposite side while drawing a large circle around. This method may be useful if the method in (1) proved difficult or especially when using a ZiNeu01 catheter rather than a ZiNeuS catheter (Fig. 4.44).

3. Before injecting the drug after foraminal balloon decompression, it is advisable to make a path to the extraforaminal area with the guidewire and give the medicine. Based on the authors' experience, adhesion might remain in the lateral area that cannot be accessed by the catheter. In this case, advancing and then withdrawing the guidewire could help to remove adhesion of the extraforaminal area.

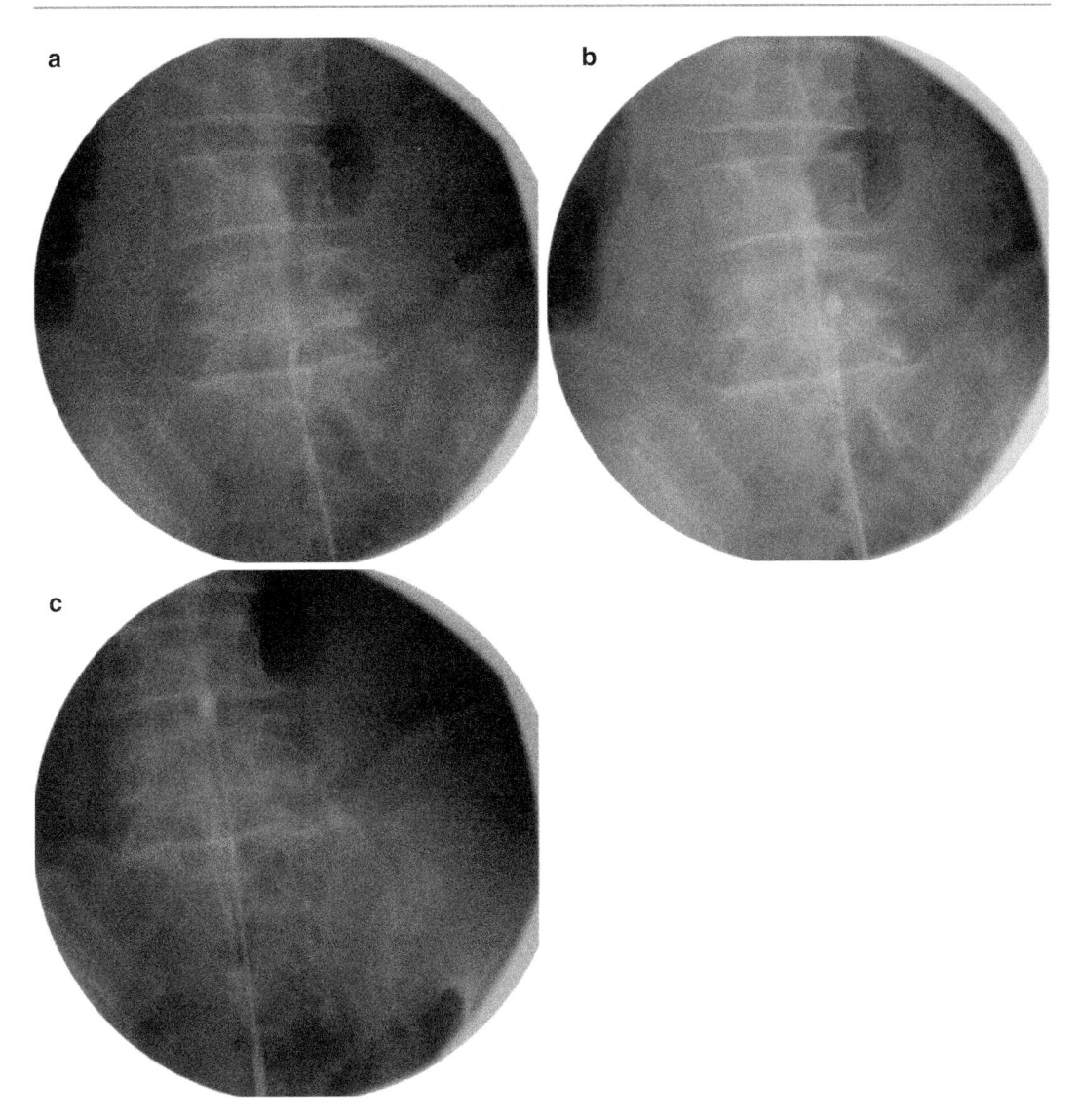

Fig. 4.38 In a patient with Rt. L5 radiculopathy, balloon decompression is performed in the (**a**) Rt. L5 foramen, (**b**) Rt. L5 preganglion, and (**c**) Rt. L4–5 retrodiscal area

In fact, when the contrast dye is injected after the trajectory has been defined by the guidewire, the dye tends to spread with greater efficacy (Fig. 4.45).

4. In cases where the procedure involving the entire intervertebral foramen is rendered difficult by severe foraminal adhesion or stenosis, a path can be created with a guidewire. A

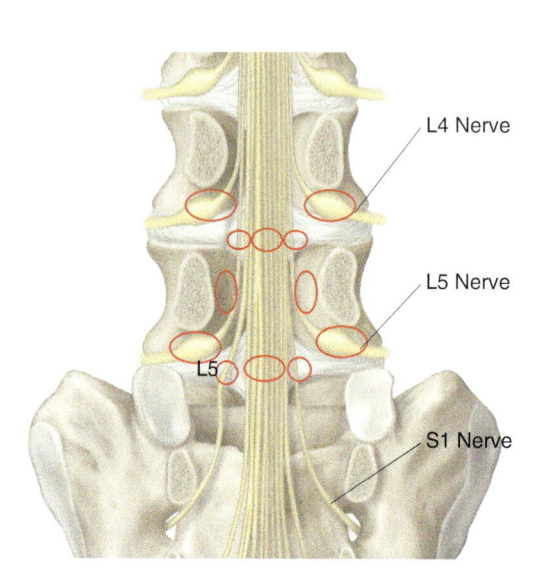

Fig. 4.39 Red circle: Areas where lesions commonly occur. These areas become the main targets for balloon decompression

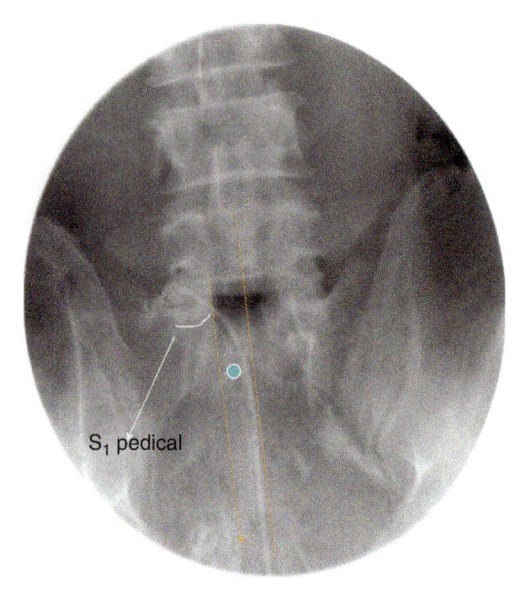

Fig. 4.41 Passing the catheter through the blue mark helps to augment the force necessary for penetrating into the intervertebral foramen

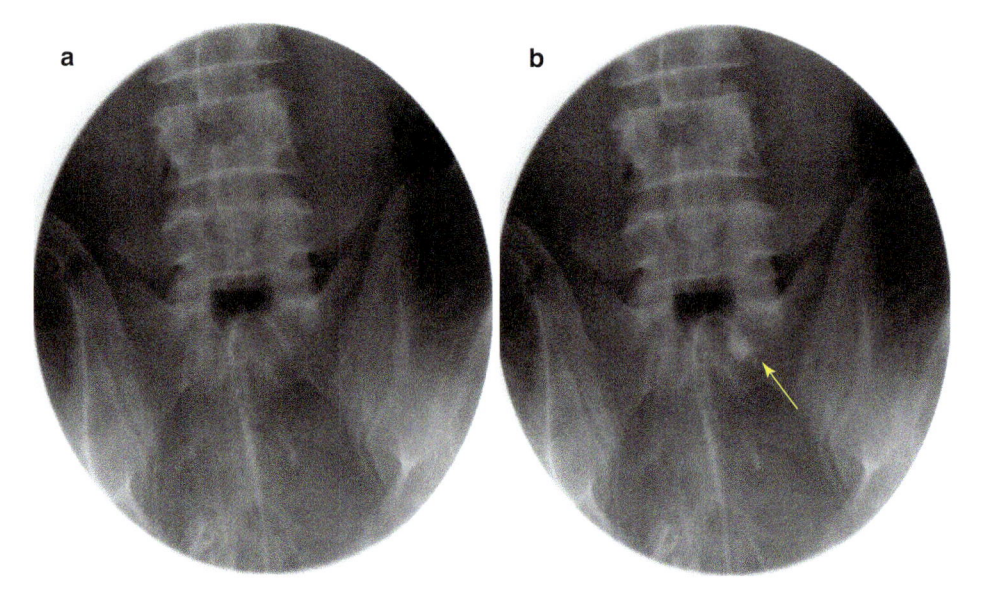

Fig. 4.40 Inflation of the balloon after inserting the catheter into the Rt. S1 foramen. Arrow: Inflated balloon

4.3 Recommended Procedure

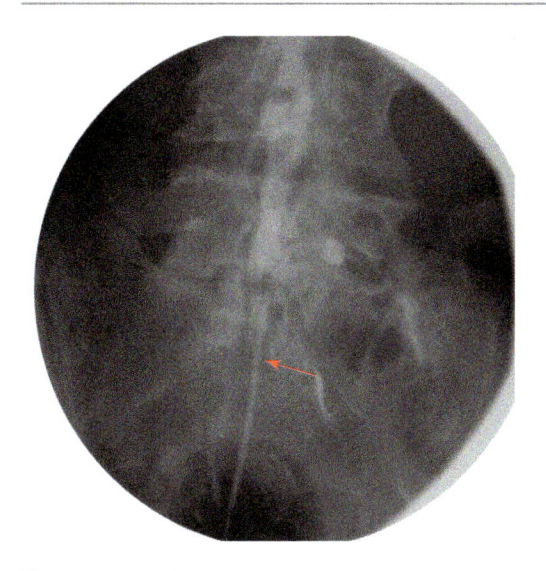

Fig. 4.42 Case in which the catheter was inserted into the midline. The catheter may not enter completely into the intervertebral foramen because the force for penetrating into the intervertebral foramen is too weak. Arrow: Catheter inserted into the midline

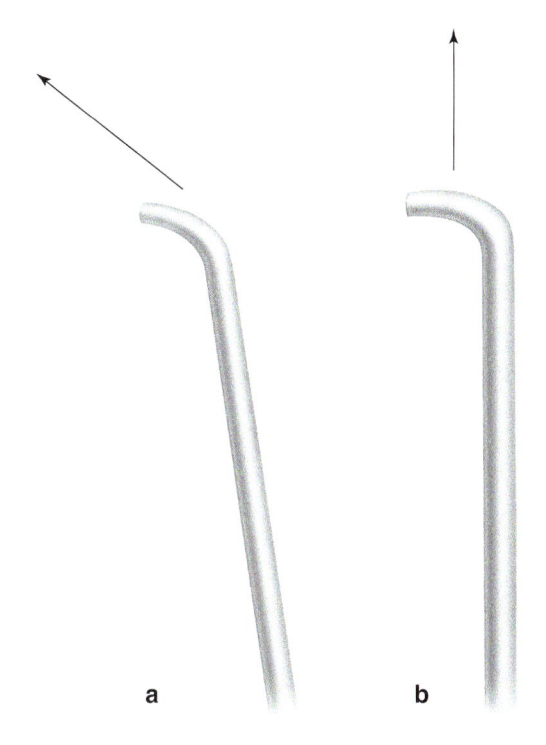

Fig. 4.43 Vector diagram of the force according to the entry angle of the catheter. (**a**) Inserting the catheter slightly to one side of the spine could increase the force necessary for penetrating into the intervertebral foramen. (**b**) When inserted into the middle of the spine, the tip tends to advance toward the head—even when bent—weakening the advance of the catheter and compromising its penetrating into the intervertebral foramen

drug-injection epidural catheter containing a reinforcing wire can then be inserted and left at the site of the lesion to attempt additional drug therapy, including hypertonic saline. Even if the balloon cannot be inserted, the best possible effort to ensure that the drug spreads efficiently into the lesion area should be made (Fig. 4.46).

5. In cases similar to (4), if the procedure should be succeeded due to a close association between the lesion in the intervertebral foramen and the patient's symptoms, the performance of an additional procedure via the transforaminal approach with the ZiNeuF catheter—instead of the drug-injection catheter—may be optimal. (This is explained in detail in the next chapter.) Considering the entry into the intervertebral foramen, employing the transforaminal approach with the ZiNeuF catheter instead of the caudal approach with the ZiNeu catheter would shorten the distance to the lesion area and allow the catheter to penetrate into the intervertebral foramen with greater force. On the other hand, a procedure whereby the caudal ZiNeu and transforaminal ZiNeuF catheters are inserted concurrently in the same patient is possible (Fig. 4.47) (Of course, the interlaminar approach could be used instead of the transforaminal approach depending on the case).

4.3.6 Entry into the Central Area

For balloon decompression in the central area, stenosis alleviation and the removal of adhesion in the retrodiscal area of the anterior epidural space are to be prioritized. As explained in Chap. 1, this is because adhesion and stenosis occur most commonly in the L4–5 and L5–S1 retrodiscal areas (Fig. 4.48).

As aforementioned, the sinuvertebral nerve, which is closely associated with low back pain, is primarily distributed in the anterior epidural space: the site at which most lesions associated with degenerative spine diseases, including disc herniation, are found. Therefore, treatment of the retrodiscal area in the anterior epidural space is paramount. However, because adhesion in the

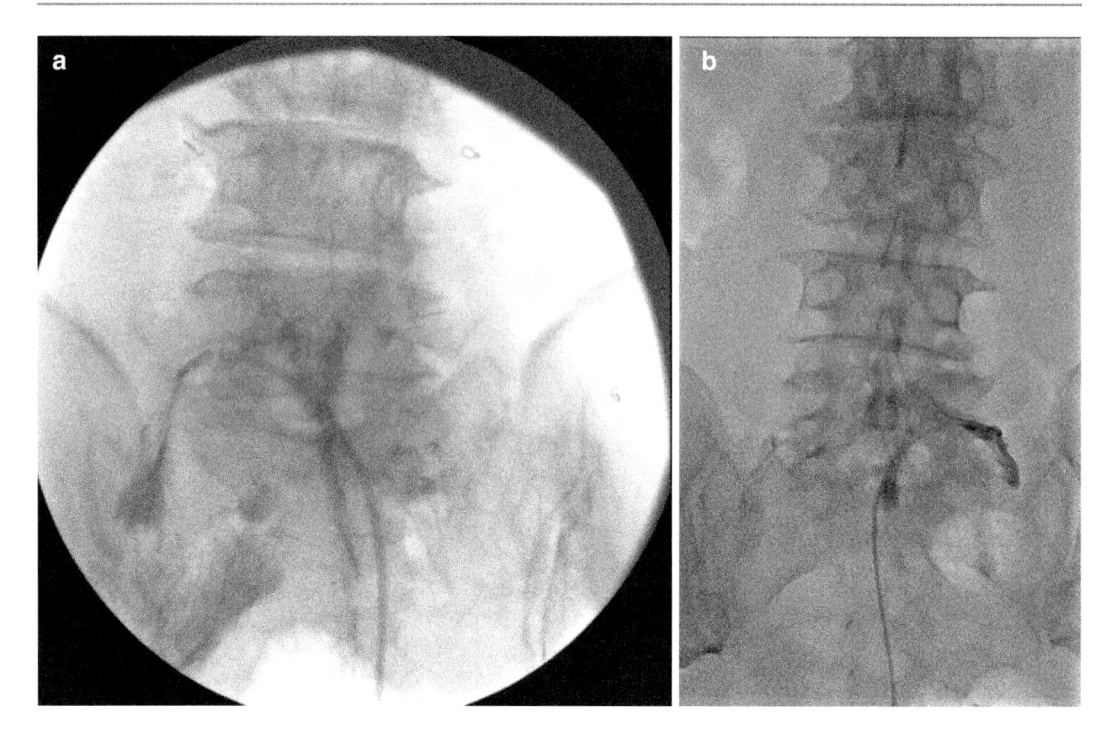

Fig. 4.44 Entry into the intervertebral foramen through the opposite side, while drawing a large circle around it

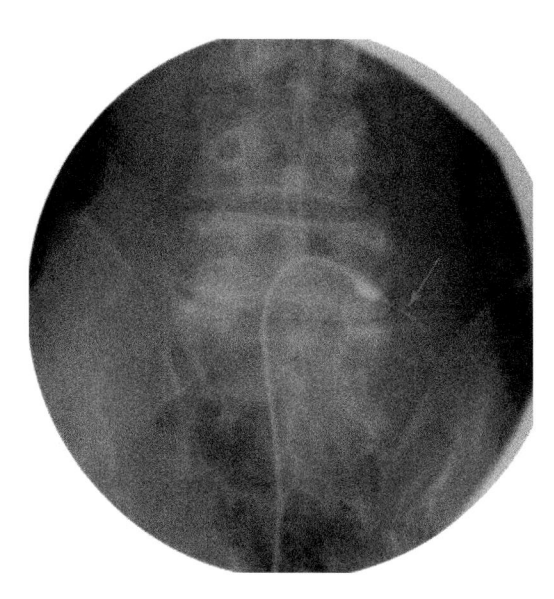

Fig. 4.45 Detaching the adhesion in the extraforaminal area with the guidewire before injecting the drug. Arrow: guidewire advanced to the extraforaminal area

posterior epidural space can also contribute to low back pain associated with movement, it is advisable to perform balloon decompression and adhesiolysis in both the anterior and posterior epidural spaces when treating the central area.

Balloon decompression in the retrodiscal area should be performed following the left-to-right division of the area into three zones (Fig. 4.49). The catheter should be moved sequentially into each zone so that it can cover a wider area.

When performing the procedures on the central area, the author uses the method of advancing the catheter past the lesion area and inflating the balloon, followed by slowly withdrawing the catheter while pulling down with the inflated balloon. When performing the procedure in the intervertebral foramen, the inflated balloon may induce traction injury to the spinal nerve as it is withdrawn; thus, it is recommended that the balloon should be pulled only when it is deflated. However, since there is virtually no risk of damaging any nerves during spinal canal procedure, the balloon can be withdrawn while inflated. This allows for the performance of the procedure across a wider area in less time.

It is important to consider that the catheter must be moved very slowly since withdrawing it quickly could be dangerous. If the patient feels severe pain, this procedure must not be performed; the initially introduced method of gradually moving the catheter while continually

4.3 Recommended Procedure

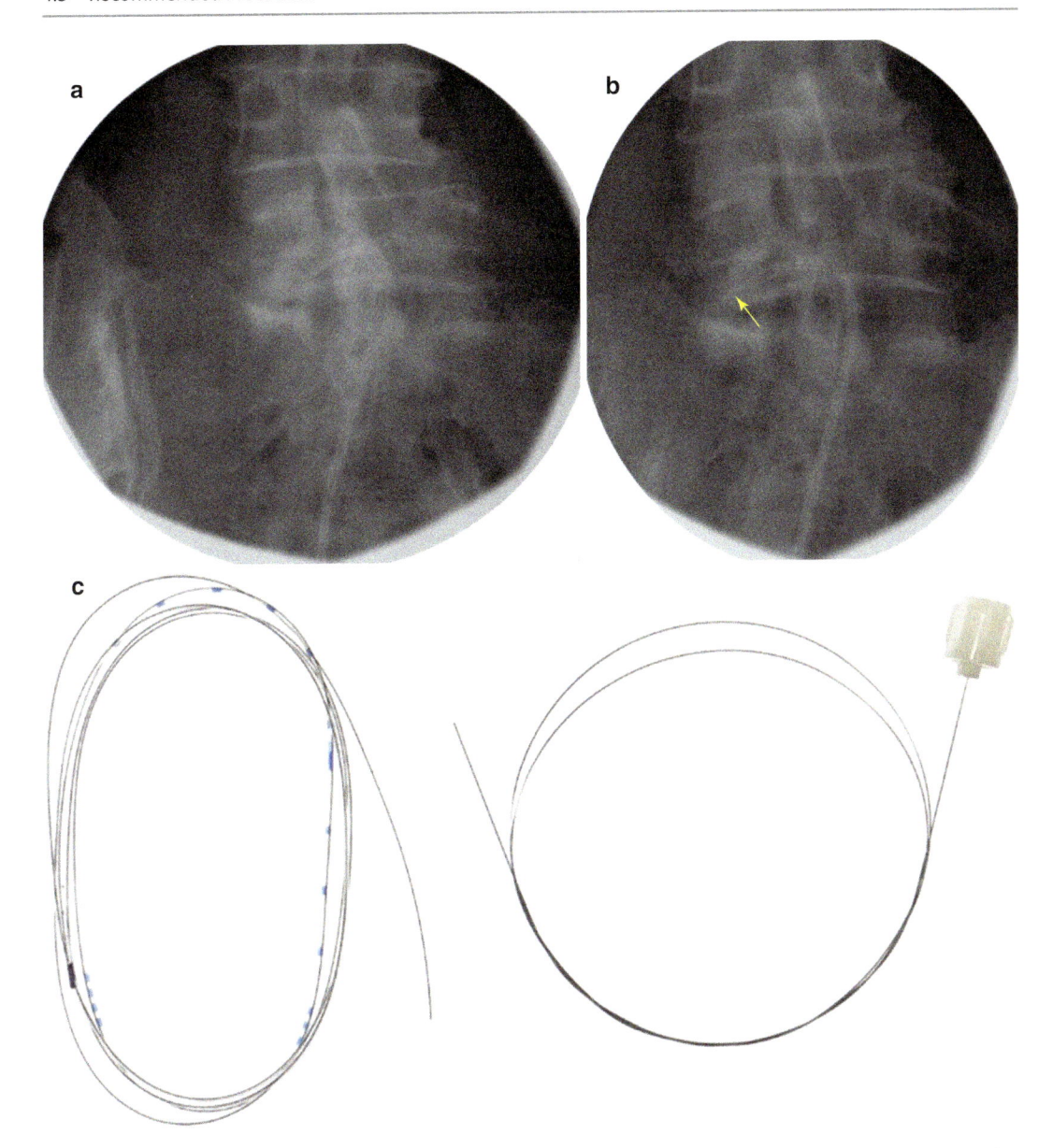

Fig. 4.46 (**a**) Case in which the catheter could not be inserted due to severe foraminal adhesion or stenosis. (**b**) Using the guidewire to create a path for drug delivery or for the drug-injection epidural catheter to pass through. A drug-injection epidural catheter containing a reinforcing wire can then be placed inside the ZiNeu catheter and thereby situated adjacent to the target area. (**c**) Drug-injection epidural catheter and reinforcing wire

inflating/deflating the balloon should be adopted instead. This bears emphasis: the balloon should never be pulled down quickly while it is inflated; it must be moved slowly (Fig. 4.50) (Video 4.1).

Procedures performed in the central area induce less pain than do those that involve the foramen. However, caution should be exercised if the patient complains of pain during the procedure. When severe central stenosis is found on MRI, presence of pain should be monitored while the catheter is moved gently from side to side to gain entry into the stenosed area. After entry is made with care, and if the patient's pain is not severe, the balloon should be inflated short of the point at which the

Fig. 4.47 The ZiNeuF catheter being inserted, while the ZiNeu catheter cannot gain entry into the intervertebral foramen—the ZiNeu catheter was used to perform the procedure in all lesion areas besides the intervertebral foramen, for which the ZiNeuF catheter was employed. White arrow: ZiNeu catheter. Yellow arrow: Inflated balloon of the ZiNeuF catheter

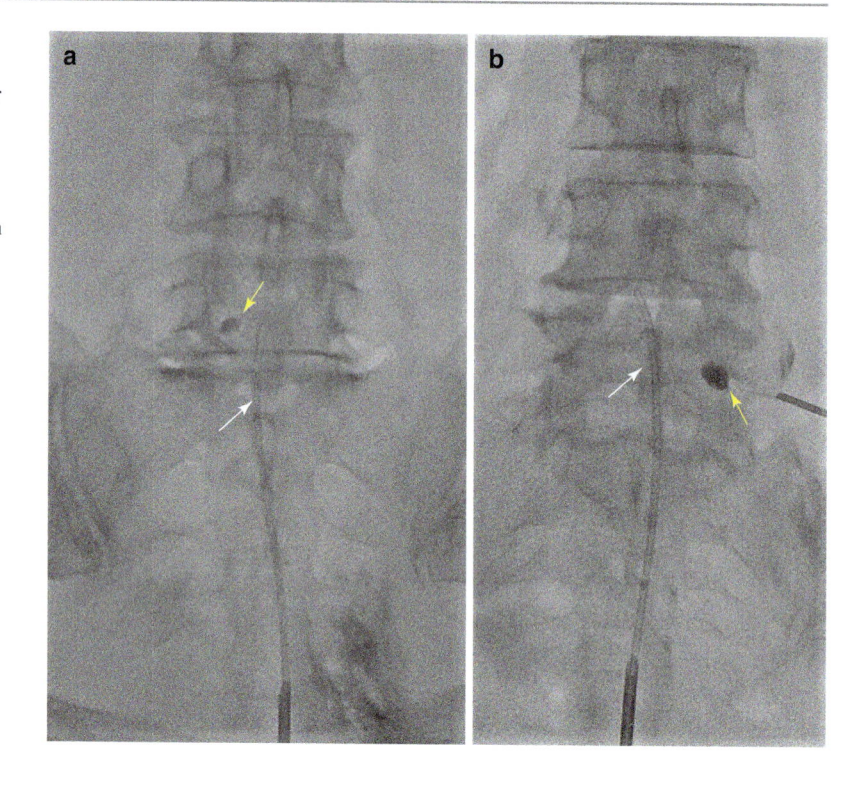

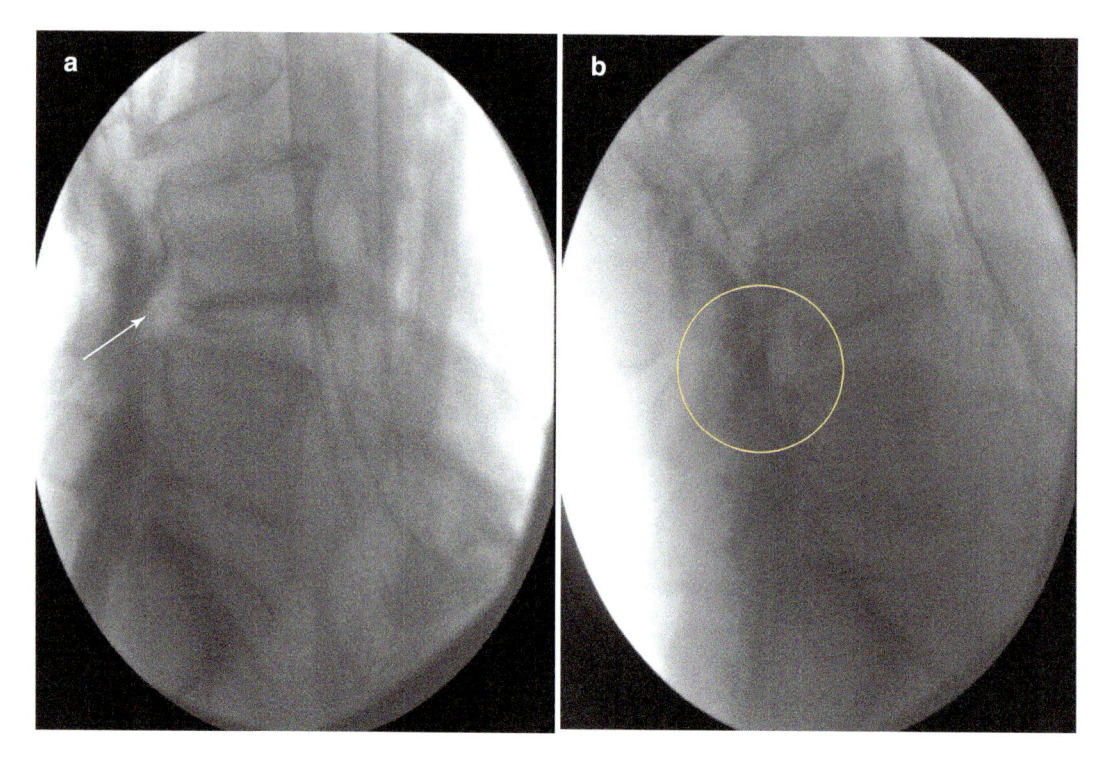

Fig. 4.48 (**a**) A patient with L4–5 central stenosis. (**b**) The performance of balloon decompression in the L4–5 retrodiscal area of the anterior epidural space. (**c, d**) Comparison of contrast dye spread in the anterior epidural space across the procedure. White arrow: Filling defect in the anterior epidural space before the procedure. Yellow arrow: The resolution of the filling defect in the anterior epidural space after the procedure. Circle: Inflated balloon

4.3 Recommended Procedure

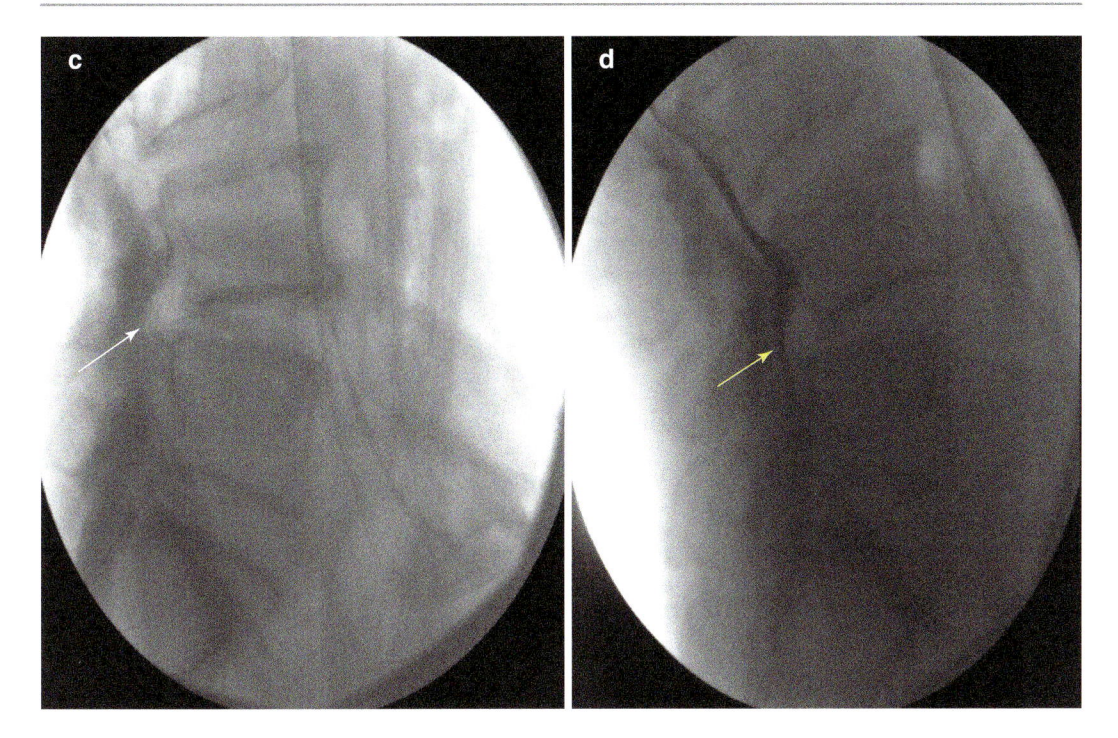

Fig. 4.48 (continued)

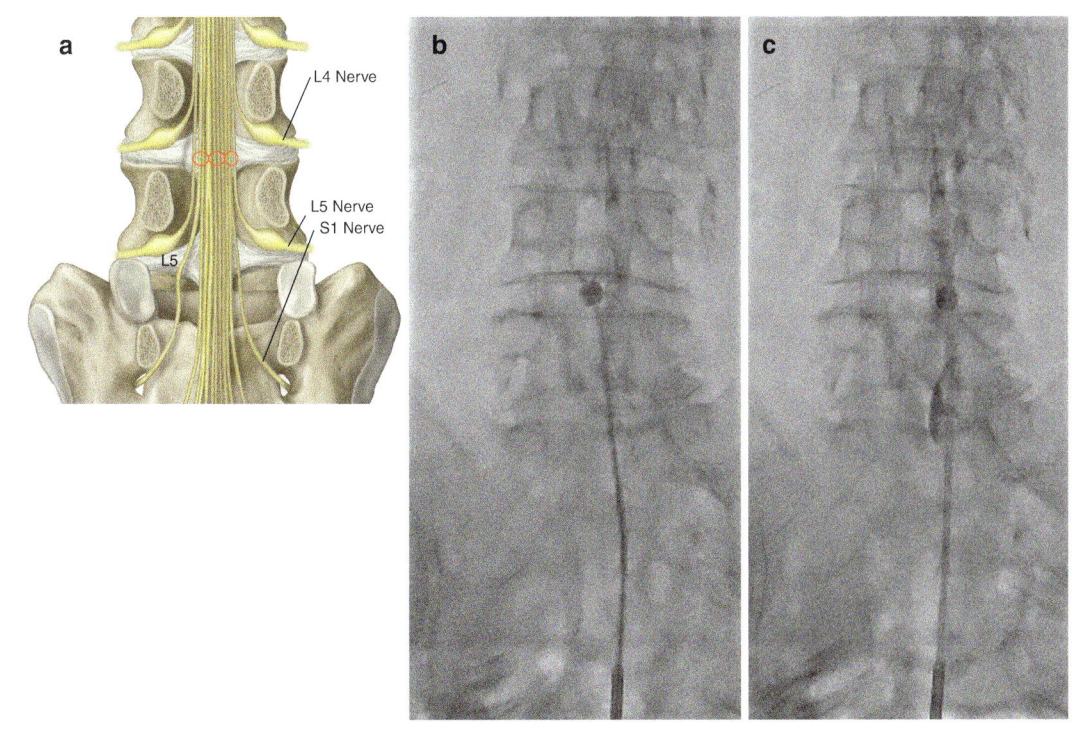

Fig. 4.49 (a) Balloon decompression in the central area—i.e., the retrodiscal area—should be performed by the left-to-right division of the area into three zones. (b, c) Balloon being inflated in both the right and left sides of the retrodiscal area. (d) Lateral view of the balloon being inflated in the retrodiscal area of the anterior epidural space. Circle: Inflated balloon

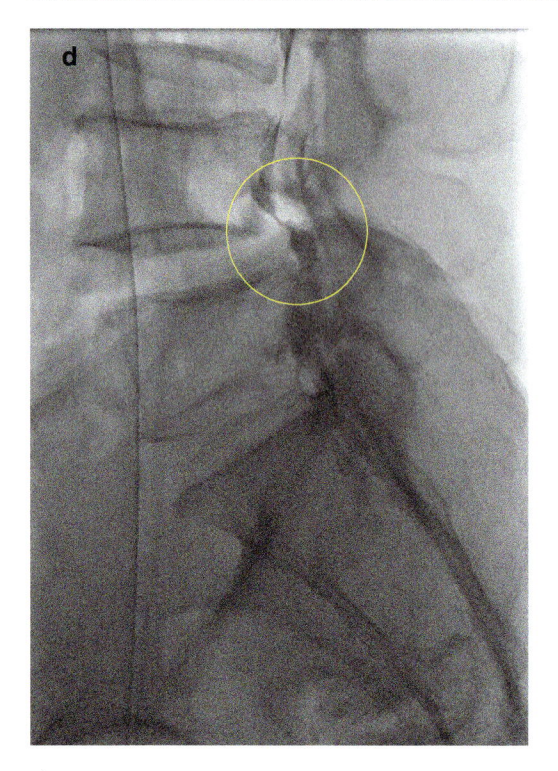

Fig. 4.49 (continued)

patient feels severe pain. If the pain is too severe, insertion of the balloon part as well as even the catheter itself could be dangerous, and the procedure should be completed with drug therapy alone. In other words, patient complaint of severe pain in an area that is typically not associated with procedure-induced pain could signal greater risk. Caution should be therefore be exercised, and the aggressive procedure should not be forced.

When performing these procedures, the insertion of the catheter is easy in some cases—despite MRI findings of severe stenosis. Hence, the feasibility of the procedure should not be determined by MRI findings alone.

When entering into the central area, MRI findings should be reviewed in advance to consider the entry angle and severity of stenosis. This will help to inform an operative plan for entry. If catheter insertion becomes difficult during the procedure, the MRI findings should be referenced for a possible solution. Indeed, the success or failure of balloon decompression is determined by the method of entry. Consider the following case example: MRI findings showed that entry into the superior aspect (toward the head) would be difficult on account of the likelihood that an L5-S1 disc protrusion in the anterior epidural space would impede catheter insertion. However, when the ZiNeu catheter tip was moved backward behind the disc protrusion in real-time lateral view, entry into the superior aspect over the protruding disc was possible. Hence, it is important to determine how the catheter should be moved by checking the MRI images before and during the procedure (Fig. 4.51).

In some cases, the excessive posterior protrusion of the disc precludes catheter insertion into the superior aspect as well as the spread of the contrast dye to toward the head (Fig. 4.52a). In such cases, inflating the balloon right below the disc could create a gap between the disc and dura (Fig. 4.52b), allowing the injected drug to flow behind the disc and ascend toward the superior aspect—i.e., the drug can be injected while the balloon remains inflated. This method can be used when entering the superior aspect is rendered difficult by the disc protrusion.

The receipt of spinal fusion may complicate the removal of severe adhesion with epidural adhesiolysis and increase the risk of dural puncture. However, during balloon decompression and adhesiolysis, balloon expansion allows effective adhesiolysis because the inflated balloon can expands the affected area smoothly, allowing for the treatment of a wider area and reducing the risk of dural puncture relative to methods that rely on only the force of the catheter to remove adhesion.

A catheter has the tendency to pass through the same trajectory each time that it is used. Using balloon adhesiolysis to remove adhesion from a wide area could make it easier to control the catheter tip and remove adhesion from nearby areas that are relatively distant from the catheter's typical trajectory.

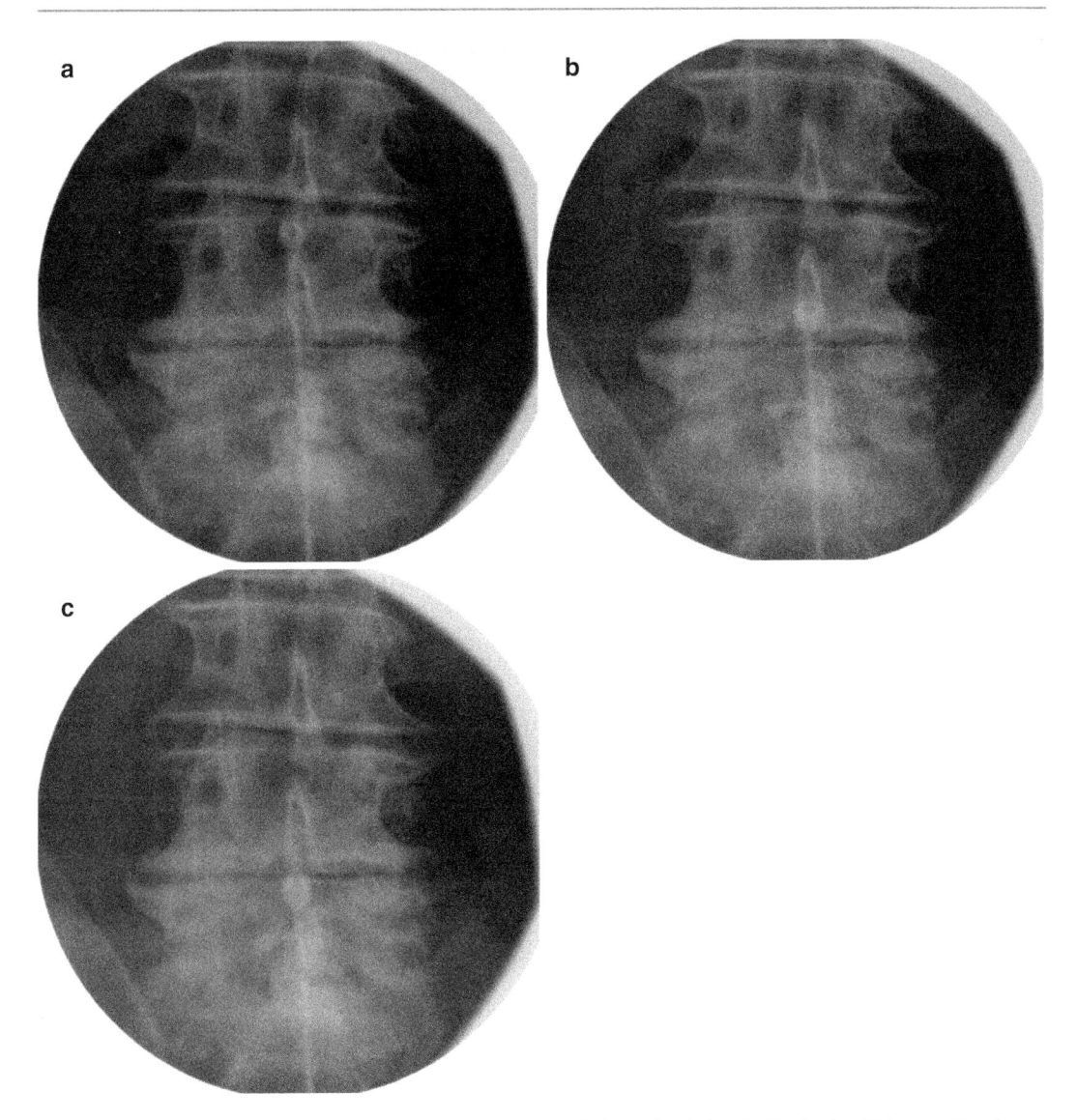

Fig. 4.50 Adhesion can be removed by slowly pulling the catheter down while the balloon is inflated, as shown in figures **a–c**. However, this must be performed slowly, and the patient's level of pain should be monitored continuously throughout

The optimal strategy would incorporate the injection of the contrast dye: As the contrast dye tends to spread more in areas where adhesion is weak—areas in which the contrast dye has spread more toward the head have a higher likelihood of featuring weak adhesion—areas to which the contrast dye has spread should be targeted for treatment. Attempting to remove the adhesion from the area with weak adhesion and gradually expanding the treatment areas with more severe adhesion could improve safety and the success rate (Figs. 4.53 and 4.54).

While detaching the adhesion, the catheter should be advanced toward the head by repeatedly moving it from side to side instead of in a straight line to reduce the risk of dural puncture (Fig. 4.55).

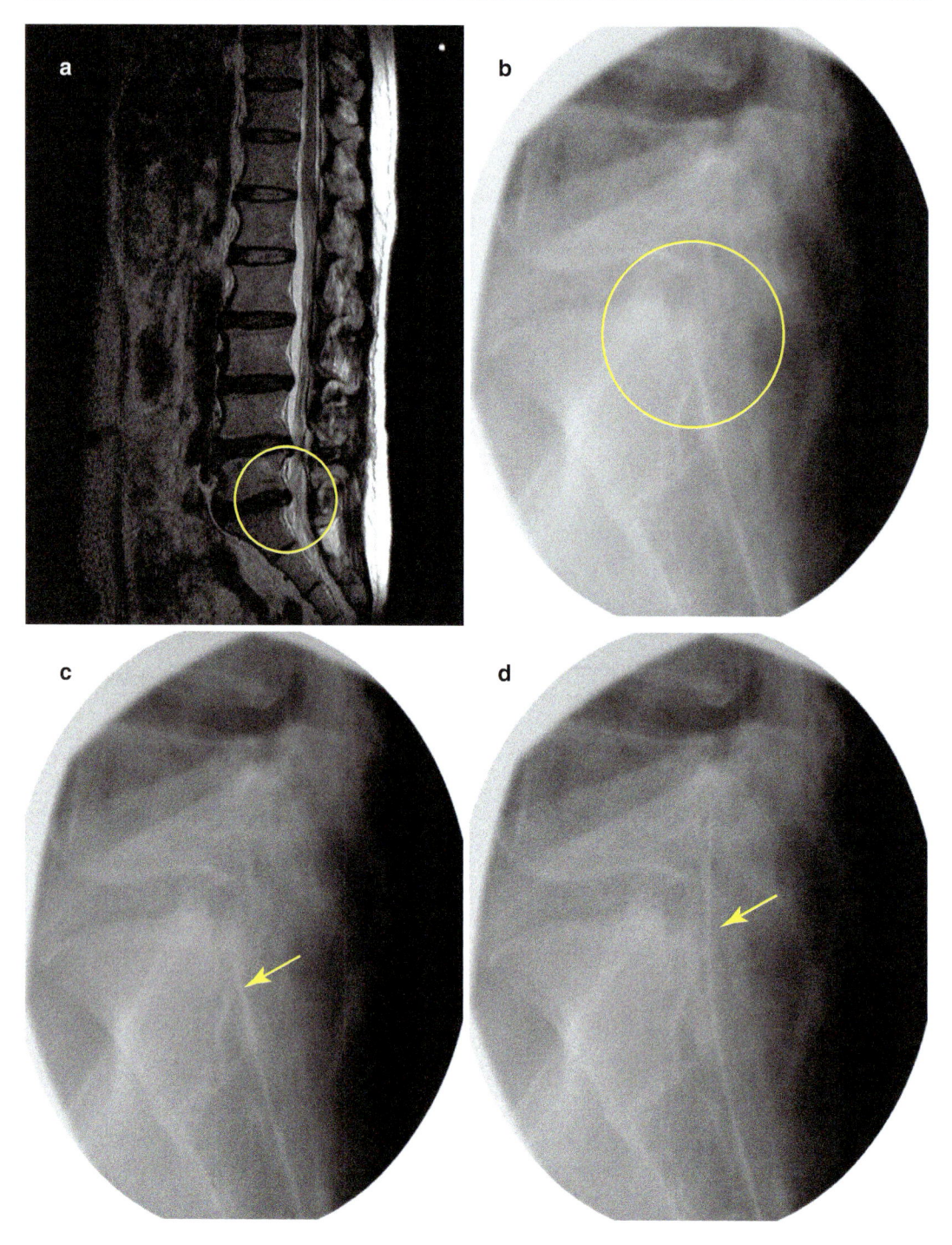

Fig. 4.51 (**a**, **b**) The catheter could not seemingly be advanced across the L5–S1 retrodiscal area due to an L5–S1 disc protrusion. (**c**, **d**) The catheter tip could cross the L5–S1 retrodiscal area when the catheter tip moved toward the back of the patient under the real-time lateral view. Circle: disc protrusion area. Arrow: ZiNeu catheter

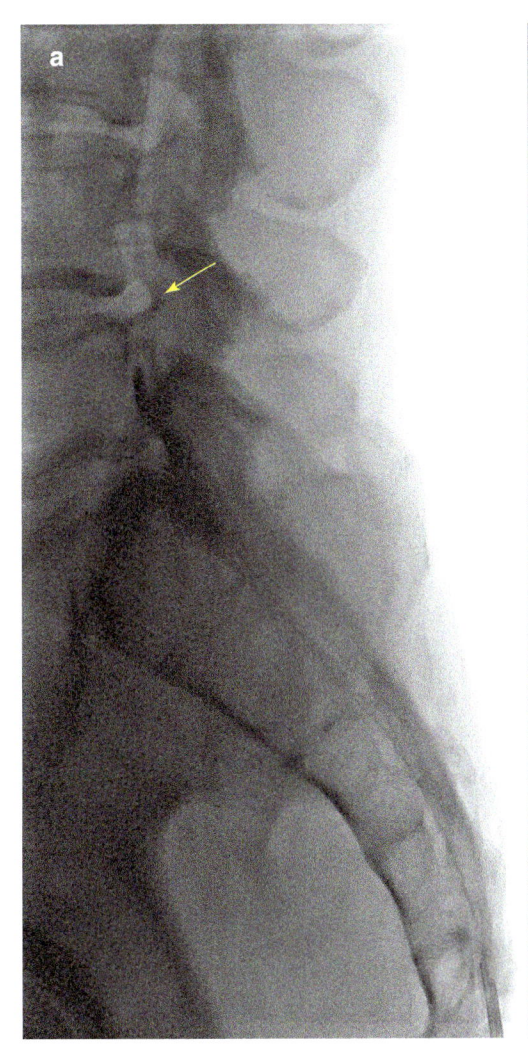

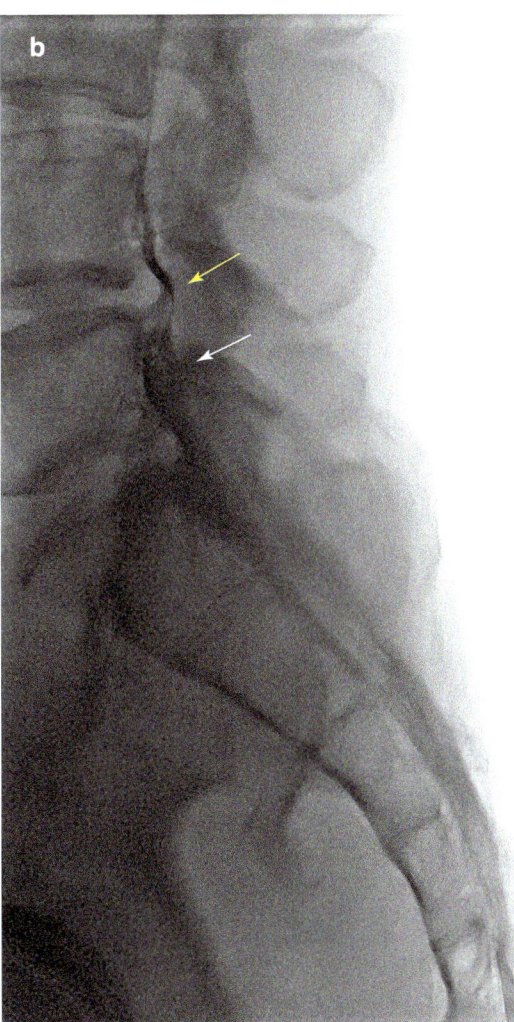

Fig. 4.52 (**a**) A case in which severe disc protrusion compromised catheter insertion and the spread of the contrast dye toward the head. (**b**) Inflation of the balloon to create a gap between the disc and dura, allowing for drug injection; the contrast dye is ascending toward the head through the gap. Yellow Arrow: disc protrusion. White Arrow: inflated balloon

4.3.7 Contrast Dye Injection

Upon completion of balloon procedure, the 100% contrast dye must be reinjected to confirm whether the dye spreads into the site of the procedure, whether dural puncture occurred during the procedure, and whether the drug is leaking into the blood vessels.

If the drug has leaked into the blood vessels, the problem may not have been resolved even if the position of the catheter tip has changed because a blood vessel that has been punctured requires time to heal. Changing the position of the catheter tip would still allow the drug to flow into of damaged blood vessel along the path created during the procedure (Fig. 4.56).

While normal saline irrigation is helpful, it is advisable to wait until the damaged blood vessel heals. However, as this may take a long time, the following can still be performed if the amount of drug that leaked into the blood vessel is not excessive: the drug can be diluted and adminis-

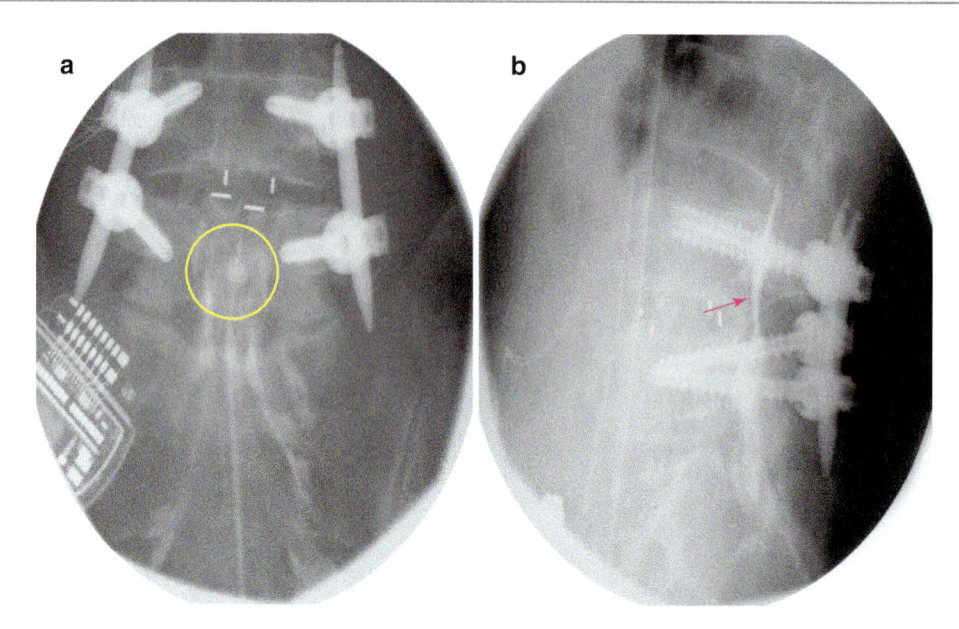

Fig. 4.53 (a) Adhesiolysis and balloon decompression performed in a patient with severe adhesion who had previously undergone spinal fusion and spinal cord stimulator implantation. (b) The expansive spread of contrast dye into the anterior epidural space after the procedure. Circle: Inflated balloon. Arrow: Dye in the anterior epidural space

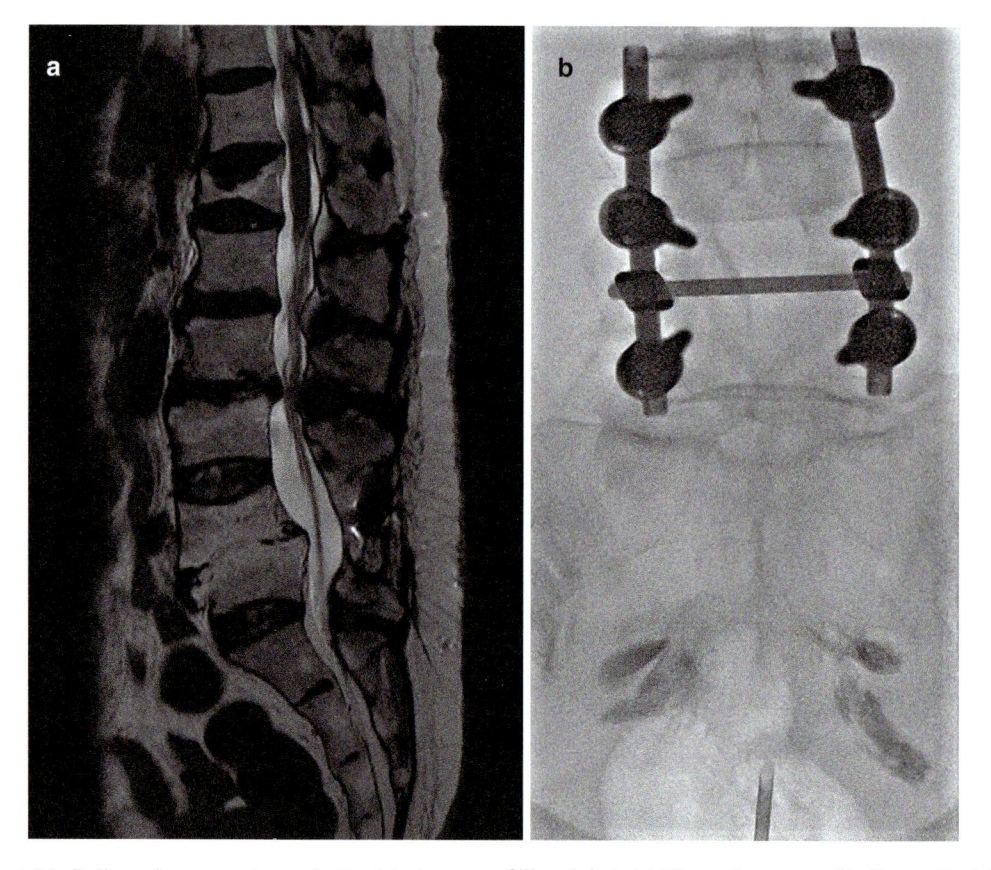

Fig. 4.54 Balloon decompression and adhesiolysis performed in a patient who had received spinal fusion. (a) MRI findings. (b) Epidurogram findings of an extensive filling defect. (c) The performance of balloon adhesiolysis. AP findings. (d) Balloon adhesiolysis being performed. Lateral findings. Circle: Inflated balloon

4.3 Recommended Procedure

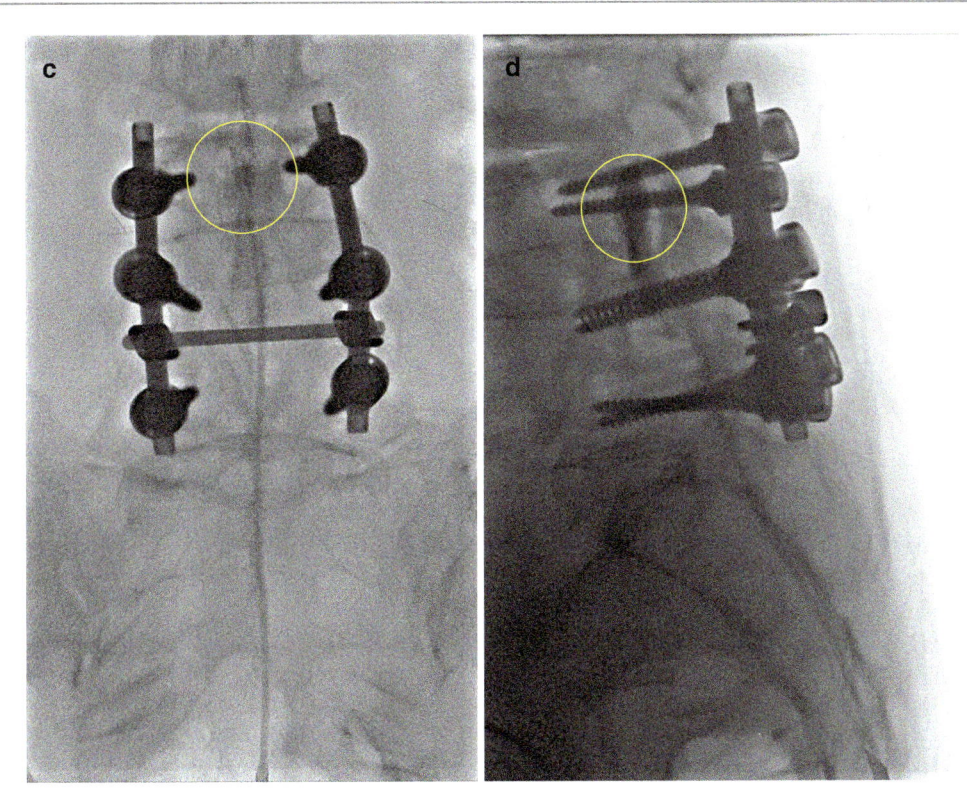

Fig. 4.54 (continued)

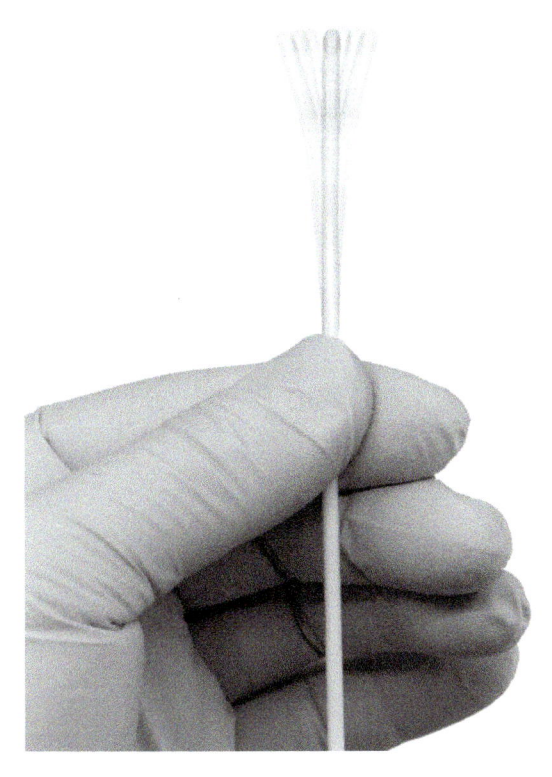

Fig. 4.55 Advancing the catheter toward the head by moving it from side to side may reduce the risk of dural puncture

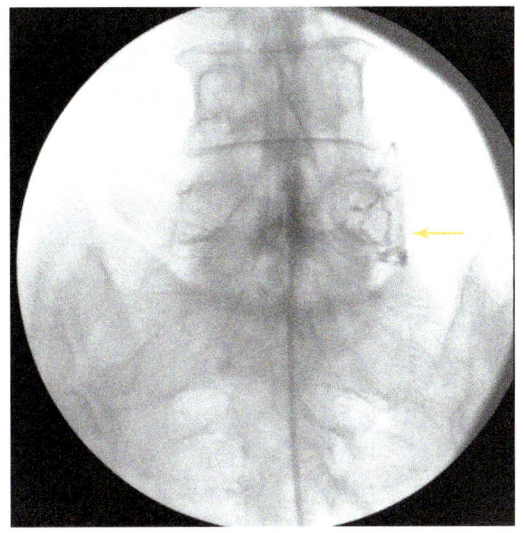

Fig. 4.56 Contrast dye flowing into the blood vessel. Arrow: Angiographic findings

tered only in small quantities, leaving the remaining portion in the drug-injection epidural catheter to be subsequently injected 30–60 min later.

However, since injecting excessive amounts of local anesthetic when there is leakage into the blood vessel could cause systematic adverse effects to the local anesthetic, caution should be exercised. In addition, if leakage into the blood vessel is suspected, particulated steroids should never be administered, as they could induce fatal complications such as an embolism.

> **Major issues associated with inflow into the blood vessel**
> 1. Inflow into the blood vessel cannot be resolved by slight changes in the position of the catheter tip.
> 2. Inflow into the blood vessel can be resolved over time as the damaged blood vessel heals.
> 3. Inflow of small amounts of local anesthetic or non-particulated steroid (e.g., Dexamethasone) is not a major problem. However, an excessive amount of local anesthetic may cause adverse systemic effects.
> 4. Never use particulated steroid (e.g., Triamcinolone) if inflow into the blood vessel is suspected.
> 5. It is safe to leave the drug-injection catheter inserted and administering the drug after more than an hour.

4.3.8 Irrigation

If the procedure is not satisfactory or epidurogram findings still show adhesion, irrigation with normal saline could be performed. In cases where advancement of the catheter was complicated by severe adhesion, the injection of a mixture of hyaluronidase and normal saline can weaken the adhesion area 3–5 min after administration and facilitate insertion.

Irrigation with higher volumes during conventional adhesiolysis can reportedly result in greater improvements. However, excessive irrigation could cause serious complications, such as intraocular hemorrhage. As balloon procedure is more effective in alleviating adhesion than are conventional methods, it demands less volume during irrigation: volumes of <100 cc per patient are recommended.

4.3.9 Injection of Therapeutic Drug and Placement of the Drug-Injection Catheter

The therapeutic drug should always be injected at volume of 2–4 cc per site after the injection of 100% contrast dye indicates that it is safe to do so.

Although there is little evidence for the capacity of hypertonic saline solution alone to help remove adhesion, it can certainly help to reduce pain and enhance the procedure's effects. Therapeutic benefits can further be maximized by leaving the drug-injection catheter in place after the removal of adhesion and alleviation of stenosis with balloon procedure; a hypertonic saline solution can subsequently be injected over 2–3 days, similar to method adopted during neuroplasty with the Racz catheter. This strategy is especially useful in cases where it is later confirmed that either the lesion has not been resolved, there is a high likelihood of recurrence, or the patient has developed neuropathic pain. Inserting a reinforcement wire inside the drug-injection catheter bolsters the strength of the catheter and makes it visible with C-arm. Hence, the tip of the drug-injection catheter could be left in place even after the ZiNeu catheter is removed (Fig. 4.57).

> **Method for leaving the drug-injection catheter at the site of lesion**
> 1. Place the tip of the ZiNeu catheter at the site of the lesion where the drug-injection catheter will be left upon completion of the balloon procedure.
> 2. Insert the drug-injection catheter with the reinforcing wire into the drug-injection hole of the ZiNeu catheter and place it adjacent to the lesion.
> 3. Retract the ZiNeu catheter alone while being careful not to change the position

4.3 Recommended Procedure

> of the drug-injection catheter. Immediately prior to the removal of the reinforcing wire from the drug-injection catheter, confirm the final position of the tip of the drug-injection catheter with C-arm; if the position of the tip of the drug-injection catheter has changed, readjust it accordingly.
> 4. Simultaneously remove the reinforcing wire, ZiNeu catheter, and the guide needle (Figs. 4.58, 4.59, 4.60 and 4.61).
>
> For further details, please refer to the procedure video (Video 4.2).

The drug-injection catheter left inside the patient's body is firmly fixed during the application of dressing to ensure that it can be maintained in place for 2–3 days. To improve protection from infection, the area from the epidural space to the skin surface could be further separated through tunneling; however, on account of time constraints, the catheter is often fixed without tunneling. If the catheter is intended to remain in place for only 2–3 days, tunneling is not required. No evidence for infections resulting from this practice has been hitherto been reported.

The dressing must be waterproof to prevent urine and feces from permeating through the gauze. It is also important to use a highly adhesive, waterproof material for application on the anus and surrounding areas. In addition, the patient should be instructed to keep urine and feces from contacting the dressing area (Fig. 4.62).

4.3.10 Drug Administration After Admission

Hypertonic saline solution should always be used with caution since injection of excessive amounts into the intrathecal space can cause complications. Although a concentration of 10% is typically used in neuroplasty, 5% is reported to be similarly efficacious. In addition, injecting 5% causes less pain and is safer.

Before every injection of hypertonic saline solution, local anesthetic should be administered in quantities of 1–2 cc higher than those required. This anesthetizes the patient ahead of time since the hypertonic saline solution itself causes pain and comprises the final confirmation of whether

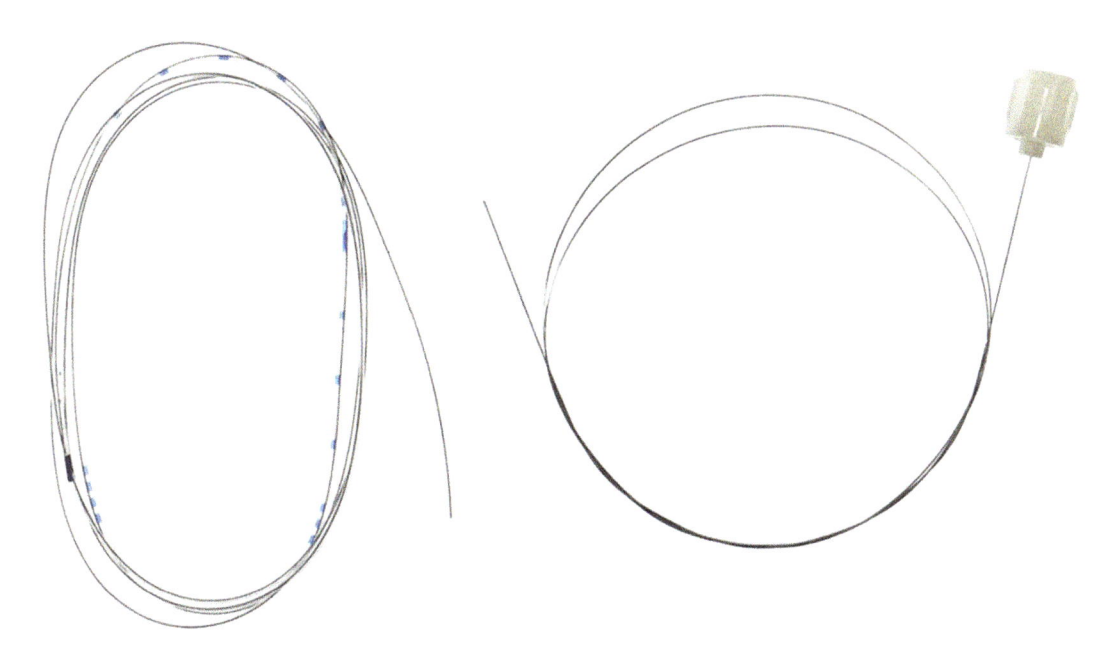

Fig. 4.57 (**a**) Drug-injection catheter. (**b**) Reinforcing wire which is placed inside the drug-injection catheter

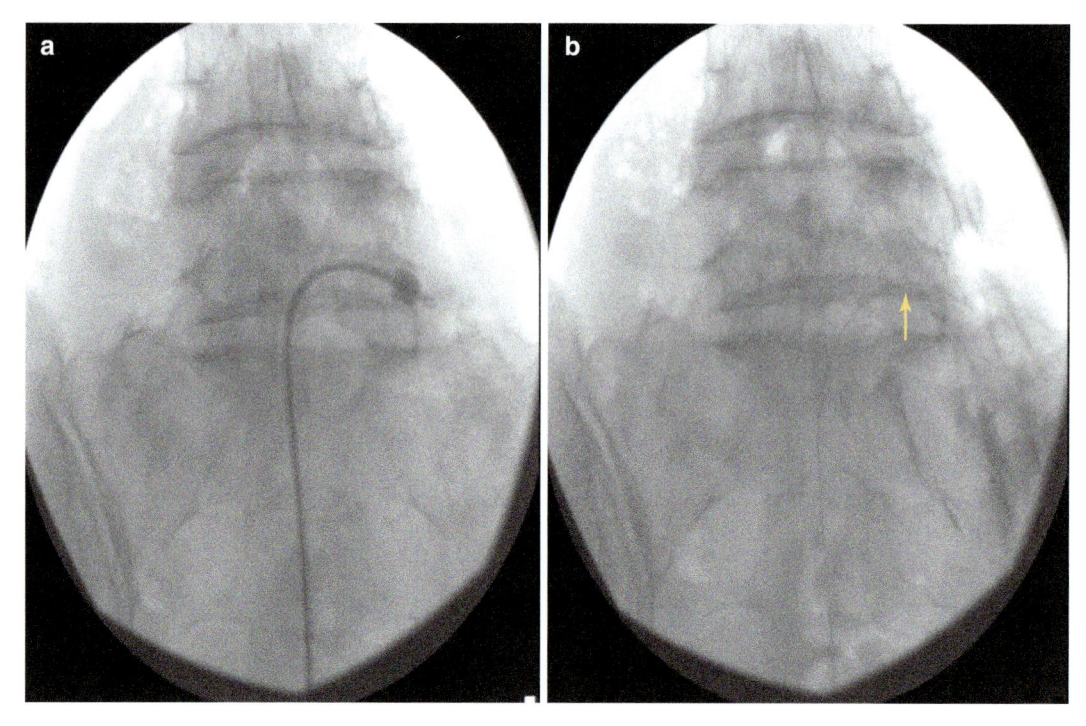

Fig. 4.58 (**a**) The performance of balloon decompression following the entry of the ZiNeu catheter into intervertebral foramen. (**b**) The insertion of the drug-injection catheter with the reinforcing wire through the ZiNeu catheter and the retraction of the ZiNeu catheter alone. The reinforcing wire allows for the identification of the drug-injection catheter's tip and the adjustment of its position. Arrow: Drug-injection catheter with the reinforcing wire

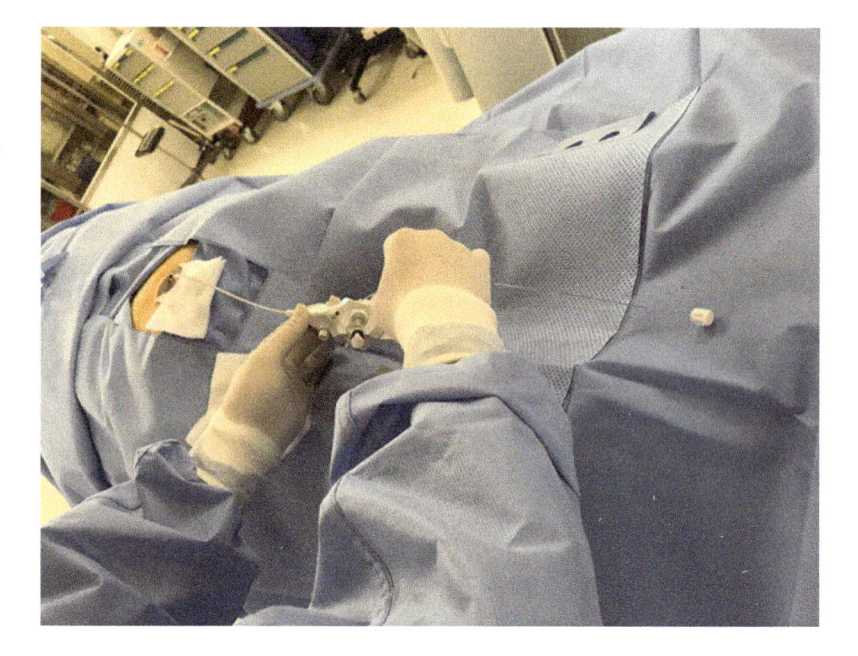

Fig. 4.59 The careful removal of the ZiNeu catheter, while the drug-injection catheter is in place at the lesion area

4.3 Recommended Procedure

Fig. 4.60 The withdrawal of the ZiNeu catheter, while the drug-injection catheter is left in place. Red arrow: Tip of the ZiNeu catheter. Blue arrow: Drug-injection catheter

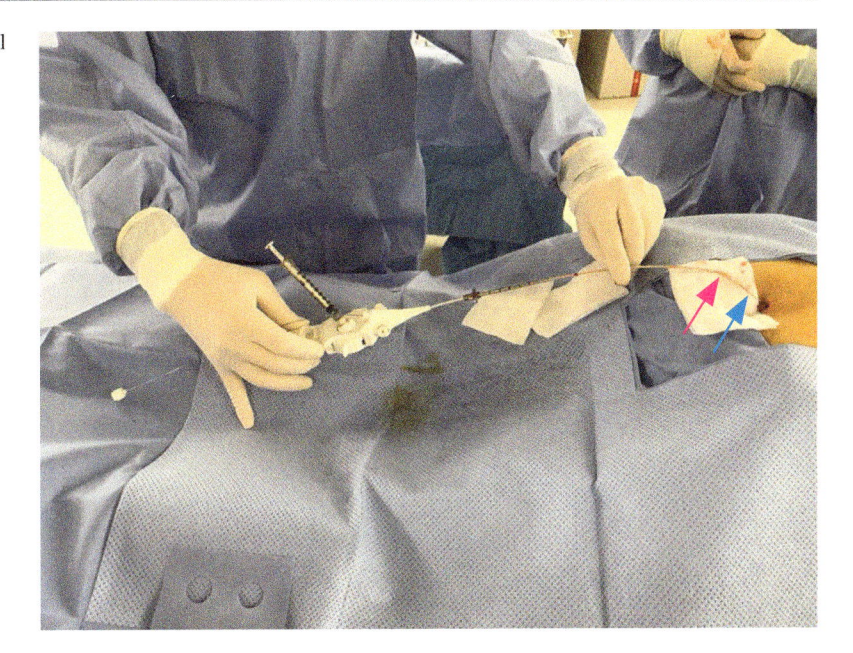

Fig. 4.61 C-arm is used to ensure that the tip of the drug-injection catheter is correctly placed at the lesion. If the position is correct, the drug-injection catheter is firmly held with the left hand to maintain the position so that catheter tip does not move, while the right hand is used to grab and remove all other materials, including the guide needle

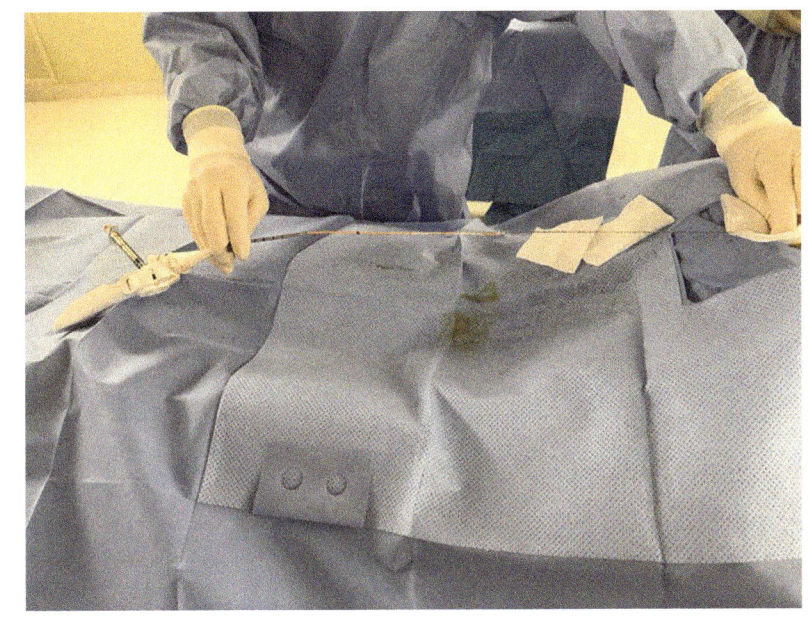

the catheter is secured inside the intrathecal space.

The administration of the hypertonic saline solution for 1–2 days is recommended if the balloon procedure did not yield satisfactory results or when neuropathic pain is suspected. While some patients may undergo inpatient treatment, others may receive the pharmacotherapy on the following day during their outpatient visits.

The authors recommend the following administration method: injecting 4 cc of 1% Lidocaine, waiting 2–3 min, and then slowly injecting 3 cc of 5% hypertonic saline solution. Using this method, the drug is administered up to 3 times a day in 2-h interval; the drug is administered up to three times on the following day.

For patients who do not have diabetes, 5 mg of dexamethasone can be administered all at once during or after the procedure. Alternatively, it can be mixed with hypertonic saline solution and administered portion-wise; however, the total amount should not exceed 5 mg.

The type and dose of the pharmacotherapy, as well as the means of administering it, may vary between physicians.

A video was prepared for the entire procedure using ZiNeu catheter. This will help you understand the procedure (Video 4.2).

Fig. 4.62 (**a**) The drug-injection catheter that was left at the lesion is fixed to the patient. (**b**) Dressing applied

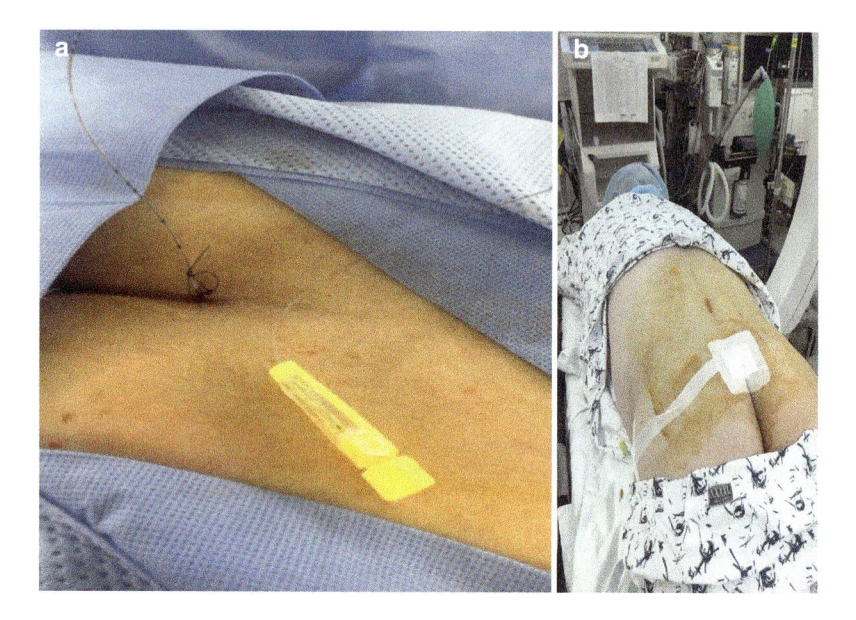

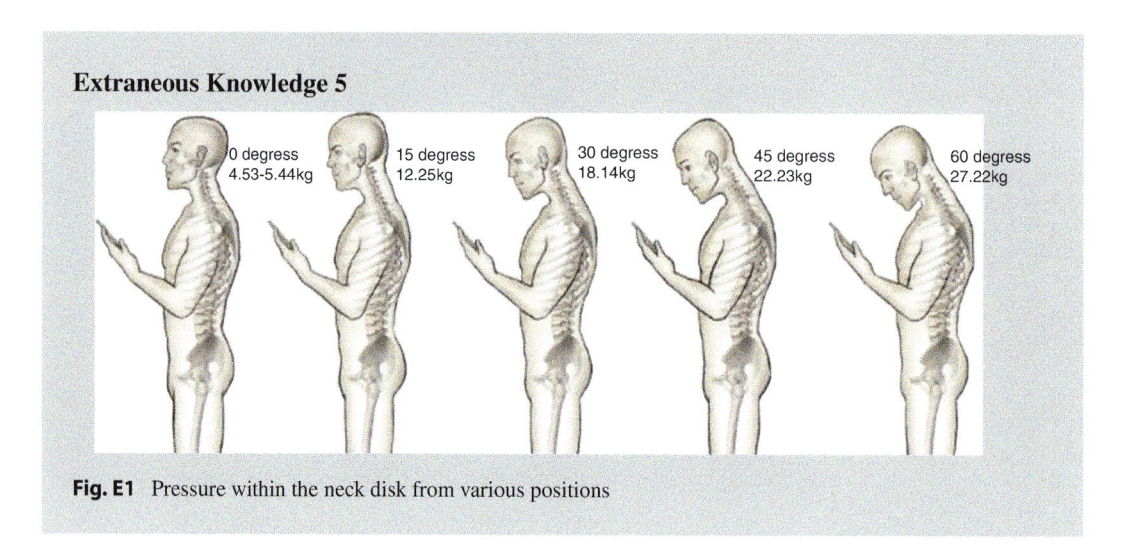

Extraneous Knowledge 5

0 degress
4.53–5.44kg

15 degress
12.25kg

30 degress
18.14kg

45 degress
22.23kg

60 degress
27.22kg

Fig. E1 Pressure within the neck disk from various positions

Methods for Executing the ZiNeuF Catheter Procedure

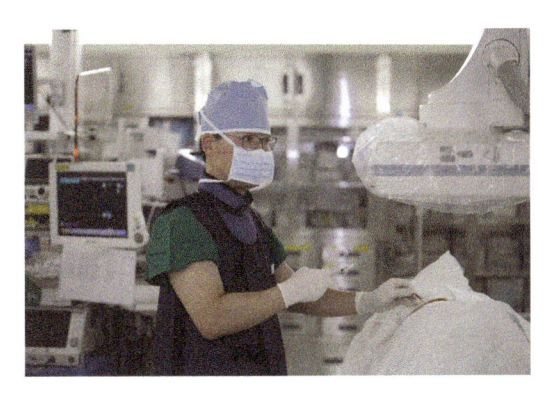

5

Image of balloon decompression being performed according to the transforaminal approach

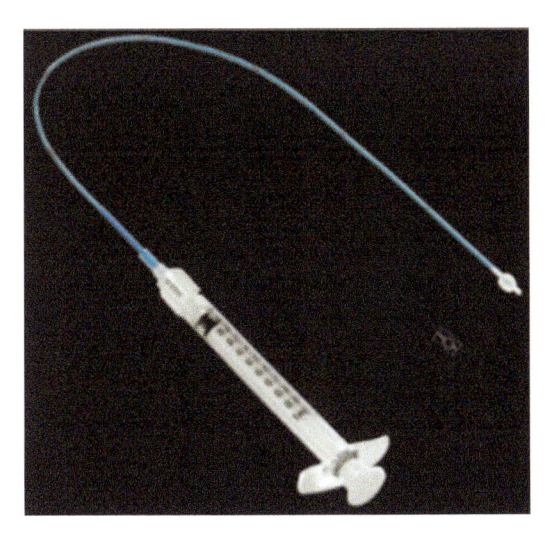

ZiNeuF Catheter

5.1 Target Diseases

- Low back and leg pain caused by chronic disc herniation
- Low back and leg pain caused by spinal stenosis
- Low back and leg pain caused by epidural adhesion
- Post-spinal surgery pain syndrome

5.1.1 Best Indications

Patients for whom conventional nerve block or neuroplasty achieved only short-lived improvements.

Patients with spinal stenosis-induced claudication.

: Cases in which the lesion is localized near the intervertebral foramen at a single level among the patients described above.

While the indications for the ZiNeuF catheter are similar to those for the ZiNeu catheter, the former was designed to allow for simple and effect approach to lesions located in the area adjacent to the intervertebral foramen rather than those situated in the central area.

Adhesion near the spinal nerves inside the intervertebral foramen is often neglected; however, it may account for the inefficacy of epidural block even in cases of moderate. Since balloon decompression can alleviate both stenosis and

© Springer Nature Singapore Pte Ltd. 2021
J. W. Shin, *Spinal Epidural Balloon Decompression and Adhesiolysis*,
https://doi.org/10.1007/978-981-15-7265-4_5

adhesion, balloon decompression could yield satisfactory results in such cases.

Regardless of the cause, balloon decompression warrants consideration in cases of foraminal adhesion, stenosis, or radiculopathy or claudication caused by a unilateral lesion in the retrodiscal area.

For patients with degenerative spinal diseases, including disc herniation, if the effect of other procedures, such as transforaminal epidural block, does not last for more than 3 months, balloon decompression is strongly recommended; it can achieve long-term improvements not only in pain but also motor functions.

5.2 Pre-Procedure Preparation

In general, the administration of antibiotics is unnecessary. However, if the procedural plan mandates leaving the drug-injection epidural catheter in place for 2–3 days after the operation for continued drug administration, antibiotics should be administered intravenously before and after the procedure—as is the case with neuroplasty—followed by the administration of anti-inflammatory analgesics and antibiotics for 3 days after the procedure.

While the patient is lying in prone position, a high pillow should be placed underneath the patient's abdomen—if possible—to reduce lumbar lordosis. If the procedure is being performed on the L5 intervertebral foramen, the success rate of the procedure could be increased by reducing lordosis to prevent the L5 intervertebral foramen from being obscured by the iliac crest.

Because the procedure does not cause severe pain, the administration of local anesthesia suffices.

5.3 Recommended Procedural Methods

5.3.1 Transforaminal Approach

The transforaminal approach can be divided into two types: the safe triangle and Kambin's triangle. If the lesion is situated near a nerve root in the intervertebral foramen, the safe triangle approach should be used; if the lesion is causing stenosis in the inferior aspect of the intervertebral foramen or is affecting the nerve root (traversing root) underneath it, Kambin's triangle approach should be used. These recommendations are informed by the difference in how the catheter is inserted in either approach (Fig. 5.1). The catheter moves along the nerve root when the safe

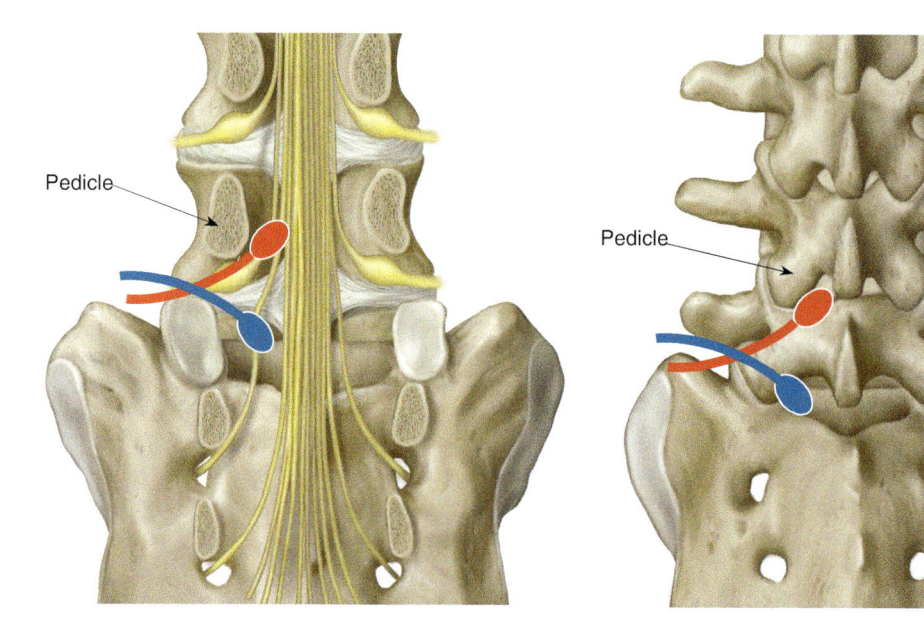

Fig. 5.1 The catheter is inserted in the direction shown in red when the safe triangle approach is used. The catheter is inserted in the direction shown in blue when Kambin's triangle approach is adopted

5.3 Recommended Procedural Methods

triangle approach is used and enters the retrodiscal area when Kambin's triangle approach is used. Therefore, the affected area must inform the selection of approach.

For either approach, the most important factor during the procedure is to keep the guide needle lying flat in the intervertebral foramen when gaining entry as much as possible; this increases the likelihood of successful catheter insertion and reduces nerve irritation.

5.3.1.1 Safe Triangle Approach

The ZiNeuF catheter is inserted along the nerve root by inserting the guide needle through the safe triangle (subpedicular area) in the intervertebral foramen (Figs. 5.2 and 5.3).

C-Arm Control

A pillow should be placed on the abdomen of the patient, and preparation for the procedure should be completed in the same manner as that for a transforaminal epidural block. Aligning the cephalad tilting of the C-arm to adjust the endplate of the target lumbar vertebra is unnecessary as it interferes with the entry of the needle in the caudal direction, as it directs the guide needle away from the nerves. If possible, it is best to insert the guide needle close to the area below the pedicle. Hence, adjusting the C-arm to 90° without any tilting is recommended (Fig. 5.4a).

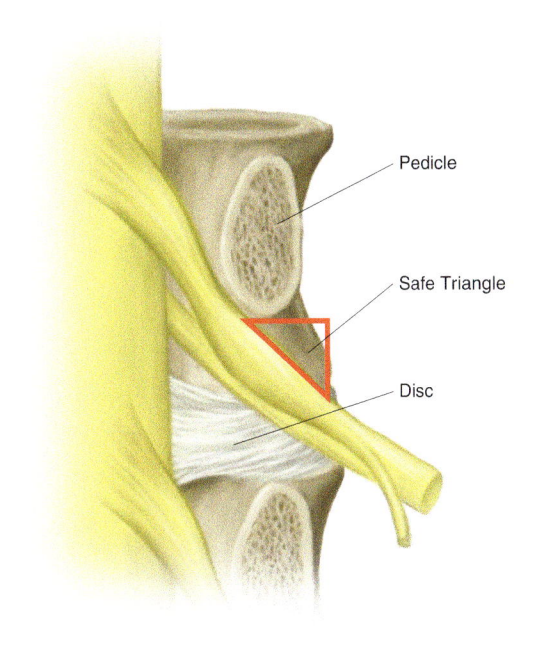

Fig. 5.2 Red triangle: The safe triangle through which the guide needle will enter

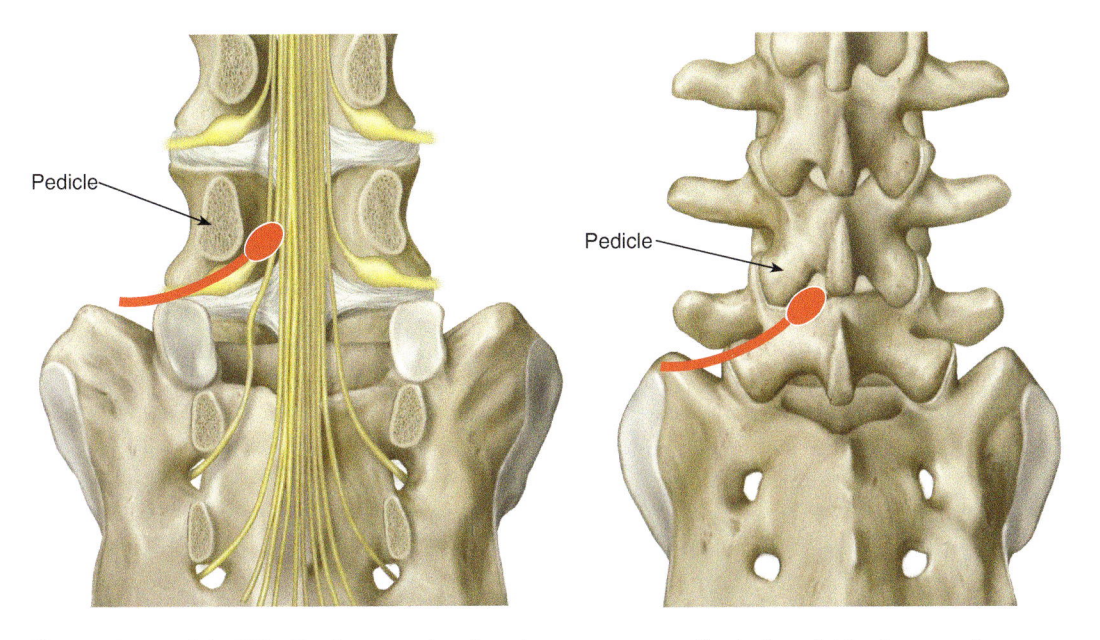

Fig. 5.3 Image of the ZiNeuF catheter entering along the nerve root according to the safe triangle approach

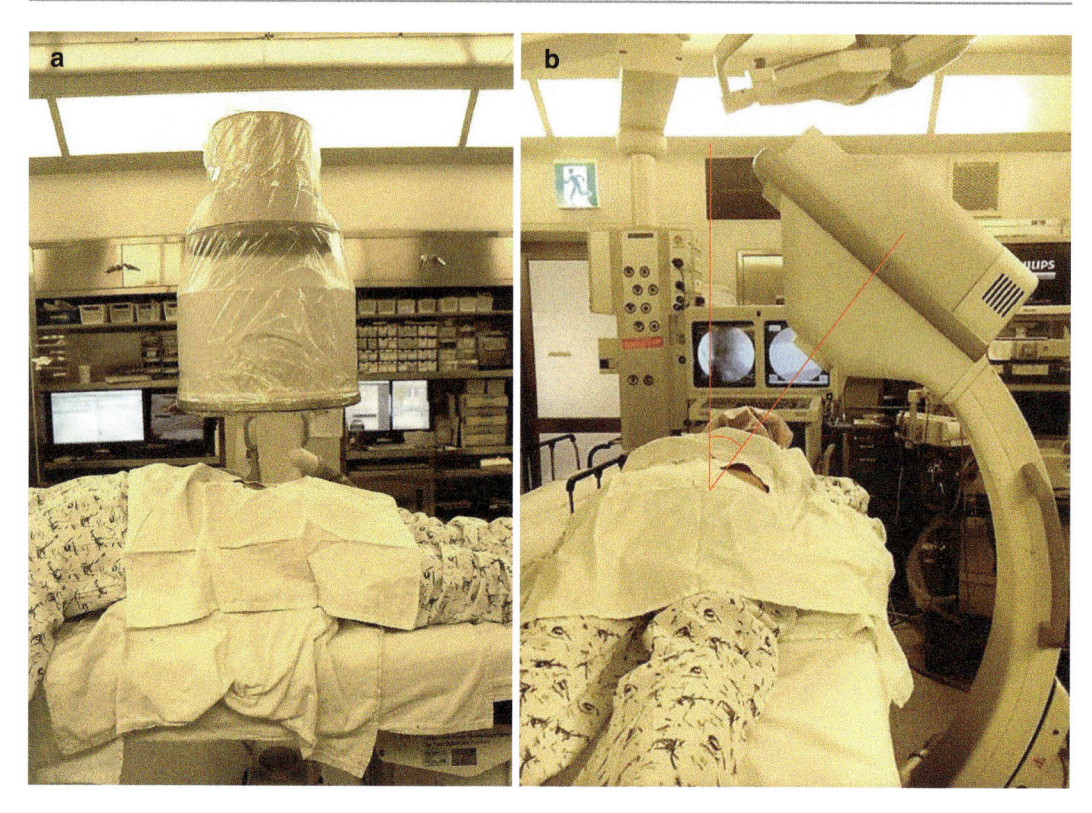

Fig. 5.4 (**a**) The C-arm angle should be adjusted to 90° to the patient without tilting. (**b**) Measurement of maximal oblique view for the guide needle to enter lying flat in the intervertebral foramen by as much as possible in this state

With respect to adopting the oblique view when entering the intervertebral foramen, it is important to find the maximal oblique view with the guide needle lying as flat as possible (Figs. 5.4b and 5.5). For example, among the figures in Fig. 5.5, Fig. 5.5b presents the most appropriate approach. If the C-arm angle is measured to be ≥30° in the maximal oblique view, the transforaminal approach is possible. A larger angle increases the likelihood of the procedure's success. If the angle is <30° in the maximal oblique view, the operator should consider employing the interlaminar approach. If entry remains difficult even in the interlaminar approach, it is advisable to use the caudal approach with the ZiNeu series catheter.

At levels above the L4 intervertebral foramen, it is easy to insert the guide needle that is lying flat since the iliac crest does not obstruct the approach. Adopting a C-arm oblique angle of 40–45° is recommended for such cases. If the angle is much larger, the catheter may be placed in the posterior epidural space, which could make the procedure itself more difficult.

Guide Needle Insertion
Either a guide needle or sheath could be used. A sheath is recommended as it entails a lower risk of balloon rupture. In the oblique view, the inferolateral area of the intervertebral foramen serves as the point of entry. Using the example of the L5 intervertebral foramen, which implies a relatively more difficult procedure, the access point at the maximal oblique view that allows entry of the guide needle into the intervertebral foramen is the area above the iliac crest and the inferolateral area of the intervertebral foramen. This permits the insertion of the needle while it lies as flat as possible (Fig. 5.6).

As indicated by the red arrow in Fig. 5.7, the guide needle should be inserted into the intervertebral foramen via the superomedial direction—i.e.,

5.3 Recommended Procedural Methods

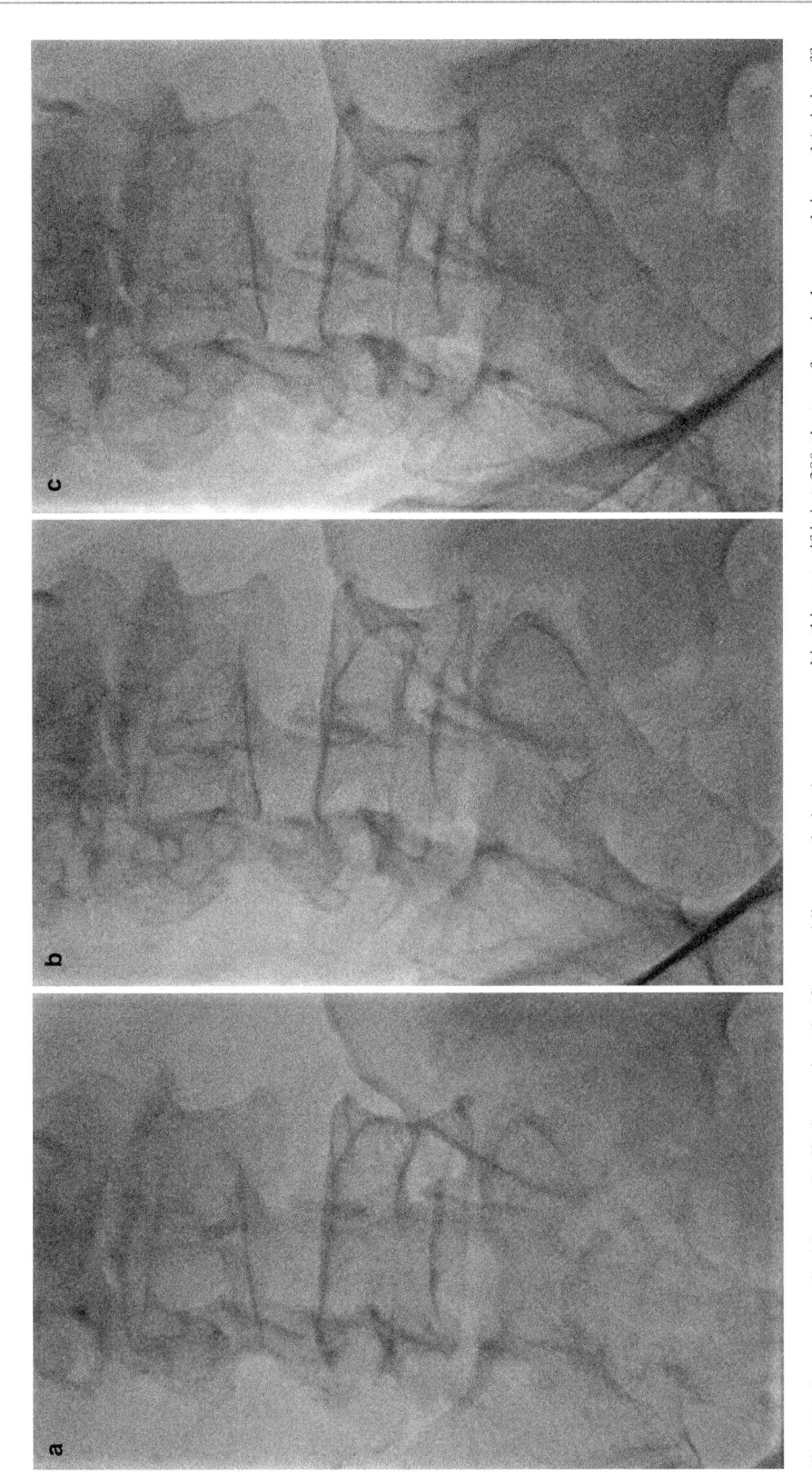

Fig. 5.5 Images acquired by gradually increasing the C-arm oblique angle in the order of **a** → **b** → **c**. The maximal oblique view that allows the guide needle to avoid the iliac crest and enter the intervertebral foramen is **b**. The C-arm angle should be measured in this state: if it is ≥30°, the transforaminal approach is used (**a** is insufficient at the maximal oblique angle, while **c** may render the entry of the guide needle into the intervertebral foramen difficult on account of obstruction by the iliac crest)

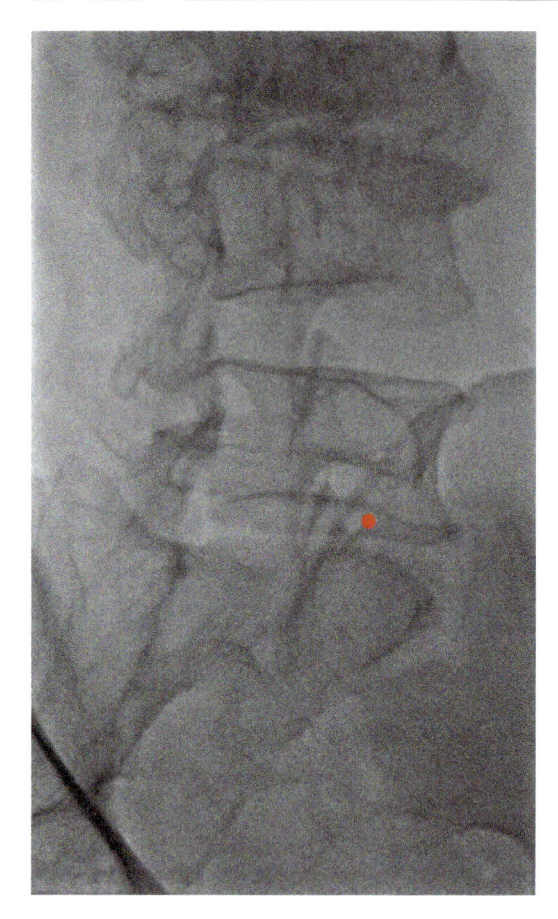

Fig. 5.6 The entry point of the guide needle (red dot) is above the iliac crest and the inferolateral area of the intervertebral foramen

the same angle as that of the nerve trajectory. In addition, the needle should be lay down as flat as possible to secure a sufficiently small angle between the intervertebral foramen and the guide needle to gain entry (Fig. 5.8a, b).

If the needle is lying too flat during procedures performed at levels above the L4 intervertebral foramen, it could be inserted too deeply and thereby cause dural puncture; hence, the needle tip should be checked in the AP view during the procedure to ensure that the guide needle does not pass the medial line of the pedicle (Fig. 5.8c).

During needle insertion, the needle must be controlled while checking the AP and lateral views to ensure that it is maintained as flat as possible and gains entry right below the pedicle. If the needle tip passes through the anterior epidural space and reaches the posterior surface of the vertebral body, the needle should be retracted by approximately 2–3 mm to allow for the catheter to pass through the needle tip. If dysesthesia or pain occurs because the needle comes into contact with nerve roots before it reaches the vertebral body, the procedure should be terminated immediately, and the needle should be retracted by 2–3 mm. The stylet should then be removed, and preparations should be made for subsequent catheter insertion.

Insertion of the Experimental Regular Epidural Catheter

If the C-arm's maximal oblique angle is over 30–35° for the needle's entry into the intervertebral foramen, there should be no impediment to the insertion of the ZiNeuF catheter. However, when attempting entry at an angle of <30°, the insertion of a regular epidural catheter should be attempted first to determine whether the insertion of the ZiNeuF catheter would be possible; if the angle is too small, the force with which the ZiNeuF catheter must be inserted could damage the balloon. If a regular epidural catheter cannot be inserted, then it is impossible to insert the ZiNeuF catheter.

If a regular epidural catheter cannot be inserted, the depth of the sheath could be adjusted, or the bevel of the needle, if a guide needle is being used, could be rotated to find the position or direction most conductive for catheter insertion. If the position at which a regular epidural catheter could be inserted to a depth of least 2–3 cm is found, the catheter should be inserted and withdrawn twice or thrice more at the same site to widen the path for the ZiNeuF catheter (Fig. 5.9).

However, the interlaminar approach (explained later) is typically used when the C-arm angle does not exceed 30°; hence, the experimental regular epidural catheter is rarely used.

ZiNeuF Catheter Insertion

The ZiNeuF catheter pass through the needle tip after slight resistance is felt upon its insertion; a suboptimal angle of entry into the intervertebral

5.3 Recommended Procedural Methods

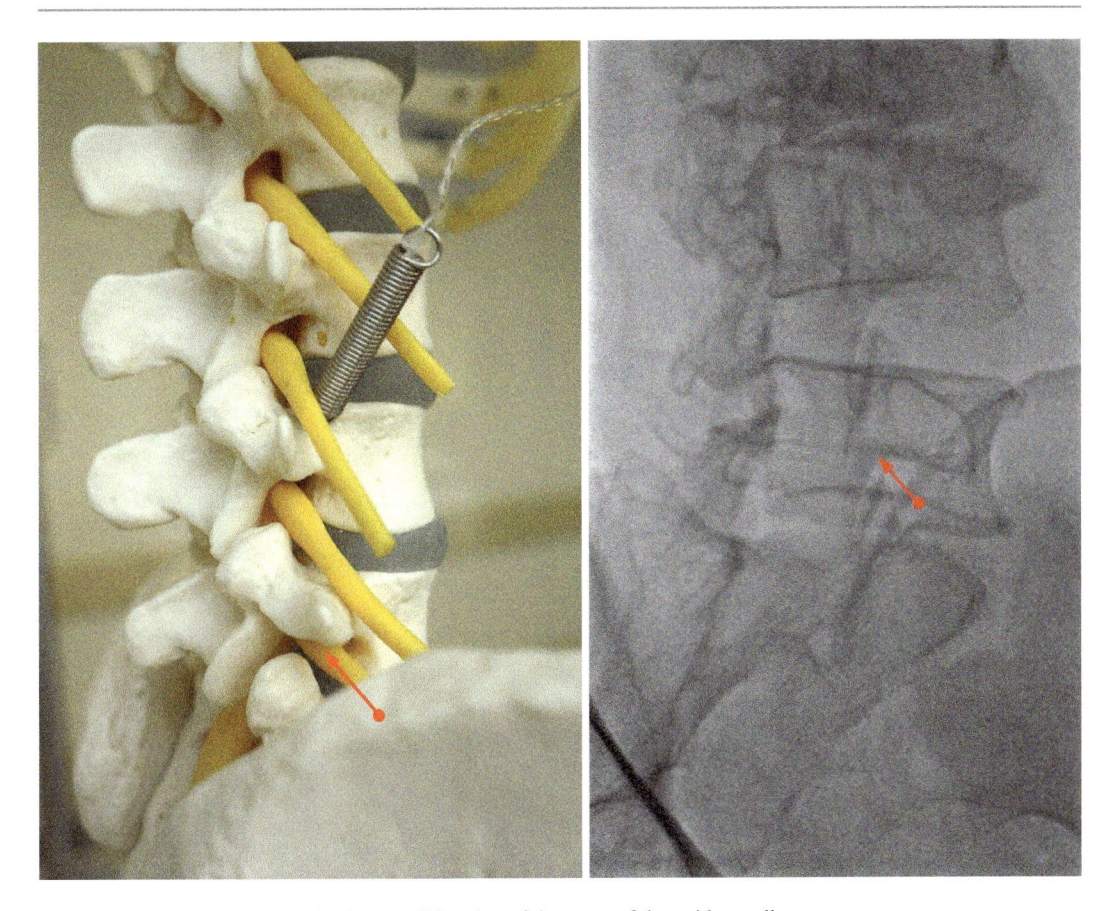

Fig. 5.7 Red dot: Entry point. Red arrow: Direction of the entry of the guide needle

foramen accounts for this resistance. If the catheter tip passes through the needle tip by 2–3 cm after resistance is met, then it can be assumed that the catheter had entered the medial aspect of the intervertebral foramen. The location and depth of insertion can be confirmed in the AP view. Because the procedure is being performed near the intervertebral foramen, there is no need for the catheter to go beyond the spinal midline (Fig. 5.10a).

As a reference, a reinforcing wire is inserted inside the ZiNeuF catheter. While the tip of the catheter is strengthened as a result, it may cause the catheter to snag and prevent its entry into the intervertebral foramen through the guide needle. Hence, it is advantageous to bend the tip slightly before insertion (Fig. 5.11a). If insertion remains difficult, the reinforcing wire can be withdrawn by approximately 0.5 cm to soften the tip and thereby facilitate insertion (Fig. 5.11b).

Balloon Decompression

If the C-arm view indicates that the position of the ZiNeuF catheter is appropriate, the guide needle or sheath is withdrawn laterally from the intervertebral foramen by approximately 2–3 cm to perform the procedure up to the extraforaminal area. Caution should be taken here to ensure that the ZiNeuF catheter is not withdrawn together with the needle or sheath; if the procedure is performed without withdrawing either, the needle tip may snag the balloon and rupture it.

If the ZiNeuF catheter is well-positioned inside the epidural space, and the needle or sheath

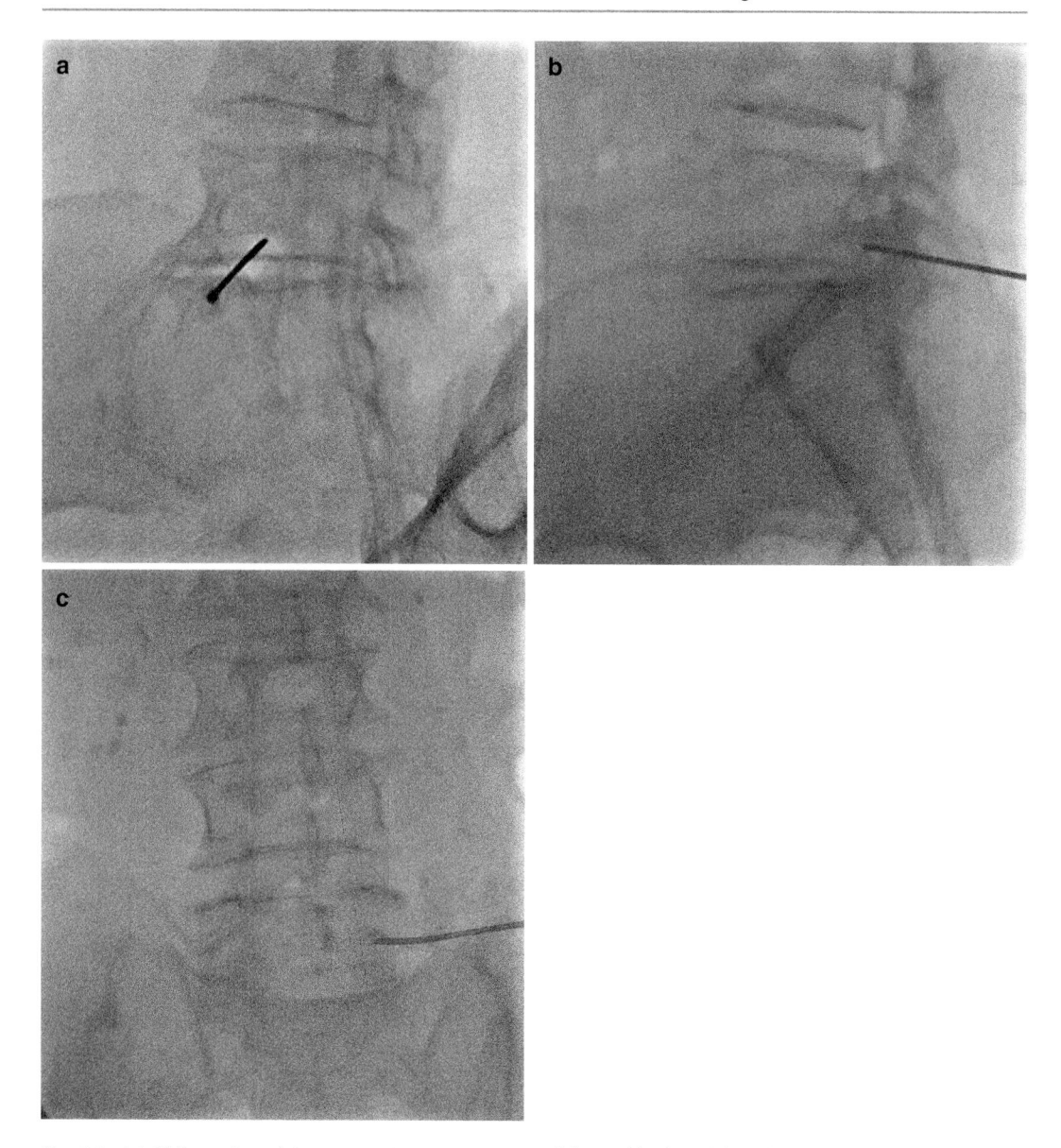

Fig. 5.8 (**a**) Oblique view of the accurate insertion of the guide needle into the intervertebral foramen via the superomedial direction. (**b**) Lateral view of the insertion of the guide needle into the anterior epidural space. (**c**) AP view of the positioning of the guide needle right below the pedicle, but before the medial line of the pedicle. Dotted line: medial line of the pedicle

5.3 Recommended Procedural Methods

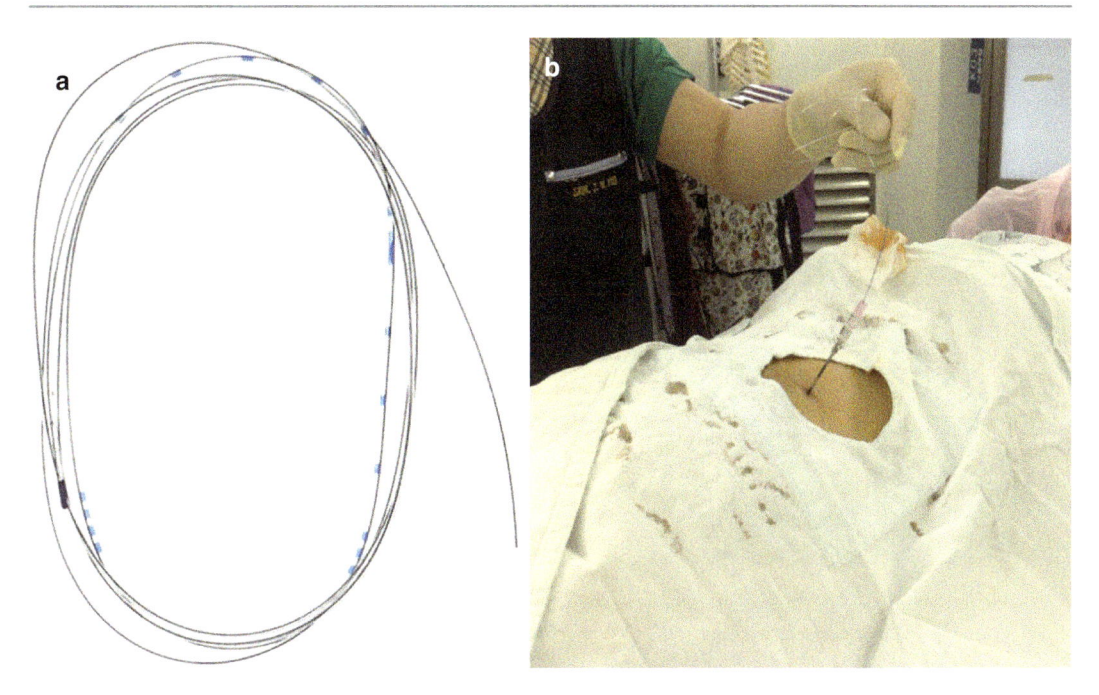

Fig. 5.9 (**a**) Regular epidural catheter. (**b**) Regular epidural catheter being inserted before inserting the ZiNeuF catheter

has been sufficiently withdrawn, the reinforcing wire should be removed: while one hand is used to pull the reinforcing wire out, the other should always hold the catheter near the hub of the guide needle to keep it steady and prevent its depth from changing (Fig. 5.12).

Because the catheter is placed inside the epidural space while its tip is bent, resistance may impede the successful removal of the reinforcing wire by just pulling on it from the end of the catheter; moreover, the position of the catheter could easily change during the attempt (Fig. 5.13). Hence, it is essential to always hold the proximal part of the catheter to keep it steady, while the other hand is used to grab the end of the reinforcing wire and pull it out.

After removing the reinforcing wire, the air inside the catheter is replaced with the contrast dye. A 5–10 cc syringe filled with approximately 2 cc of contrast dye is connected to the ZiNeuF catheter. When the plunger forcefully pulled back, the air inside the balloon catheter is expelled. Typically, when the plunger is released after the air is expelled all at once upon the application of strong negative pressure with the syringe in the erect position, the contrast dye automatically flows into the syringe. In other words, when the plunger is released after applying strong negative pressure, the catheter automatically fills with the contrast dye (Fig. 5.14).

If strong negative pressure is not applied, the air inside the catheter may not be expelled com-

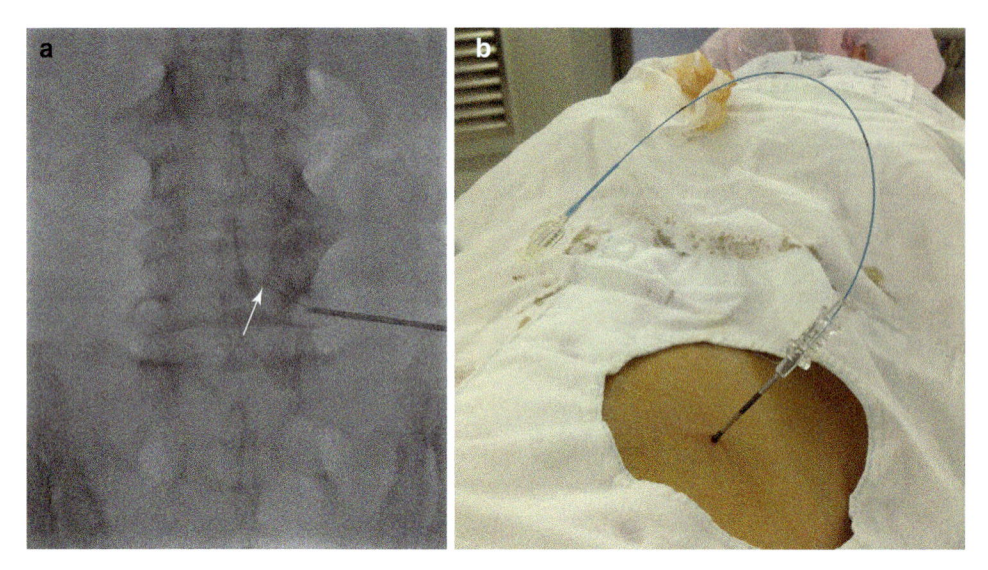

Fig. 5.10 (**a**) When the ZiNeuF catheter is inserted to a depth of 2–3 cm past the needle tip, the trajectory and extent of the catheter entry can be confirmed in the AP view. The operator should ensure that the catheter does not pass the midline. Arrow: Insertion of the ZiNeuF catheter. (**b**) The ZiNeuF catheter being inserted

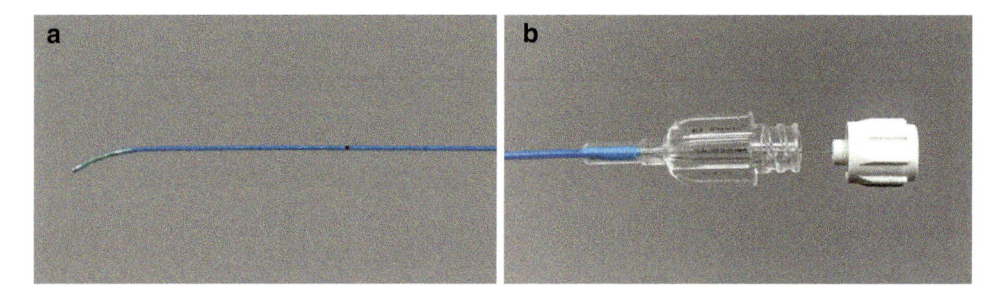

Fig. 5.11 Two methods for facilitating catheter insertion. (**a**) Insert the catheter after bending the tip slightly. (**b**) Insert the catheter after softening the tip by withdrawing the reinforcing wire by approximately 0.5 cm

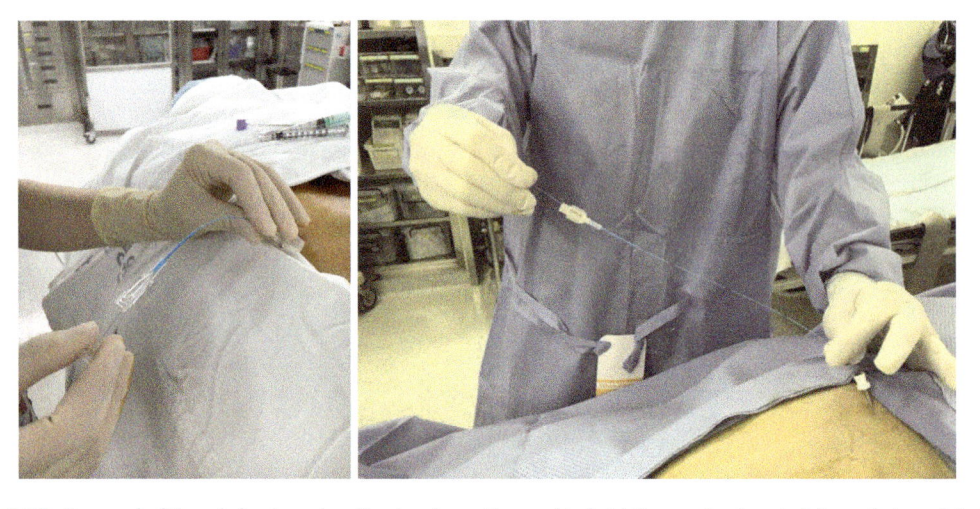

Fig. 5.12 Removal of the reinforcing wire. One hand must be used to hold the proximal part of the catheter, while the other grabs the end of the reinforcing wire to pull it out

5.3 Recommended Procedural Methods

pletely upon releasing the plunger. This could lead to the retention of air inside the balloon during balloon decompression and consequently complicate the determination of the extent of balloon dilation in the C-arm images. In severe cases, air retention could suggest the false impression of balloon rupture. The application of strong negative pressure is therefore essential when expelling air from the catheter (Fig. 5.15).

Once air inside the ZiNeuF catheter has been replaced with the contrast dye, a 1 cc Luer lock syringe filled with 0.1 cc of contrast dye is connected to the ZiNeuF catheter (Fig. 5.16).

Balloon decompression is performed by dividing the entire intervertebral foramen into two to three zones. The balloon is continually inflated and deflated as it is gradually withdrawn between zones (Figs. 5.17, 5.18 and 5.19).

Balloon decompression in the perineural area could apply pressure to nerves along the procedural trajectory and consequently inflict pain. Hence, the balloon should be gradually inflated short of the point of pain intolerance; once this threshold has been reached, the procedure should be paused for 3–5 s, after which the balloon should be deflated. Initially, the procedure is

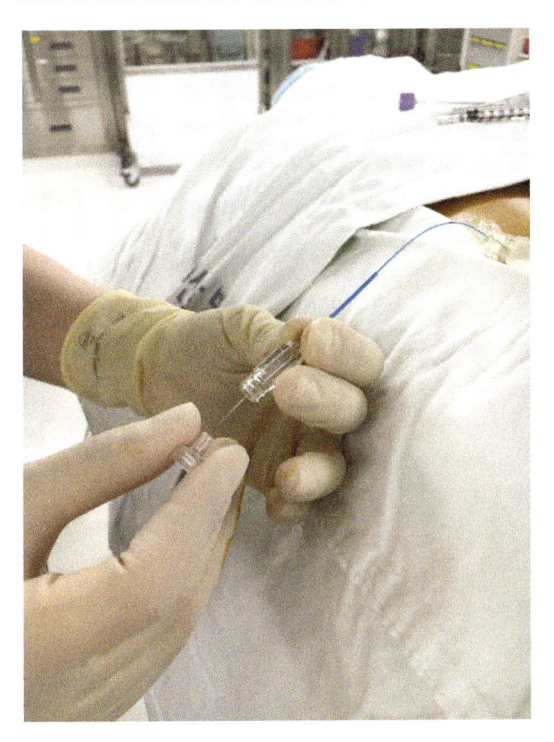

Fig. 5.13 Improper removal of the reinforcing wire. As shown in the figure, only holding the end of the ZiNeuF catheter when pulling out the reinforcing wire—without keeping it steady with the other hand—often results in the unsuccessful removal of the wire

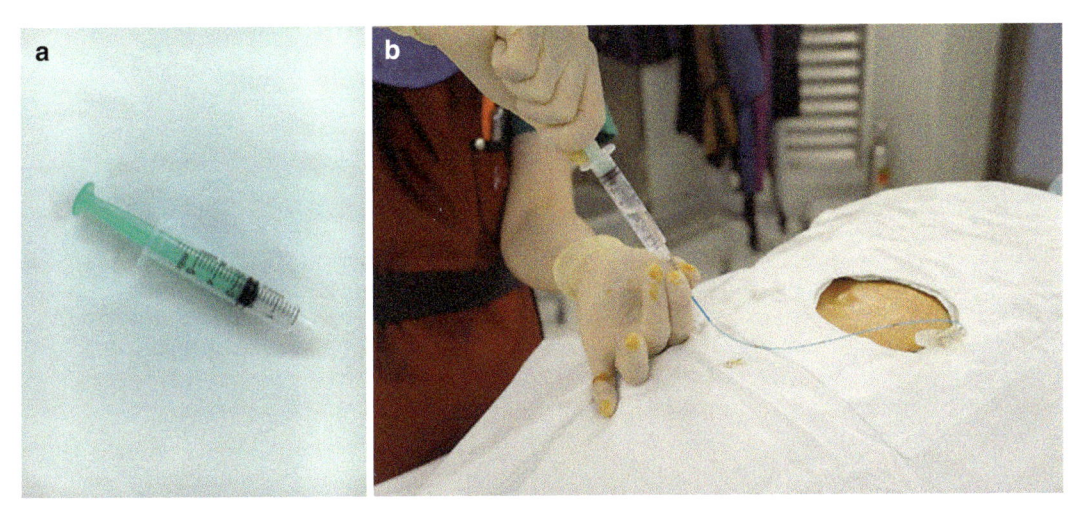

Fig. 5.14 (**a**) A 5 cc syringe filled with approximately 2 cc of contrast dye. (**b**) Image of the air inside the ZiNeuF catheter being expelled upon the application of strong negative pressure. (**c**) Image of the contrast dye filling the catheter when the plunger is released

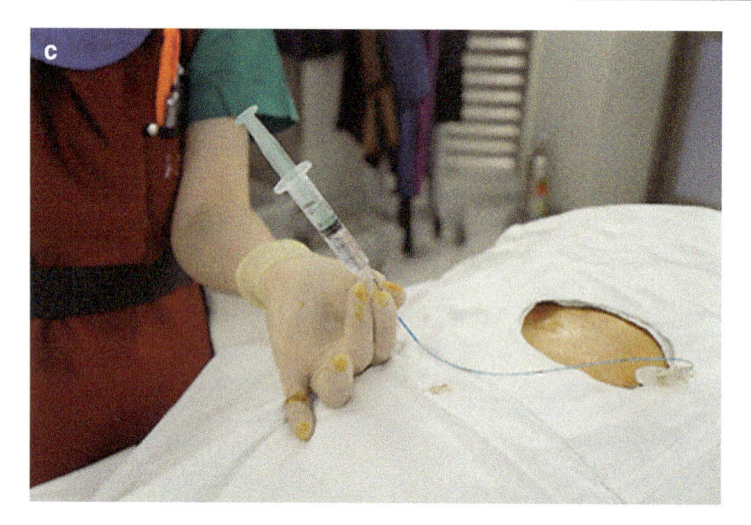

Fig. 5.14 (continued)

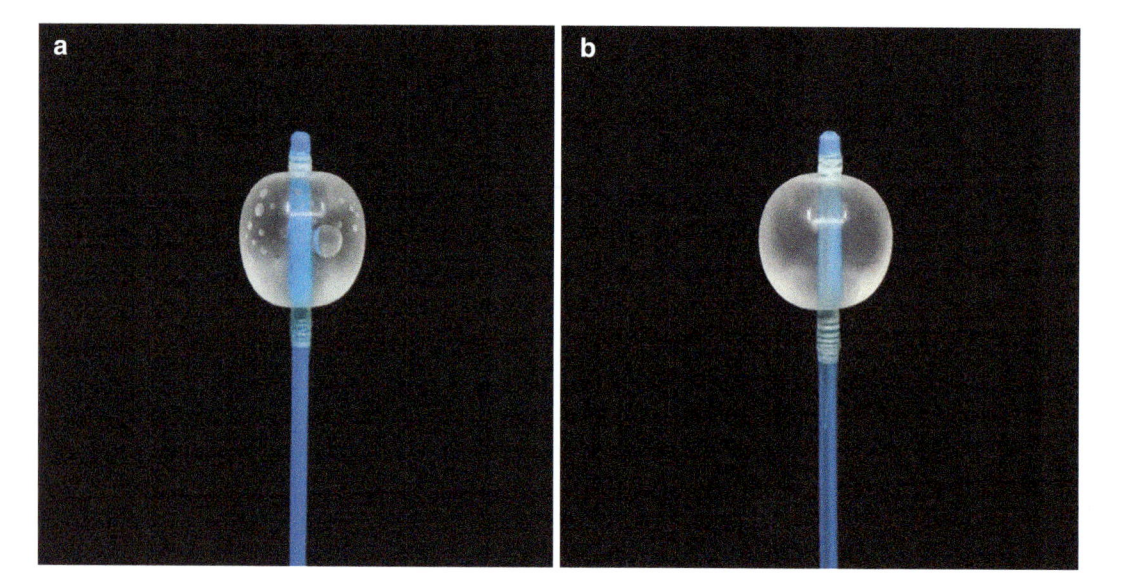

Fig. 5.15 (**a**) Air has remained in the inflated balloon because the air in the catheter was not expelled completely. (**b**) Image of an inflated balloon without air, as the air inside the catheter was completely removed

performed on the entire target site by slowly injecting 0.05 cc of contrast dye under the C-arm view. The catheter is then deflated and withdrawn; it must be moved while the balloon is deflated. After performing the procedure across the entire affected area, the catheter is reinserted at its initial position, and the procedure is performed once more with up to 0.1 cc of contrast dye. If 0.1 cc is used to inflate the balloon in the initial procedure, the balloon may rupture on account of its inelasticity when it is first used; this can also cause severe pain. Using only 0.05 cc during the first procedure and fully inflating the balloon with 0.1 cc thereafter improves the elasticity of the balloon and reduces the likelihood of balloon rupture. In addition, expansion of the perineural area during the initial procedure reduces pain inflicted during the second procedure because of increased free space. However, as aforementioned, if the patient complains of

5.3 Recommended Procedural Methods

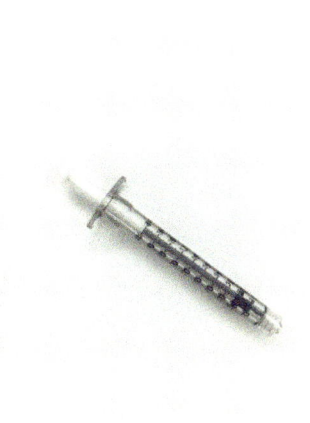

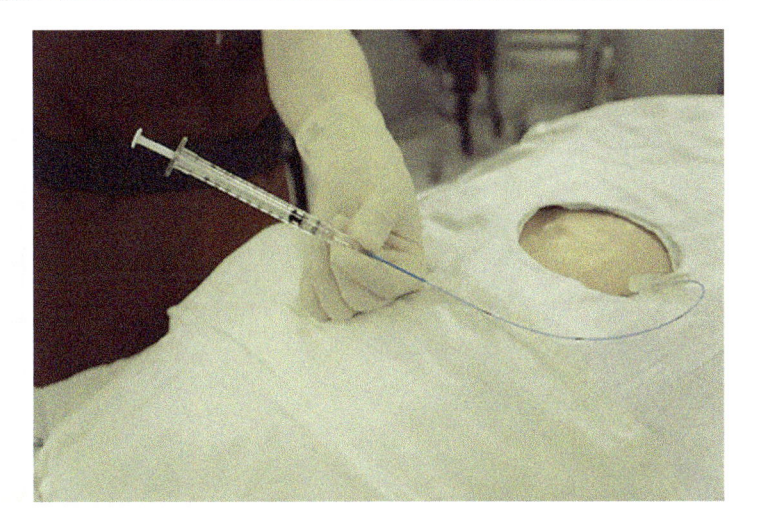

Fig. 5.16 A 1 cc Luer lock syringe filled with 0.1 cc of contrast dye is connected to the ZiNeuF catheter

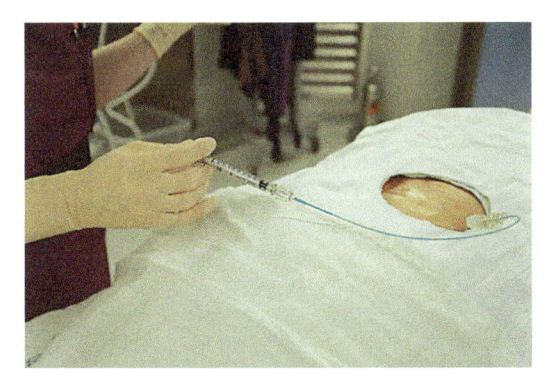

Fig. 5.17 The performance of balloon decompression

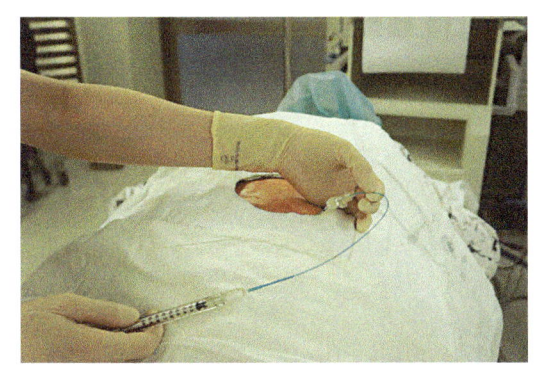

Fig. 5.18 Transition from one zone to another while the balloon is gradually withdrawn in its deflated state

intolerable pain during balloon inflation, the procedure must be ceased without any further inflation of the balloon. The balloon is then deflated and withdrawn.

If the patient does not complain of severe pain after the inflation of the balloon with 0.1 cc of contrast dye, up to 0.2–0.3 cc of contrast dye can be administered to fully inflate the balloon once more to more than 15 mm; balloon rupture at this point is nonproblematic, and the potential increase in stenosis alleviation and adhesion removal achievable with this increase in inflation warrants its attempt. In other words, this method prescribes the stepwise increase in the size of the balloon to achieve a greater improvement effect (Figs. 5.20 and 5.21).

When the catheter is reinserted after the initial procedure, it can be done so without reinforcing the wire inside. As free space has already been created by balloon decompression, the reentry could be easily executed with the catheter alone.

If the reinforcing wire is reinserted into the same catheter used during balloon compression, the wire may cause undesired balloon inflation by pushing the contrast dye remaining inside the catheter to the balloon portion. If it becomes necessary to reinsert the reinforcing wire, the catheter must be removed completely from the

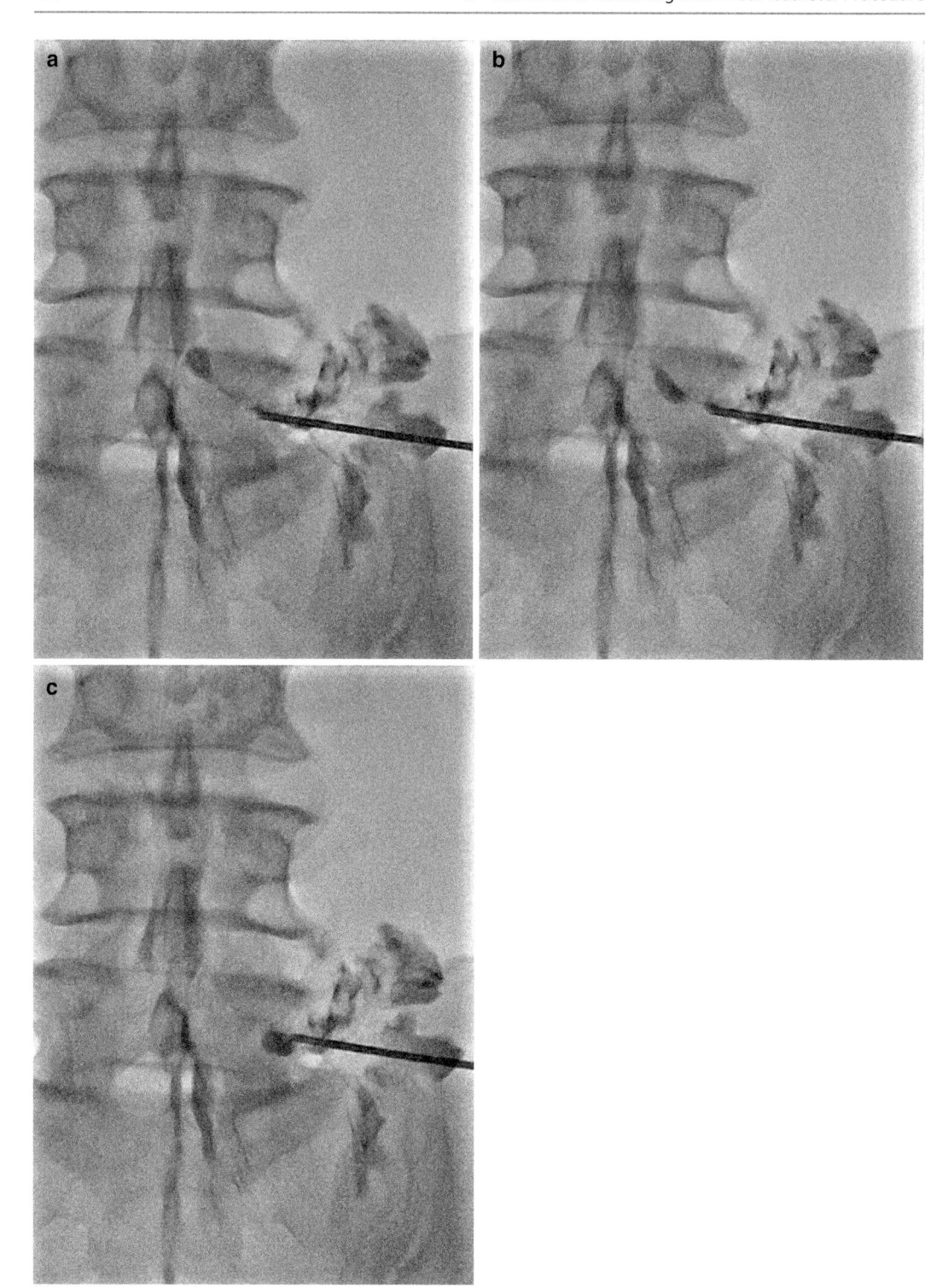

Fig. 5.19 The procedure is performed by gradually withdrawing the catheter from the medial aspect (**a** → **b** → **c**) while repeatedly inflating and deflating the balloon

5.3 Recommended Procedural Methods

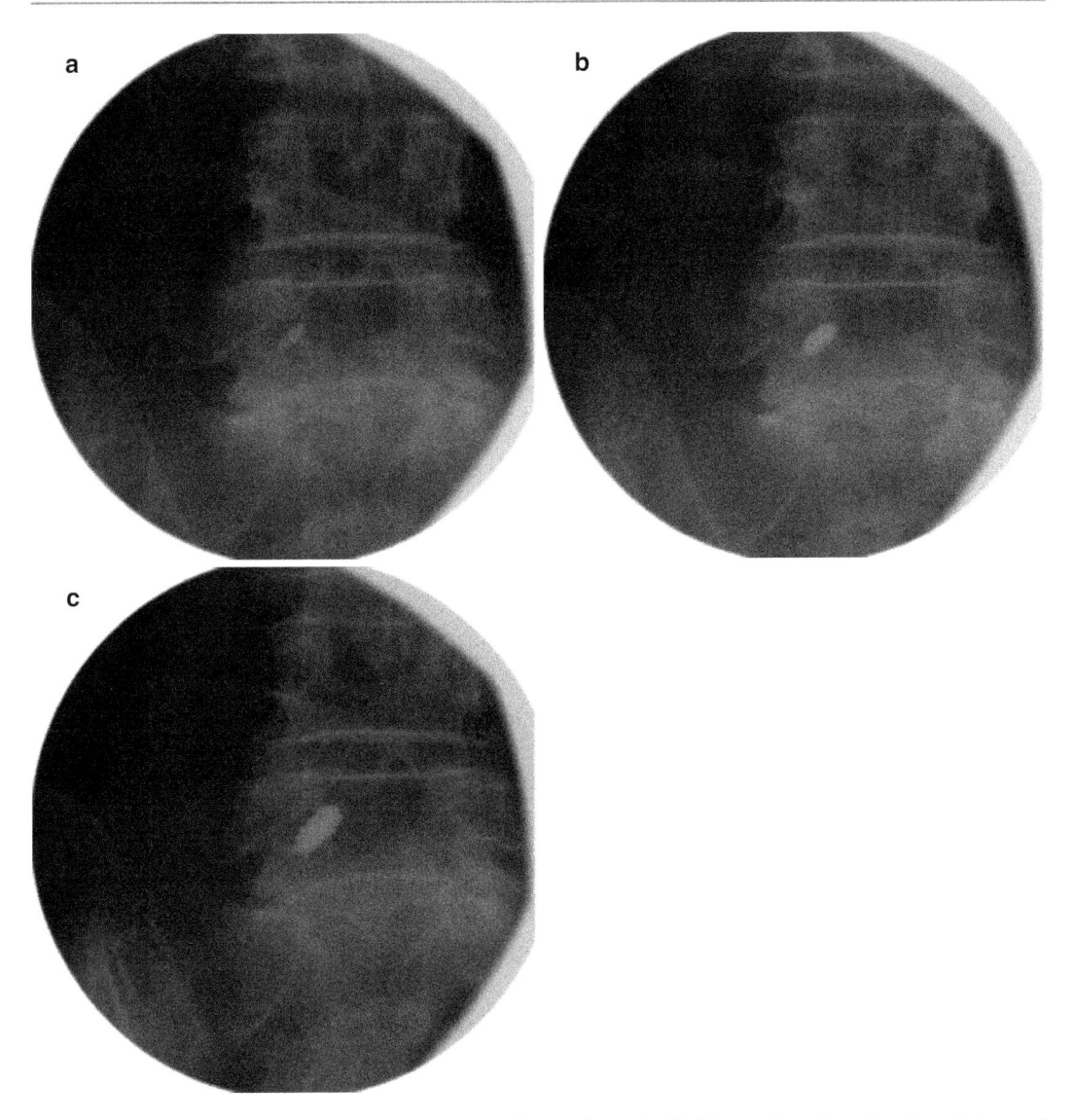

Fig. 5.20 When pain is not severe, the procedure could be performed in three steps. (**a**) Procedure performed using 0.05 cc of contrast dye. (**b**) The procedure is then performed with 0.1 cc after reinserting the catheter, and (**c**) again with ≥0.2 cc

patient's body, and the wire should be inserted slowly while the balloon section is pressed down with the thumb and index finger. This allows the wire to be inserted without inflating the balloon. The slow insertion of the wire is essential to the successful performance of this step.

When completely removing the balloon catheter from the body, the balloon section may snag on the needle tip. Pulling the catheter forcibly in such cases can cause it to break. Hence, the catheter should be pulled carefully while the bevel of the needle is rotated. If the problem persists, the needle and catheter should be removed concurrently. Using a sheath reduces the likelihood of encountering this difficulty.

Reinsertion of the Guide Needle

As aforementioned, the needle or sheath should be retracted slightly before the balloon is inflated when performing balloon decompression up to

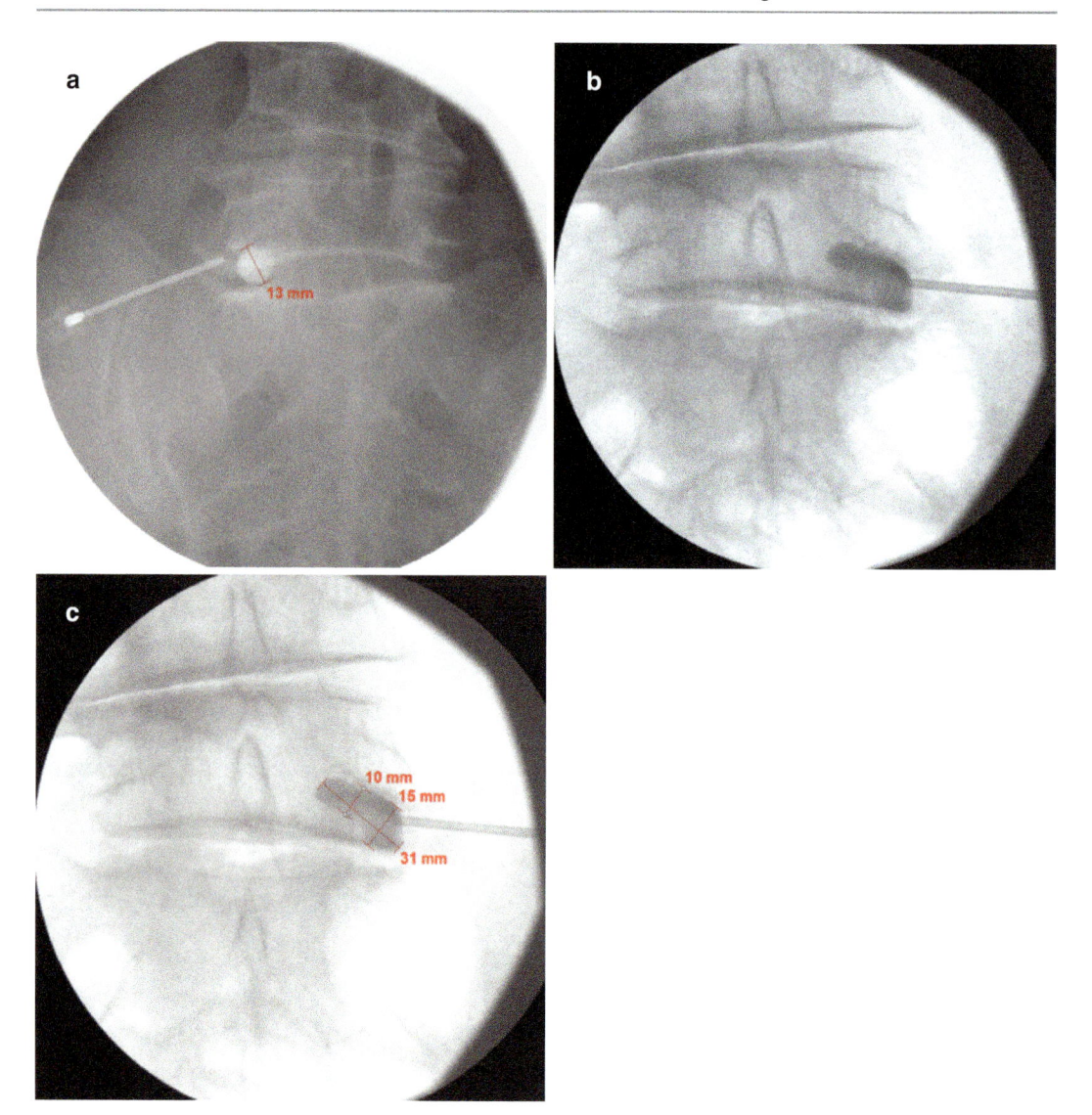

Fig. 5.21 (a) By injecting up to 0.2 cc of contrast dye, the balloon can be inflated up to a diameter of 13–15 mm. (b, c) The space within the entire intervertebral foramen expands as the balloon inflates with the injection of 0.3 cc of contrast dye. The balloon adopts the shape of the space and extends to a length of up to 30 mm

the extraforaminal area. Upon completion of balloon decompression, the guide needle or sheath is reinserted at the site at from which it was retracted. If the patient complains of dysesthesia or pain, the process should be halted immediately. Once the guide needle is reinserted at its previous position, the contrast dye is used to check for abnormalities. Steroids and local anesthetics are then injected, and the needle or sheath is removed to complete the procedure (Fig. 5.22).

Post-Procedural Care

The patient should be notified that he or she may experience pain or discomfort for 2–3 days after balloon decompression. Pain may occur during the procedure if physical irritation is applied to an area with neuritis caused by spinal disc herniation or stenosis; such pain may persist for 2–10 days following the procedure. Hence, post-procedural pain management should be attended carefully. Although pain subsides within

5.3 Recommended Procedural Methods

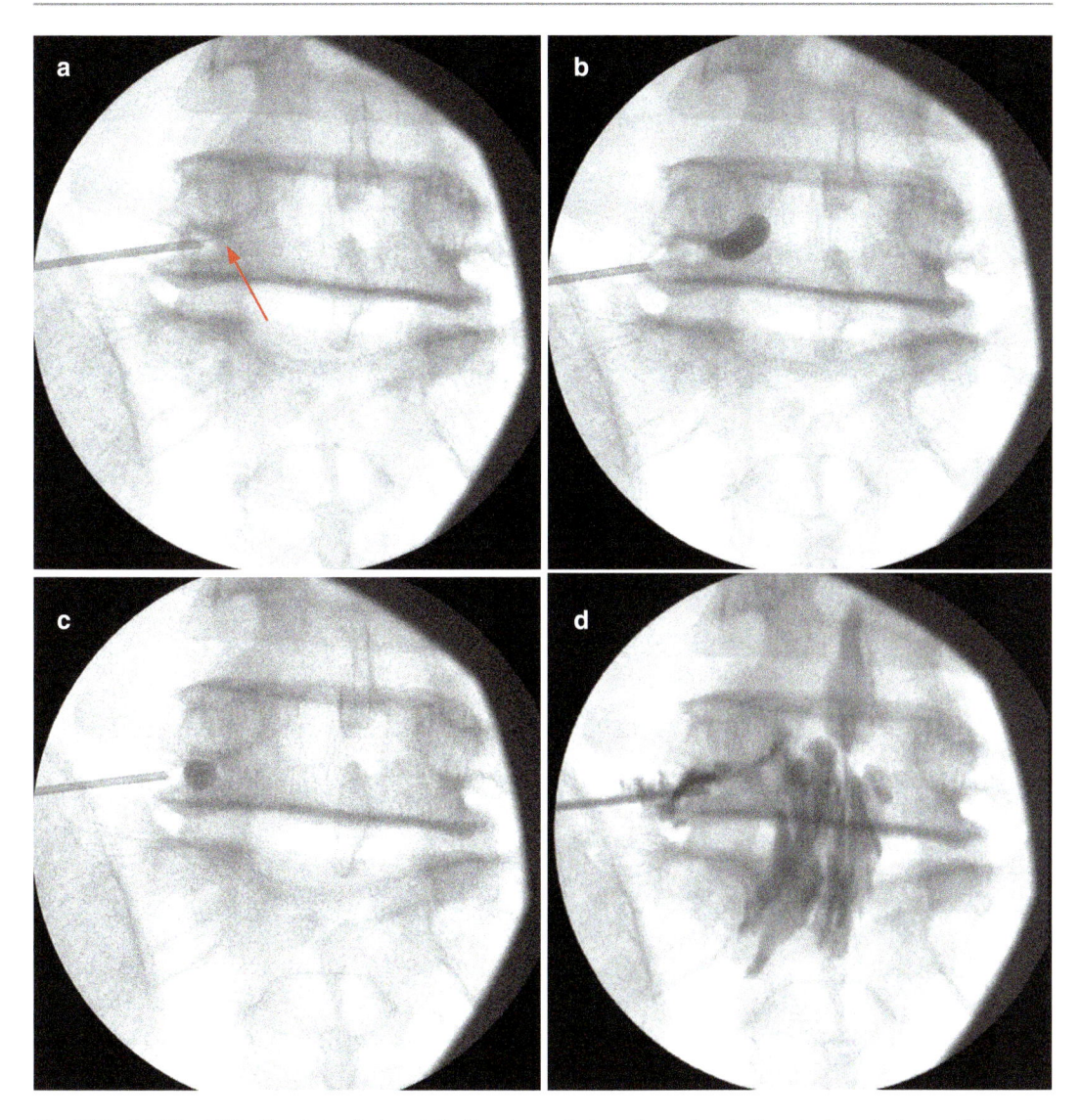

Fig. 5.22 (**a**) The ZiNeuF catheter is inserted after the guide needle is placed. Arrow: ZiNeuF catheter. (**b**, **c**) The performance of balloon decompression after the guide needle is performed up to the extraforaminal area. (**d**) The dye spread is checked after the guide needle is reinserted at its original position (compare the location of the needle tip)

2–10 days after the procedure, and symptoms present before the procedure improve in most cases, some patients may experience overly severe pain or pain that persists for more than 10 days. In such cases, epidural block using local anesthetic could be helpful in reducing pain. The local anesthetic used in epidural block helps to reduce the hyper-excitability of nerves. Whether it should be used together with steroids should be determined according to the patient's condition.

As in the use of the ZiNeu catheter, balloon decompression using the ZiNeuF catheter can induce excellent improvement in pain and walking distance. If the patient's ability to walk improves noticeably, the patient should be encouraged to engage in even more walking. While patients are instructed to engage in walking for at least 1 h each day, they are also advised to pay attention to pain and rest before they attempt to exercise again if it is felt.

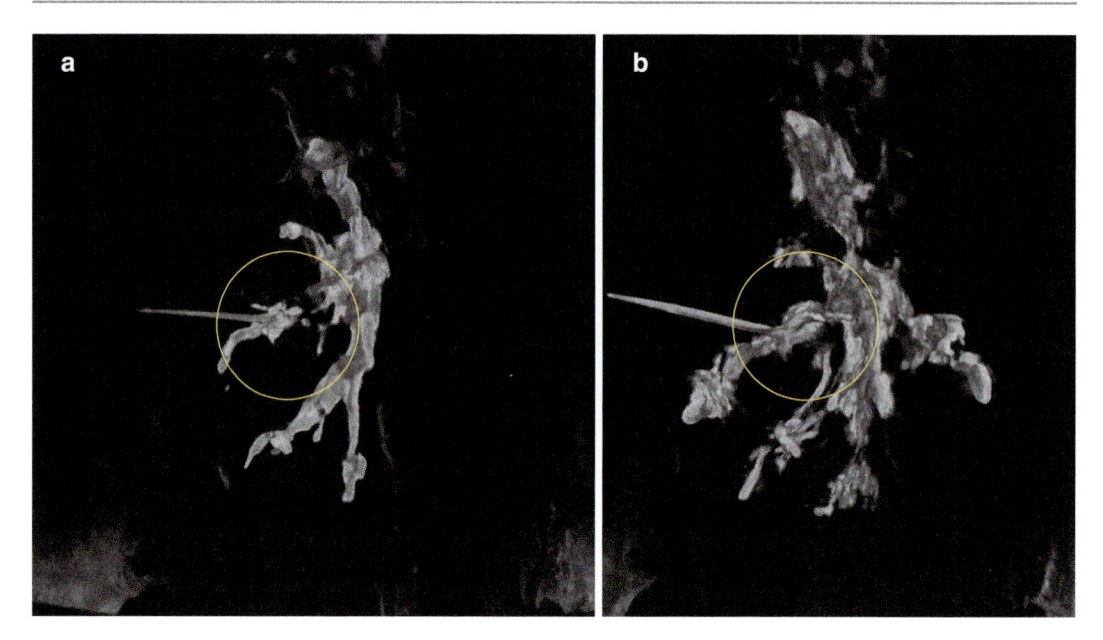

Fig. 5.23 A 3D reconstructed view of the findings derived from the spread of the dye before and after balloon decompression in a patient with foraminal stenosis. (**a**) Contrast dye findings before the procedure. (**b**) Contrast dye findings after the procedure. Circle: Filling defect in the intervertebral foramen was resolved after the procedure

As explained in the Introduction, the balloon decompression procedure not only helps to remove adhesion and but also helps to improve blood circulation by the expansion of marginal free space in the stenotic area. As a result, the patients' capacity to walk also increases. However, the patients must continually engage in a sufficient amount of walking to maintain or achieve greater improvement (Fig. 5.23).

5.3.1.2 Kambin's Triangle (Retrodiscal) Approach

When the lesion is situated in the retrodiscal area or the inferior aspect of the intervertebral foramen, the catheter must be inserted into the retrodiscal area to treat the area directly. This mandates the insertion of the guide needle according to Kambin's triangle approach (Fig. 5.24).

By using Kambin's triangle approach, the ZiNeuF catheter can be inserted directly into the retrodiscal area (Fig. 5.25).

C-Arm Control

Kambin's triangle approach requires the same method as does the discogram procedure: the superior and inferior endplates of the disc at the level where the procedure is being performed are aligned parallel to the X-ray beam, and the oblique view is adjusted to align the superior articular process of the inferior vertebral body on the central part of the disc. For the C-arm oblique view angle, 40–45° is appropriate. The entry points include the retrodiscal area and lateral aspect of the superior articular process (Fig. 5.26).

Guide Needle Insertion

After anesthetizing the entry points with a local anesthetic, the guide needle is inserted using the tunnel view. The insertion depth of the needle is adjusted in the lateral view, and an attempt is made to insert the needle tip up to the retrodiscal area by referencing the sagittal view of the patient's MRI images. The insertion should be executed carefully: if it is too deep, the guide needle may penetrate through the disc. An experienced operator may be able to feel the needle tip contacting the disc.

The needle tip should be inserted toward the superior endplate of the vertebral body—right below the disc—to allow the catheter to slip

5.3 Recommended Procedural Methods

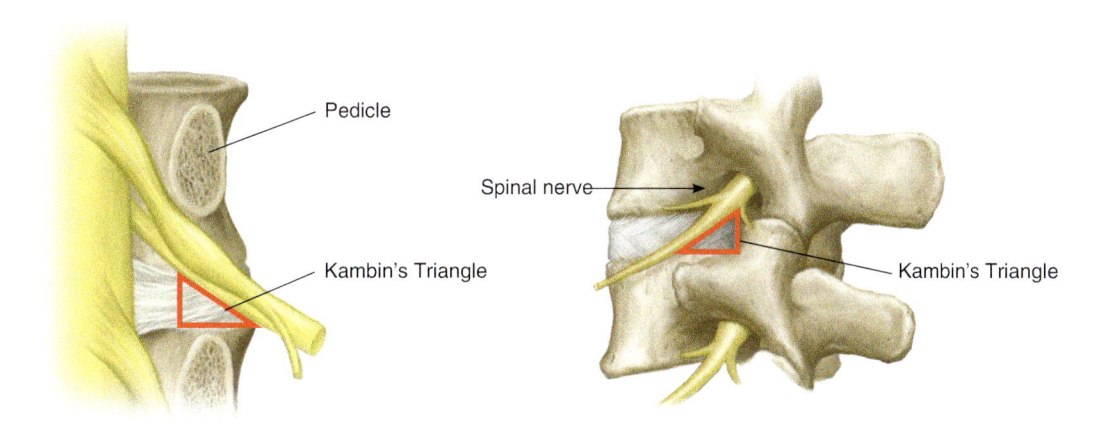

Fig. 5.24 Location of the Kambin's triangle

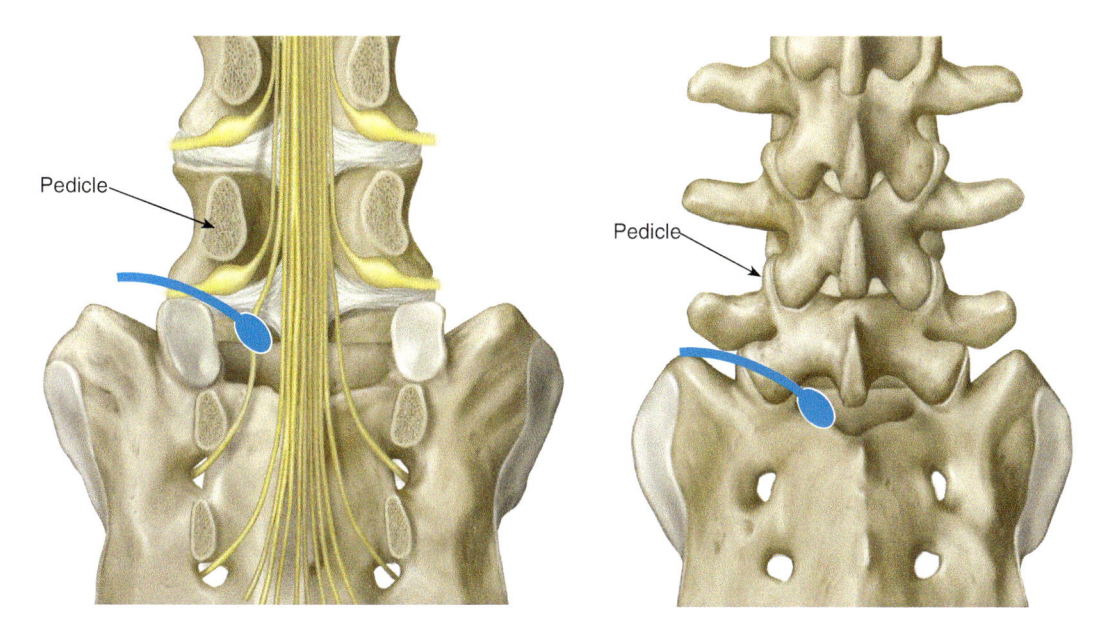

Fig. 5.25 The insertion of the ZiNeuF into the retrodiscal area according to Kambin's triangle approach

through to the retrodiscal area. In other words, retrodiscal lesions often cause problems involving traversing nerves that run down inferior levels; thus, the needle should be inserted slightly below the retrodiscal area to allow the catheter to pass through the area where the disc comes into contact with the traversing nerves (Fig. 5.27).

Insertion of the ZiNeuF Catheter
Once the needle reaches the superior endplate of the vertebral body at the lower part of the retrodiscal area, the stylet is removed, and the ZiNeuF catheter is inserted. After the catheter passes through the guide needle tip, the catheter is inserted to an additional depth of 2–3 cm. It is ideal to insert the catheter while it is oriented toward the lower level (Fig. 5.28).

Balloon Decompression
After removing the reinforcing wire and eliminating the air inside the catheter according to the method used in the safe triangle approach, the

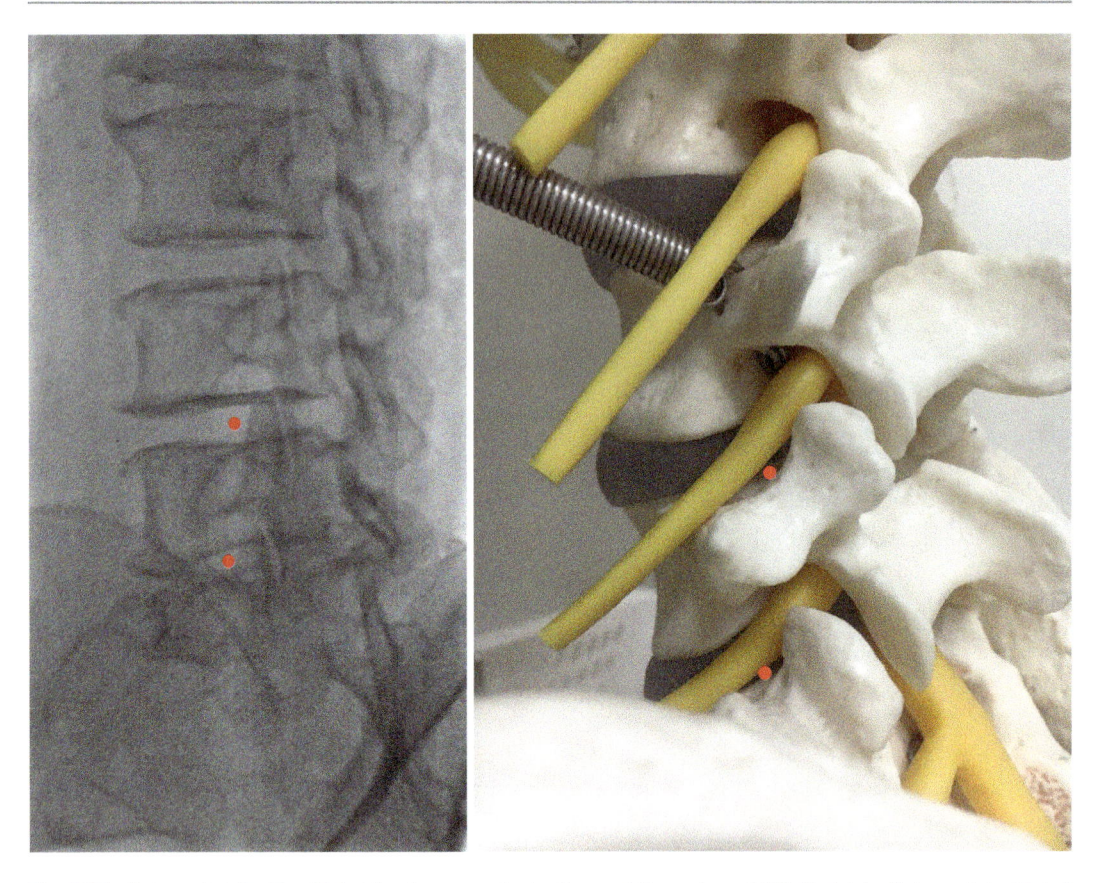

Fig. 5.26 Entry points for Kambin's triangle approach at a C-arm oblique view of 45°. Red dots: Entry points at L4–5 and L5–S1 levels

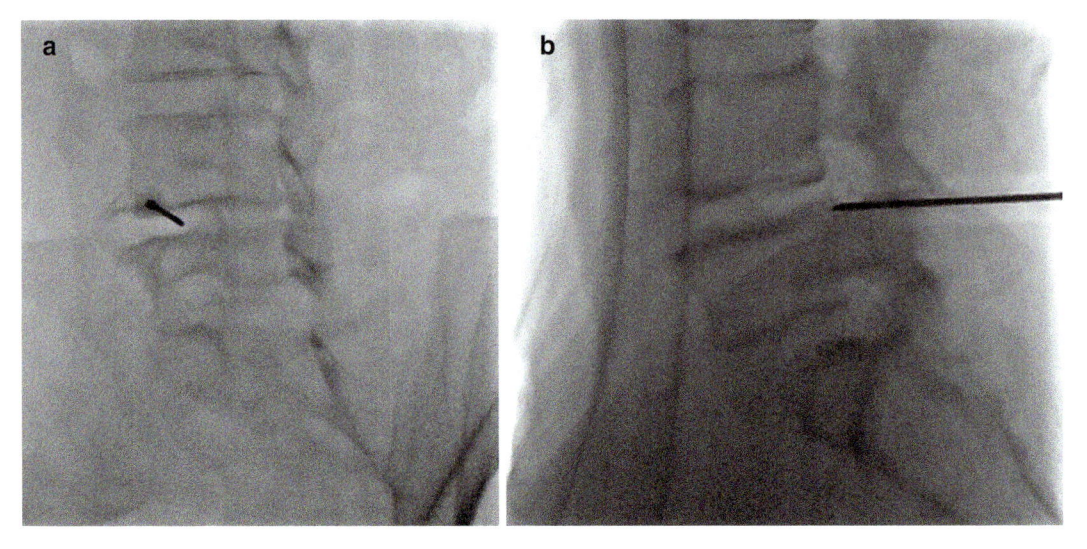

Fig. 5.27 (**a**) The needle is inserted toward the lateral aspect of the superior articular process using the tunnel view. (**b**, **c**) Insert the needle up to the retrodiscal area by referencing MRI images

5.3 Recommended Procedural Methods

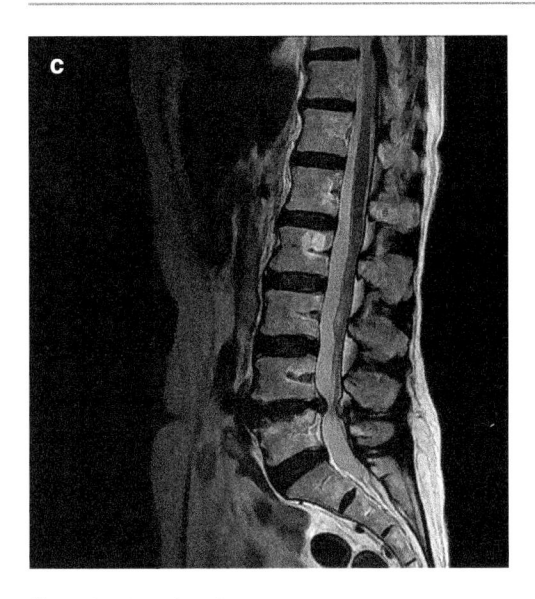

Fig. 5.27 (continued)

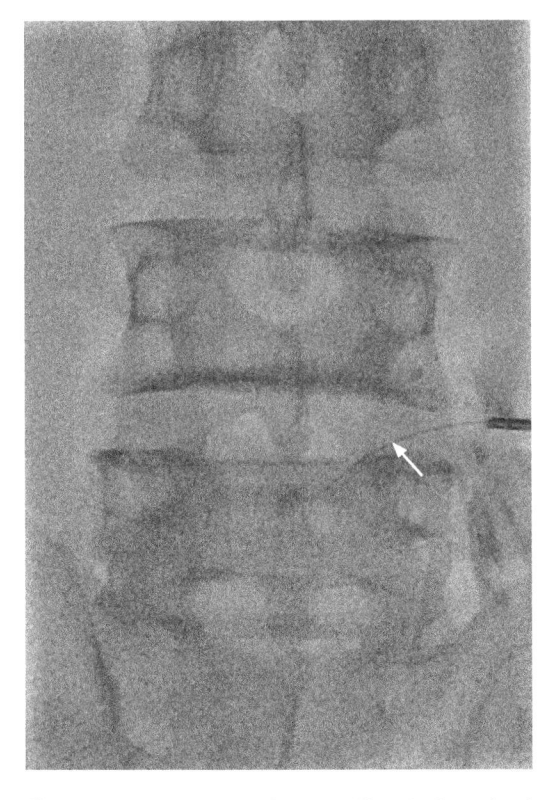

Fig. 5.28 ZiNeuF catheter is inserted into the lower level through the L4–5 retrodiscal area. Arrow: ZiNeuF catheter

procedure is performed twice or thrice across the entire retrodiscal area. The amount of contrast dye injected is increased stepwise—from 0.05 cc, through 0.1 cc, to 0.2 cc—to increase the balloon size in a stepwise manner and thereby expand the area (Fig. 5.29).

Balloon decompression performed according to the method shown in Fig. 5.29 can expand the inferior aspect of the intervertebral foramen, relieve the compression of traversing nerves in the retrodiscal area, and remove adhesion, thereby maximizing the effect of the administered drug.

Case 1 A 45-year-old male patient whose MRI findings showed Lt. S1 root compression caused by Lt. L5–S1 disc extrusion. The primary symptom was Lt. S1 radiculopathy (Fig. 5.30). Despite undergoing two rounds of S1 root block within 1 year of the symptom onset, an improvement from the procedures lasted only 3–7 days. Accordingly, transforaminal Lt. L5-S1 retrodiscal balloon decompression was performed with the ZiNeuF catheter (Fig. 5.31). At 13 months following the procedure, the patient has continued to do well and has experienced no recurrences.

Case 2 A 62-year-old female patient visited the pain clinic for Lt. L5 radiculopathy that had begun 5 months prior. Despite three rounds of the transforaminal epidural block at another hospital, her symptoms did not improve. The MRI findings revealed a Lt. L4–5 sequestrated disc (Fig. 5.32). Accordingly, a transforaminal Lt. L4–5 retrodiscal balloon decompression with the ZiNeuF catheter was planned. However, the needle was inserted too deeply and penetrated through the disc. Balloon decompression was performed without recognizing this fact (Fig. 5.33a). Because there was no pain during balloon inflation and the appearance and location of balloon inflation were abnormal, the catheter was removed, and the contrast dye was injected and spread into the disc.

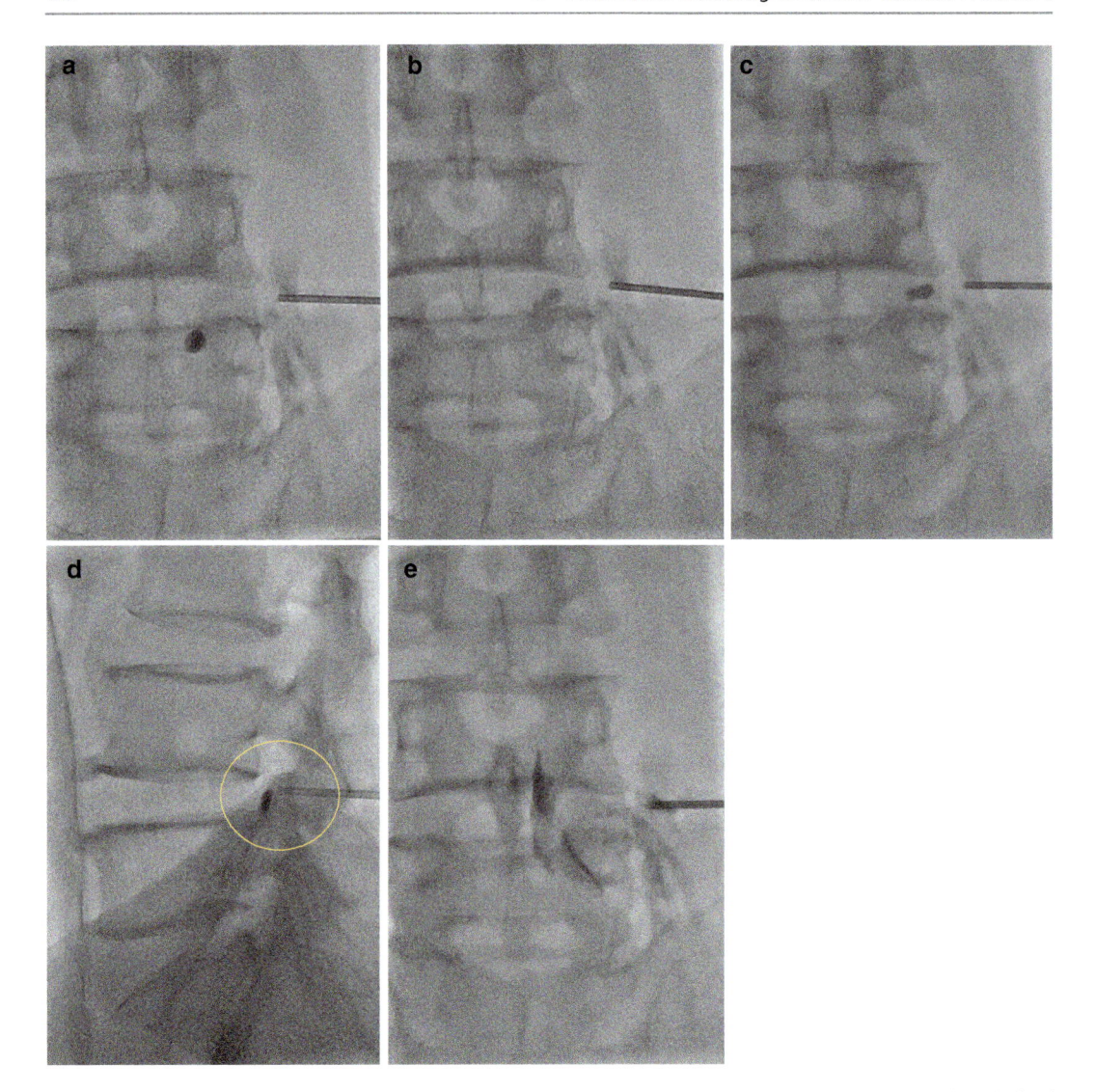

Fig. 5.29 Transforaminal retrodiscal balloon decompression. (**a–c**) The entire retrodiscal area is divided into three zones, and the procedure is performed by gradually withdrawing the catheter while continually repeating the inflation and deflation of the balloon. (**d**) Lateral view of the balloon inflated in the retrodiscal area of the anterior epidural space. Circle: Inflated balloon. (**e**) Findings derived from the spread of the contrast dye after balloon decompression. The contrast dye spread well to the area expanded by ballooning along the traversing nerve and anterior epidural space. This is an ideal contrast dye finding

The guide needle was subsequently retracted slightly, and the catheter was reinserted to gain entry into the retrodiscal area. Balloon decompression was then performed again (Fig. 5.33b). The patient was discharged without any problems. She reported ≥80% improvement at the 3- and 6-month follow-up visits. As of the 15-month follow-up, she had experienced no recurrence of follow-up.

Reference

Types of Catheters Used for the Transforaminal Approach

There are two types of balloon catheters that can be used for the transforaminal approach: ZiNeuF and ZiNeuF03. The former is a 2F catheter which, while thin, lacks a separate drug-injection port. The ZiNeuF03 catheter is a 3F catheter that feels some-

5.3 Recommended Procedural Methods

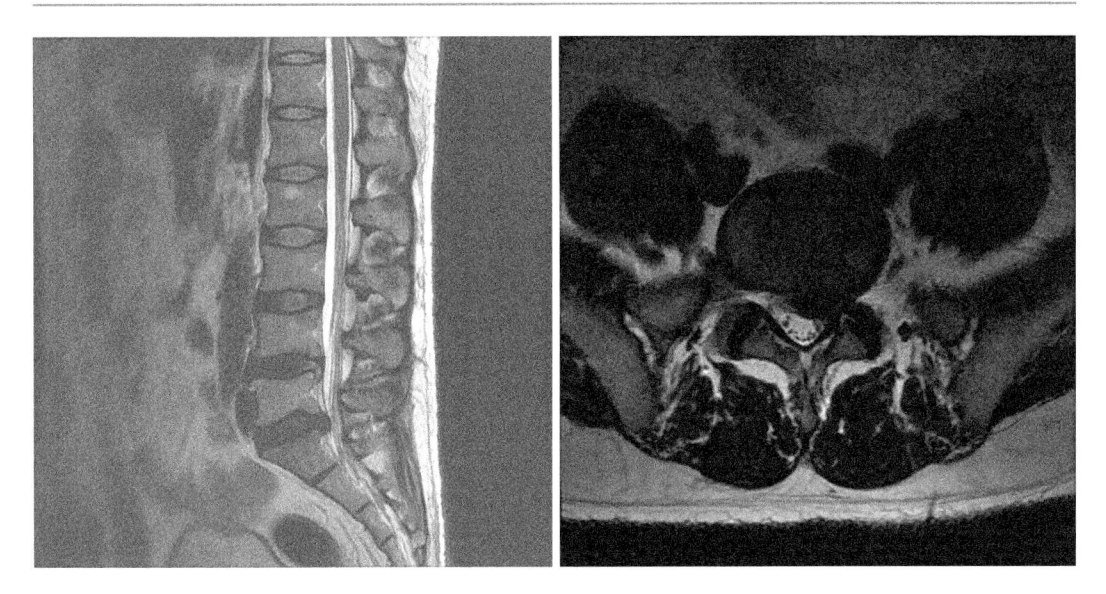

Fig. 5.30 MRI findings. Lt. L5–S1 extrusion with Lt. S1 root compression

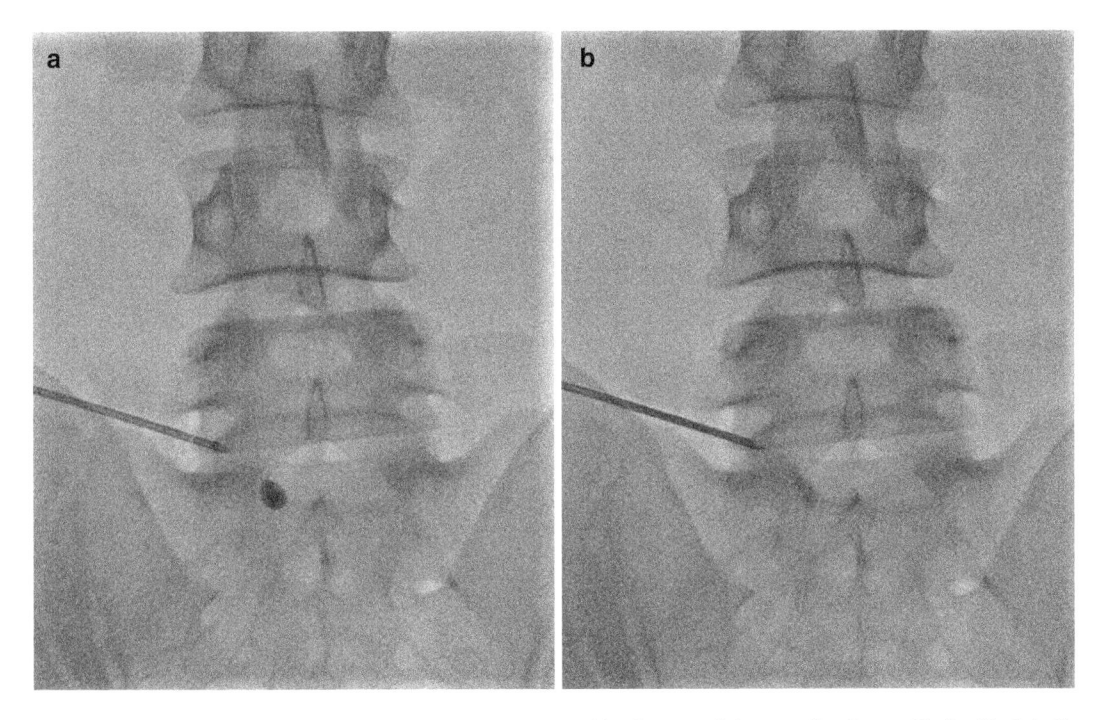

Fig. 5.31 (**a, b**) The AP view of balloon decompression being performed while the catheter is gradually withdrawn from the retrodiscal area. (**c**) The lateral view of balloon decompression being performed in the anterior epidural space of the retrodiscal area. Circle: Black indicates the inflated balloon. (**d**) Contrast dye spread findings after balloon decompression

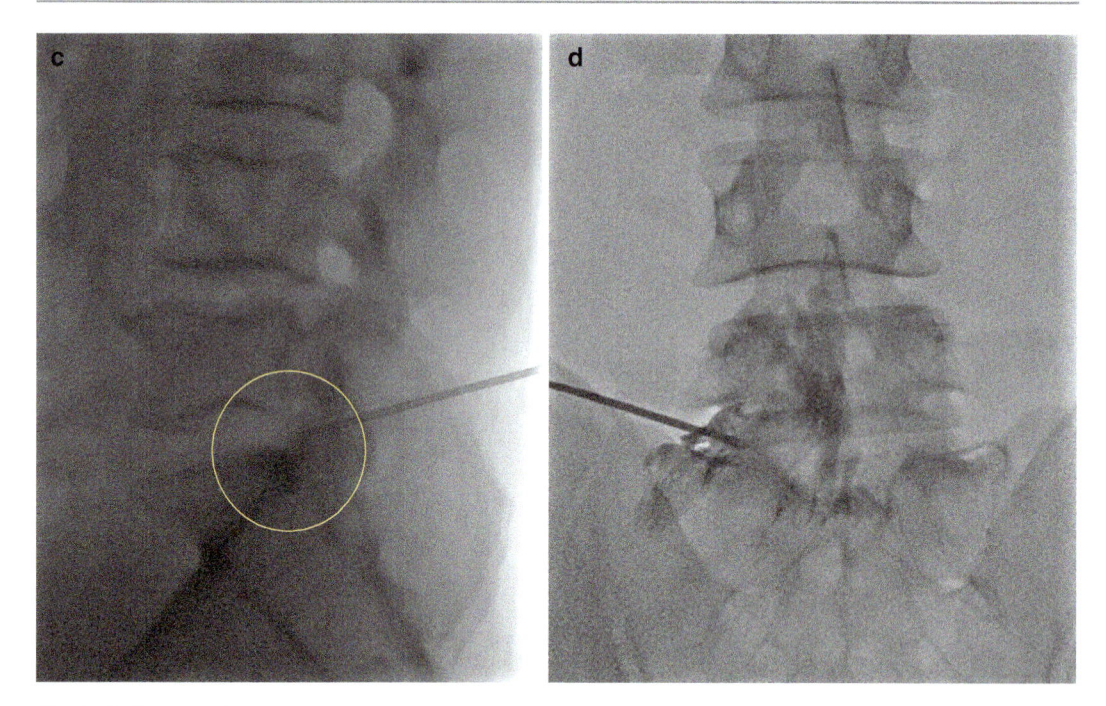

Fig. 5.31 (continued)

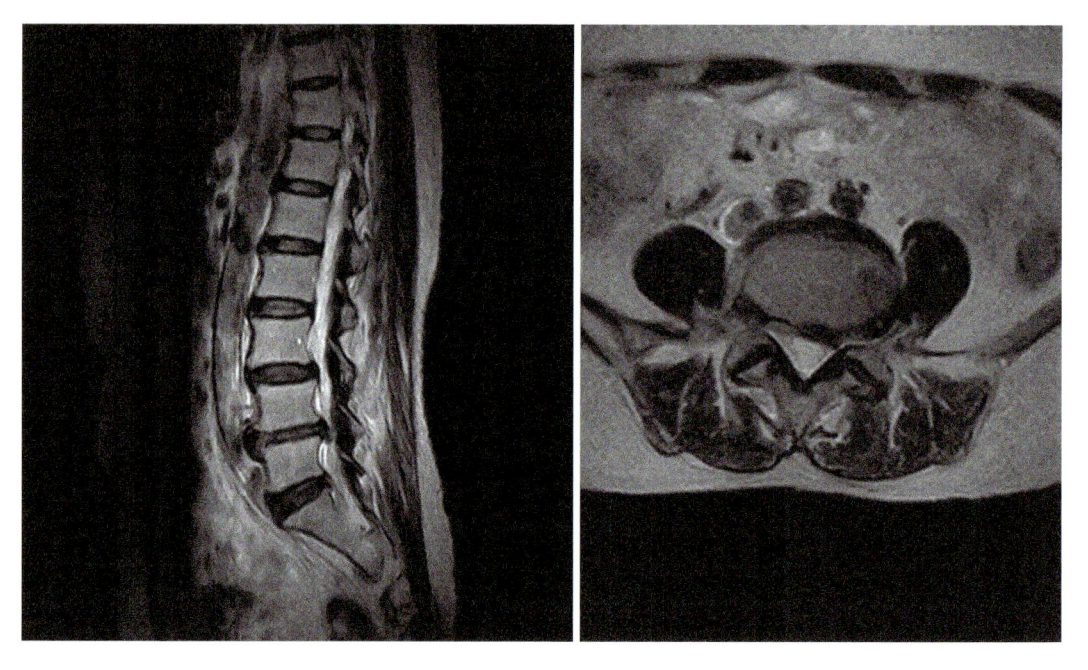

Fig. 5.32 MRI findings. Lt. L4–5 inferior sequestrated disc

what thicker, but because it features separate balloon and drug ports, it allows for the drug to be injected simultaneously with balloon decompression.

If the ZiNeuF catheter is used for the transforaminal approach, the drug must be administered with the needle after the catheter has been

5.3 Recommended Procedural Methods 125

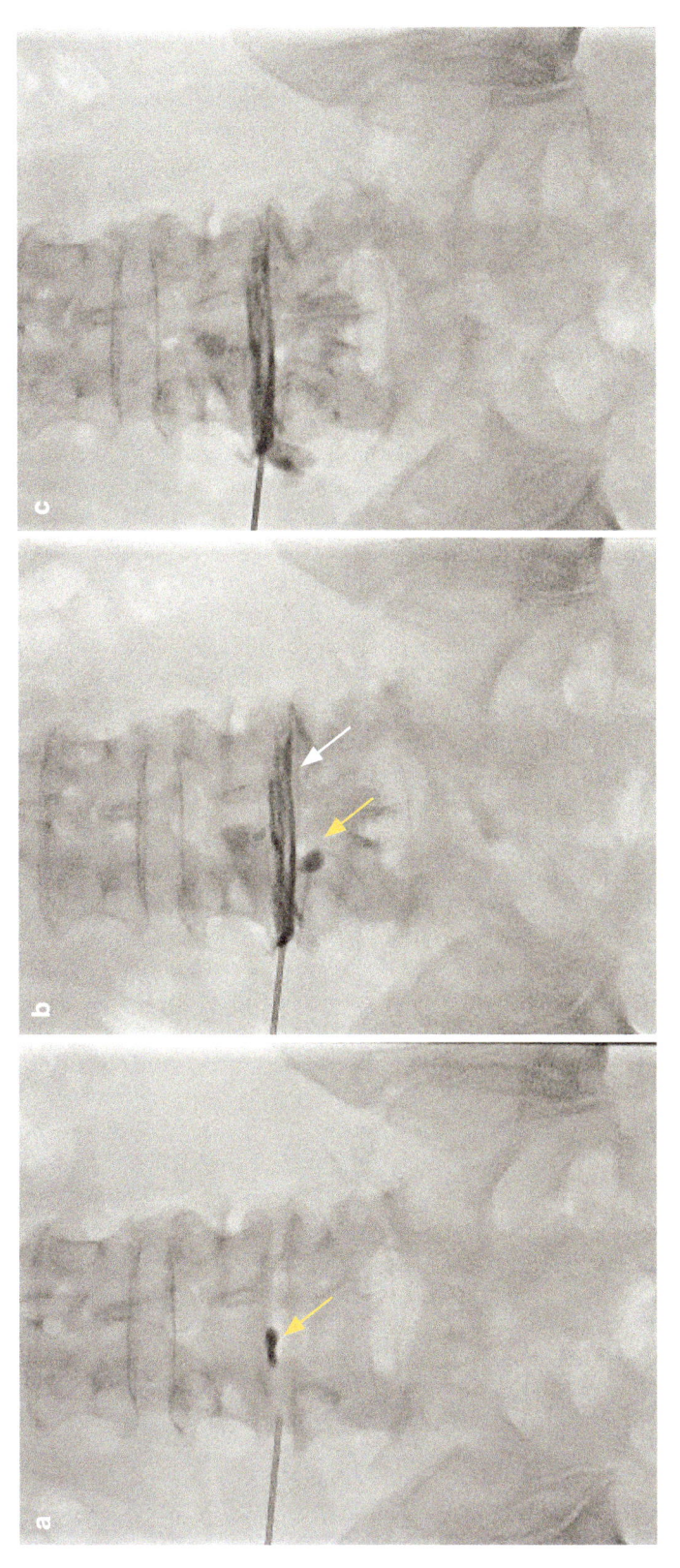

Fig. 5.33 Lt. L4–5 transforaminal retrodiscal balloon decompression. (**a**) Balloon being inflated inside the disc. (**b**) The performance of balloon decompression in the retrodiscal area after the catheter had been reinserted. Contrast dye findings inside the disc were also seen. (**c**) The findings obtained from the contrast dye spread after balloon decompression. Yellow arrow: Inflated balloon. White arrow: Discogram findings

removed. Some operators think that this is not good because it cannot administer the drug directly to the affected area. However, because the actual distance between the needle tip and affected area is small and there is little room for the drug to leak into areas apart from the affected area, injecting the drug through a needle could help to deliver the drug to the affected area in terms of supplying a sufficient amount of drugs for the lesion. In several cases, the 3F ZiNeuF03 catheter failed to delivered sufficient drug to the affected area due to the backflow of the drug through the needle when it was injected after transforaminal insertion of the catheter. This is because severe stenosis or adhesion in the affected area could increase the pressure in that area when the drug is injected, which causes the drug to backflow toward the needle, which has lower pressure. Although each operator may have a different preference, the 2F ZiNeuF catheter may be more appropriate for the transforaminal approach, while the 3F ZiNeuF03 catheter may be better suited to the interlaminar approach, which will be explained later.

When Kambin's Triangle Approach Is Impossible

In cases of severe disc herniation-induced stenosis in the inferior aspect of the intervertebral foramen, performing balloon decompression in the retrodiscal area via Kambin's triangle approach is impossible (Fig. 5.34). This is because Kambin's triangle approach entails a high likelihood of disc penetration. In such cases, if the lesion is in the retrodiscal area, the ZiNeu series catheter should be used with the caudal approach.

5.3.2 Interlaminar Approach

5.3.2.1 Retrograde Interlaminar Ventral Approach

When approaching the L5 intervertebral foramen, catheter insertion becomes difficult if the guide needle cannot be advanced while lying flat due to the iliac crest. In such cases, the catheter could be inserted relatively easily by using the interlaminar approach—i.e., if the C-arm angle is $\geq 30°$ after the maximum oblique view possible for insertion into the intervertebral foramen is found, then the transforaminal approach is possible. If an angle of $\geq 30°$ cannot be attained because of the iliac crest, adopting the interlaminar approach is recommended (Fig. 5.35).

With this method, even if the catheter is initially inserted into the posterior epidural space, it approaches the anterior epidural space in the intervertebral foramen. Therefore, it is referred to as the interlaminar ventral approach.

The following outlines the use of the retrograde interlaminar ventral approach for insertion into the L5 intervertebral foramen:

After cephalically or caudally tilting the C-arm to find the position with the best view of the interlaminar space in the target area (Fig. 5.36), the needle being inserted is placed the patient's back. The angle that would allow access into the superior aspect of the L5 intervertebral foramen—the area just below the L5 pedicle—through the interlaminar space is estimated in AP view (Fig. 5.37a). The intersection between this angular line and the line extending from the midline of the pedicle on the opposite side is set as the entry point, and the target point for needle insertion is at the intersection of this angular line and the area at which the interlaminar space begins. After inserting the needle at the insertion point, the epidural space is found using the loss of resistance technique while inserting the needle toward the target point (Fig. 5.37b).

As confirmed by the CT images in Fig. 5.38, inserting the needle with the midline of the pedicle as the entry point allows for the attainment of an angle appropriate for the interlaminar approach.

To reiterate, the guide needle can be placed easily in the epidural space by adopting a mode

5.3 Recommended Procedural Methods

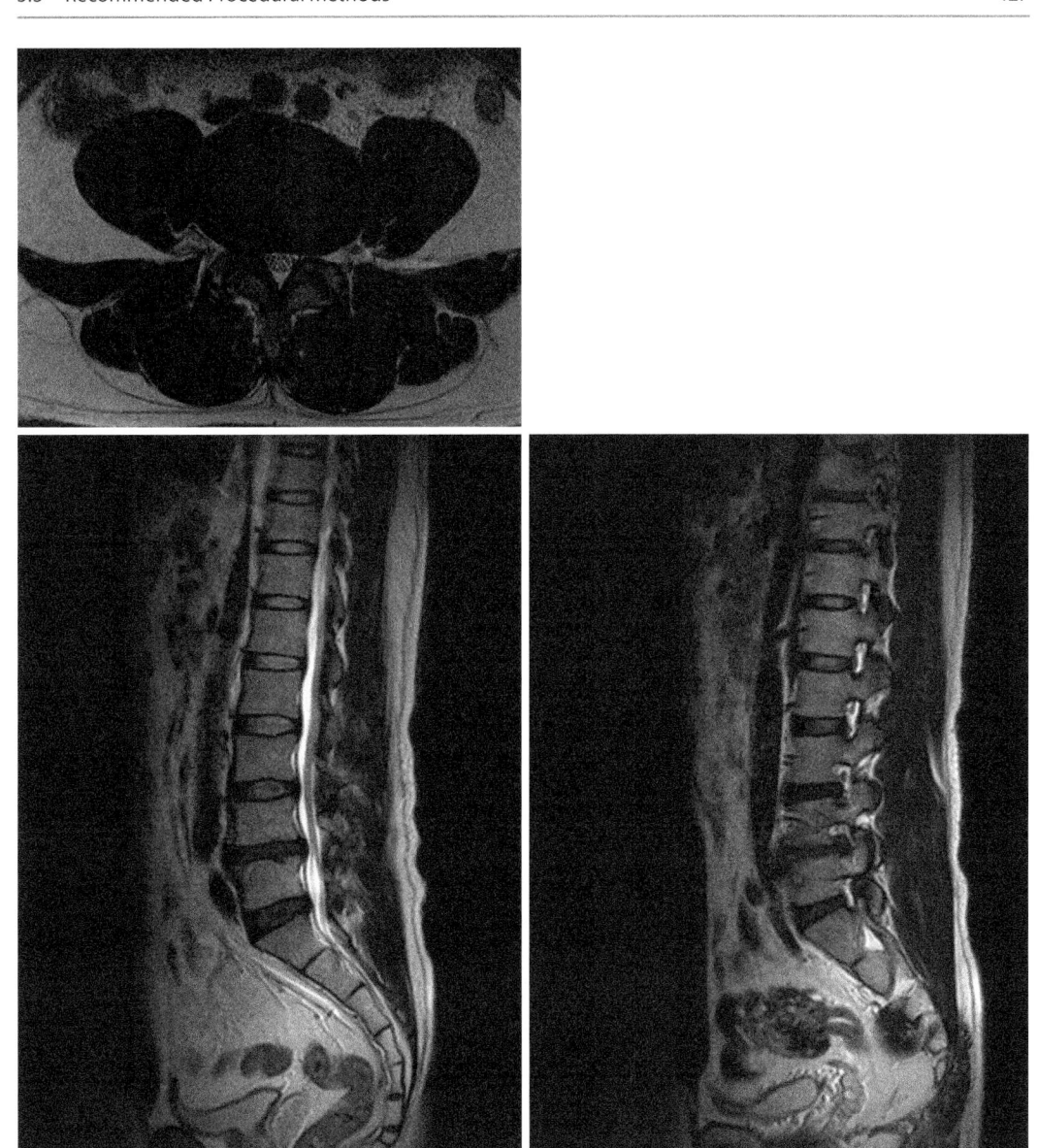

Fig. 5.34 MRI findings. Extraforaminal and foraminal stenosis caused by Rt. L4–5 extruded disc. Adopting Kambin's triangle approach to gain entry into the inferior aspect of the L4–5 intervertebral foramen is precluded by the extruded disc

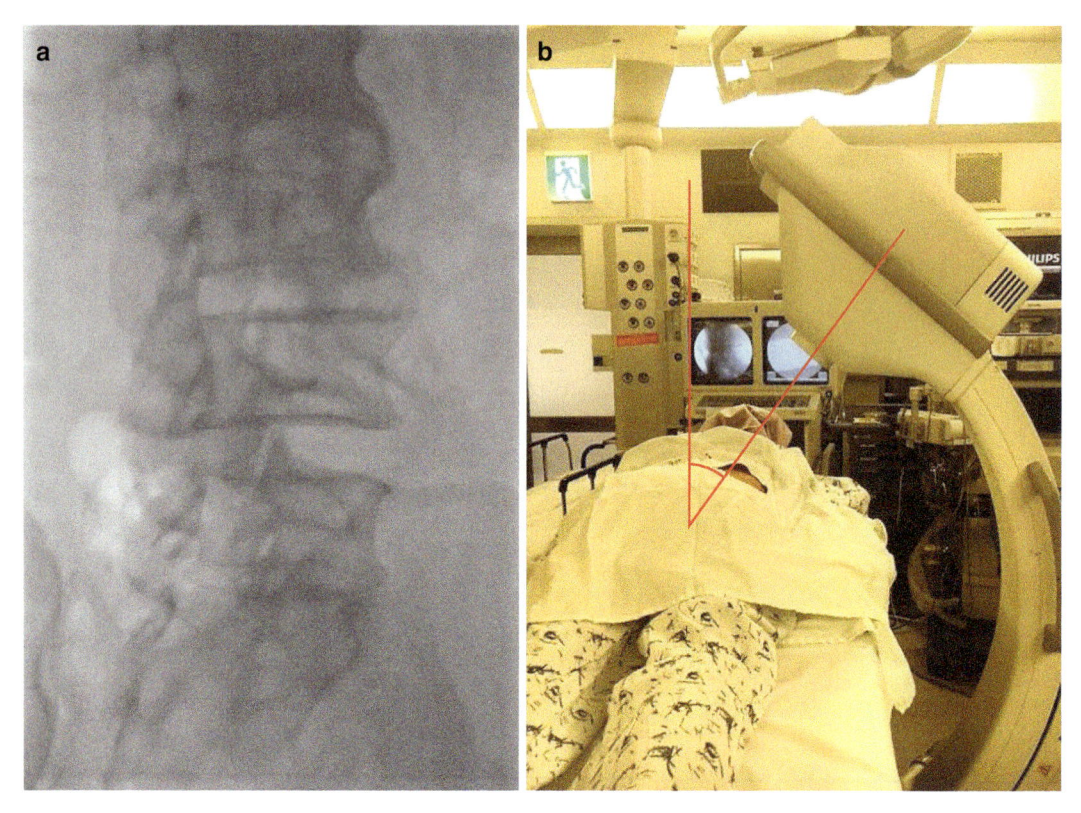

Fig. 5.35 (**a**) Maximum oblique view possible for insertion into the intervertebral foramen. (**b**) If the C-arm angle is ≥30°, then the transforaminal approach is possible. If an angle of ≥30° cannot be attained because of the iliac crest, then the interlaminar approach should be used

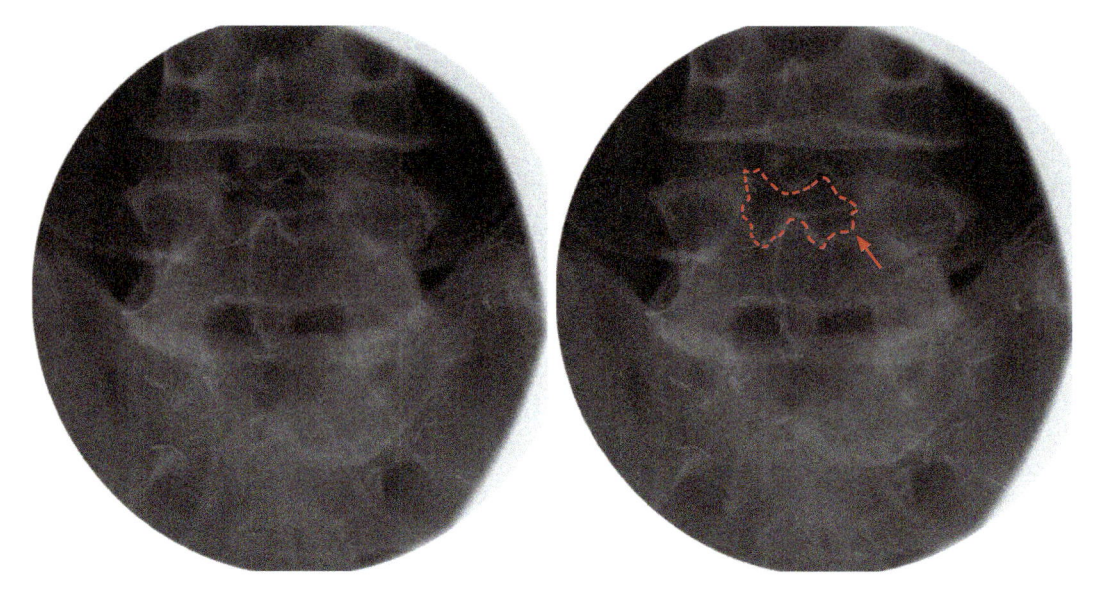

Fig. 5.36 The C-arm is controlled through cephalically or caudally tilting to find the best view of the L4–5 interlaminar space. Arrow: interlaminar space

5.3 Recommended Procedural Methods

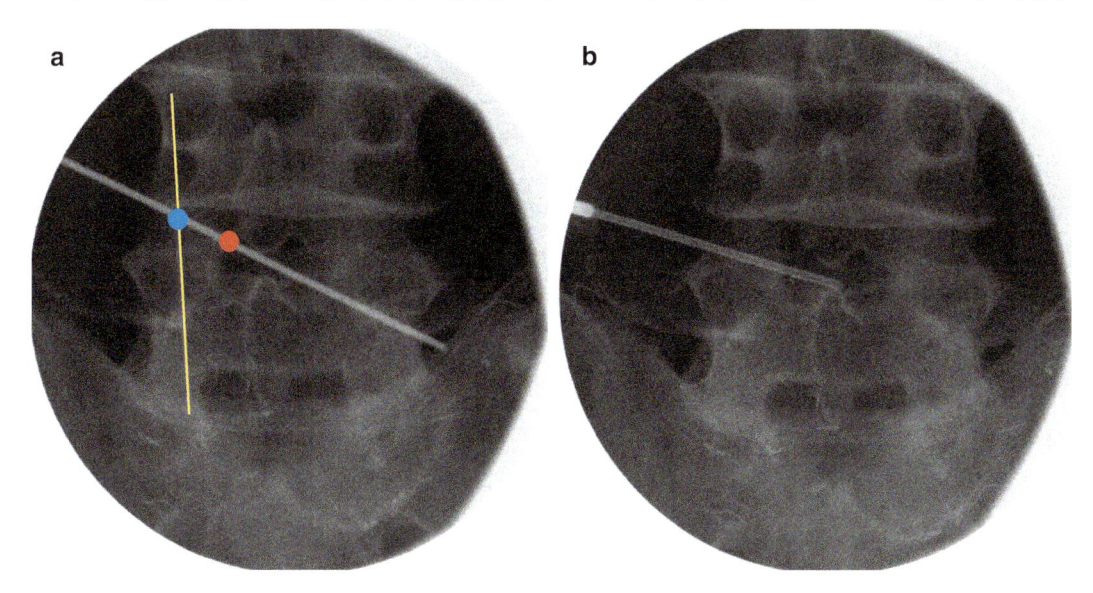

Fig. 5.37 (**a**) The needle is placed on the back of the patient before being inserted. The insertion angle is estimated in the AP view. The intersection between this angle and the line extending from the midline of the pedicle on the opposite side is set as the entry point (blue dot), and the intersection of this angle and the area at which the interlaminar space begins is set as the target point (red dot). (**b**) The needle is inserted and placed in the epidural space

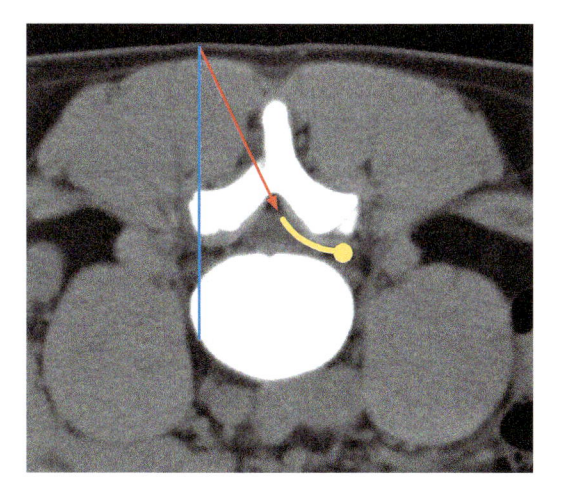

Fig. 5.38 CT images reveal the angle at which the needle is inserted (red arrow) for the interlaminar approach at the midline of the pedicle (blue line). The entry of the catheter (yellow color) into the intervertebral foramen when inserted at this angle

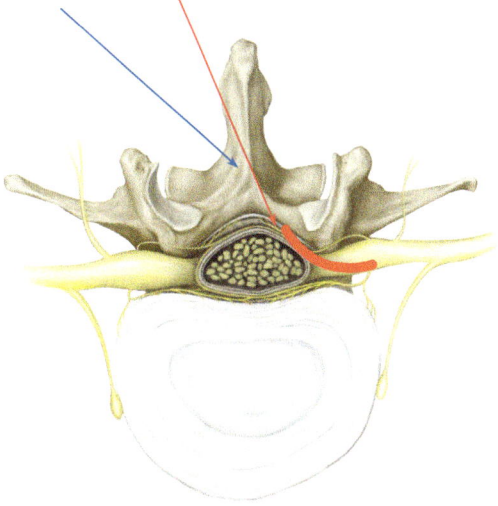

Fig. 5.39 The proper entry angle (red arrow), improper entry angle (blue arrow), the catheter (red line)

of entry similar to the red arrow shown in Fig. 5.39. Based on the belief that entry into the intervertebral foramen would be easier by laying it flat, operators tend to acquire the habit of laying the guide needle flat; however, as shown by the blue arrow in Fig. 5.39, this could complicate finding the epidural space as well as accessing the epidural space.

When employing the interlaminar approach, it is important to consider that the tip of the guide needle inside the epidural space must be placed

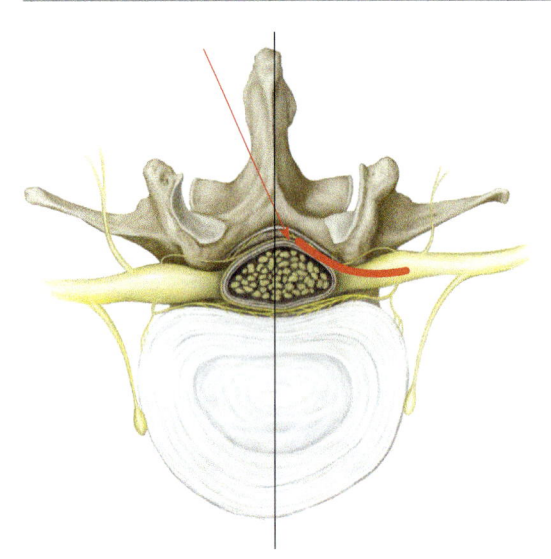

Fig. 5.40 The guide needle (red arrow) is placed inside the epidural space beyond the midline (black line): the catheter (red line) has been placed into the intervertebral foramen on the affected side

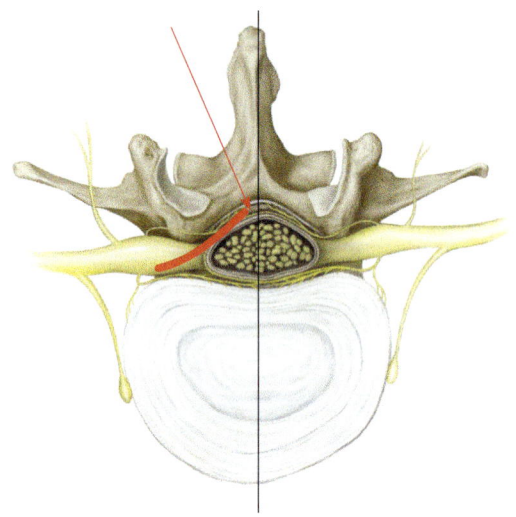

Fig. 5.41 The guide needle (red arrow) is placed inside the epidural space without passing the midline (black line): the catheter (red line) is inserted into the intervertebral foramen on the opposite side

beyond the spinal midline. The center of the dura, which wraps around the spinal nerves, has a bulging oval shape on the posterior surface. Therefore, if the tip of the guide needle does not extend beyond the spinal midline, advancing the catheter to the affected side becomes difficult. It is thus advisable to place the needle in the epidural space with its tip extended slightly beyond the midline. A three-dimensional conception of the needle's trajectory is thus needed for successful insertion (Figs. 5.40 and 5.41). If the needle tip reaches the epidural space without extending beyond the midline, the ZiNeuF catheter could be inserted first. If the catheter is inserted into the side opposite to the lesion, the catheter should be removed, and the needle should be retracted slightly outside the epidural space. Then, the needle is further laid down and reinserted into the epidural space using the loss of resistance technique. Because it is reinserted while lying flat, there is a greater likelihood of its extension beyond the spinal midline.

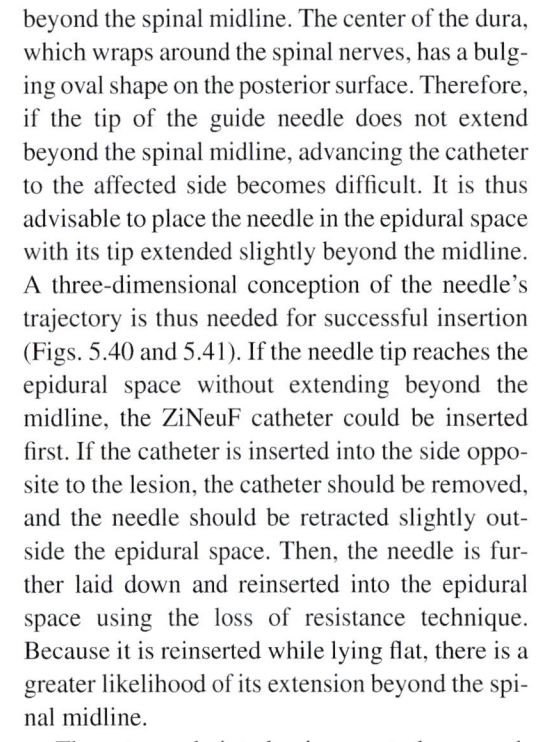

The retrograde interlaminar ventral approach involves inserting the catheter into the extraforaminal area, removing the reinforcing wire, filling the inside of the catheter with the contrast dye, and performing the procedure by gradually pulling the catheter from the lateral to the medial direction while repeatedly inflating and deflating the balloon as explained earlier (Fig. 5.42).

Although the ZiNeuF catheter could be used for this procedure, the ZiNeuF03 catheter is more suitable: its separate drug-injection ports allow the drug to be injected with the catheter in place.

With the transforaminal approach, it is advisable to inject the drug after removing the catheter, as the distance between the needle tip and affected area is short. The distance between the target intervertebral foramen and needle tip is lengthened when the interlaminar approach is adopted, and the epidural space, which features little resistance, spans this distance. Hence, when the drug is injected through the needle, the drug spreads mostly into the epidural space preceding the intervertebral foramen, impeding drug flow into the intervertebral foramen (Fig. 5.43a). When 2F catheter is used in the interlaminar approach, the balloon should be overinflated to induce its rupture and allow for the drug to be injected through the balloon port (Fig. 5.43b). Alternatively, the catheter may be removed, the balloon ruptured, and then, the catheter must be reinserted into the

5.3 Recommended Procedural Methods

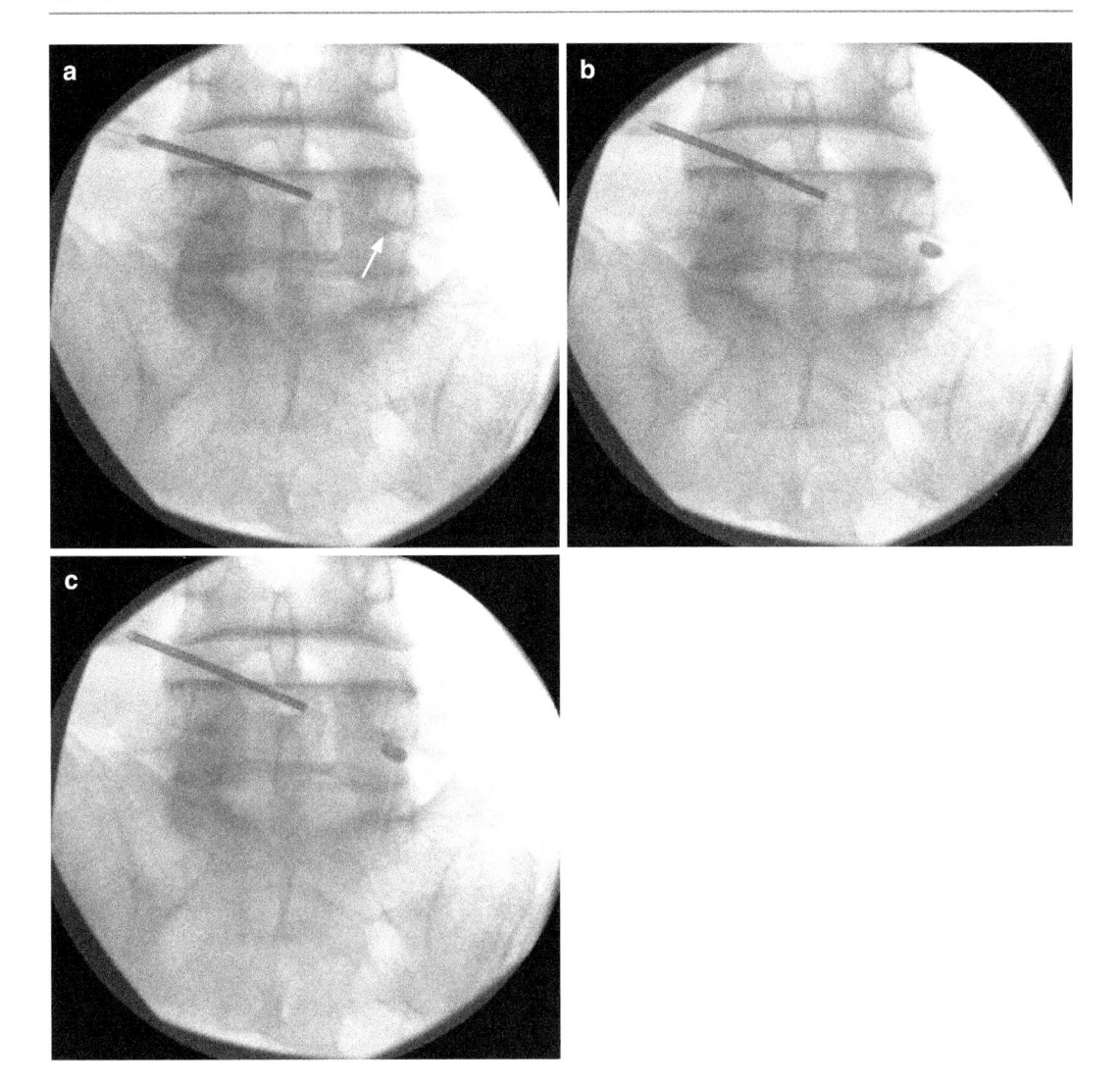

Fig. 5.42 Retrograde interlaminar ventral approach. (**a**) The ZiNeuF catheter is inserted into the extraforaminal area. (**b → c**) Image of the balloon being inflated as it is gradually withdrawn from the extraforaminal area to the medial aspect of the intervertebral foramen. Arrow: ZiNeuF catheter

target area with reinsertion of the reinforcing wire; the drug may then be injected the drug after the reinforcing wire is removed. However, the 3F ZiNeuF03 catheter has a separate drug-injection port at its distal end that allows the drug to be injected with the catheter in place. Therefore, the ZiNeuF03 catheter is optimal for the interlaminar approach. However, because the 3F catheter and its guide needle are relatively thick, catheter insertion may be more difficult. Because each operator may have his or her own preference, each operator should try both catheters and choose that with which he or she is more comfortable. The author prefers the 3F ZiNeuF03 catheter for the interlaminar approach.

5.3.2.2 Same Level Interlaminar Ventral Approach

Unlike the previous methods, there is a way to enter the same level of the interlaminar space.

The angle by which entry can be made into the superior aspect of the L5 intervertebral foramen on the opposite side after passing through the same level in the interlaminar space is estimated

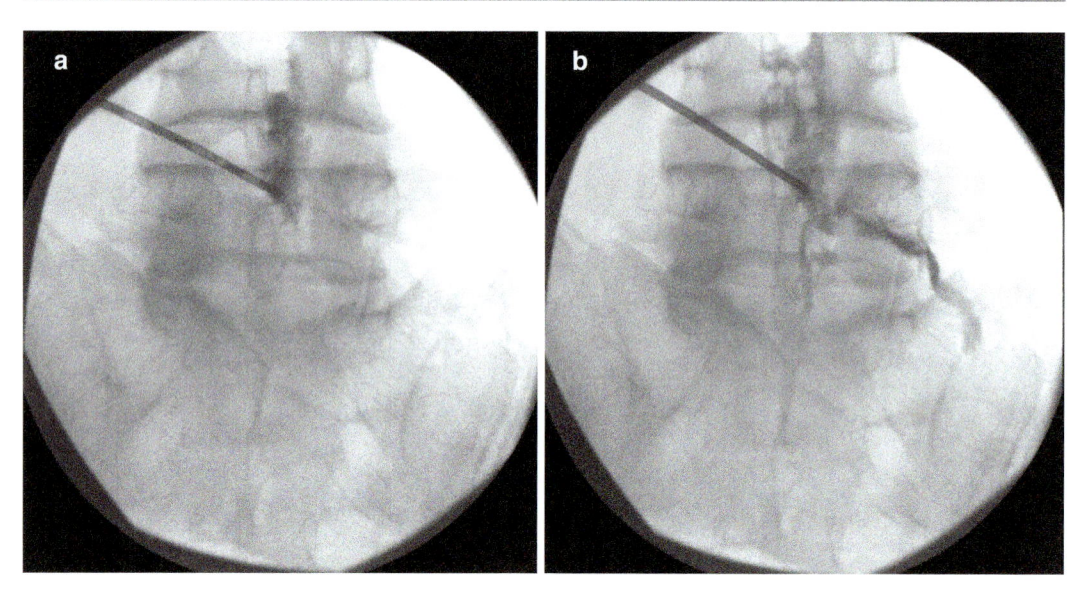

Fig. 5.43 (**a**) When the drug is injected with a needle in the interlaminar approach, the drug does not spread into the intervertebral foramen. Rather, it spreads only into the epidural space near the intervertebral foramen. (**b**) The balloon in the ZiNeuF catheter was overinflated and ruptured. The drug was injected to allow for its spread into the intervertebral foramen

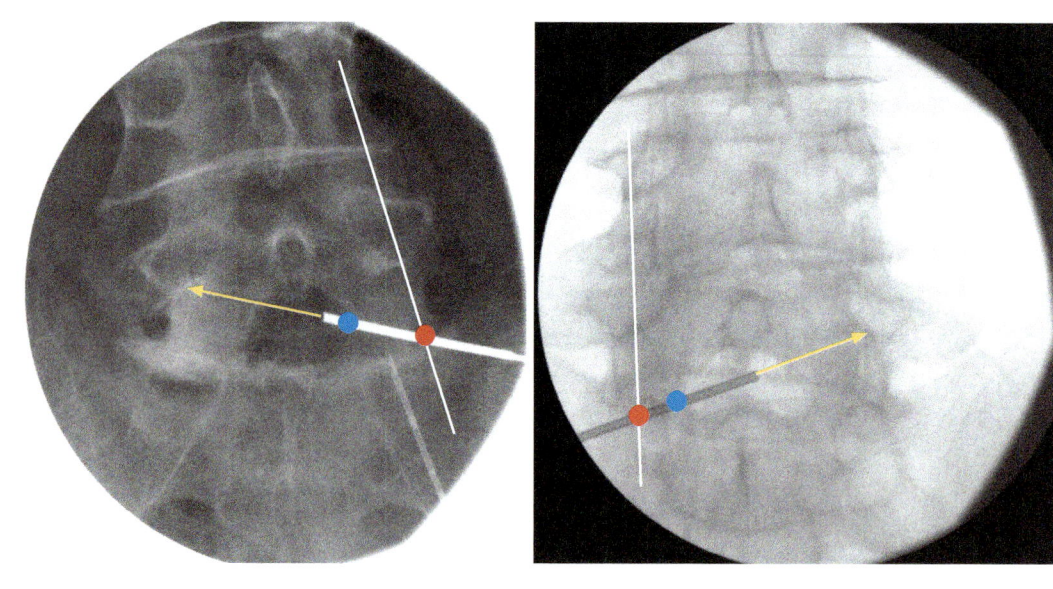

Fig. 5.44 Same level interlaminar ventral approach. The intersection between the angle that allows entry into the superior aspect of the L5 intervertebral foramen on the opposite side after passing through the same level in the interlaminar space and the line connecting the midline of the pedicle is the entry point (red dot). The area where the entry angle reaches the first interlaminar space is the target point (blue dot). When the needle tip reaches the epidural space, it needs to extend slightly beyond the midline

with the guide needle, and the intersection between this angle and the line connecting to the midline of the pedicle is set as the entry point. The area at which the entry angle reaches the first interlaminar space is the target point. The remaining steps are the same as those used for the retrograde interlaminar ventral approach (Fig. 5.44, 5.45 and 5.46).

5.3 Recommended Procedural Methods

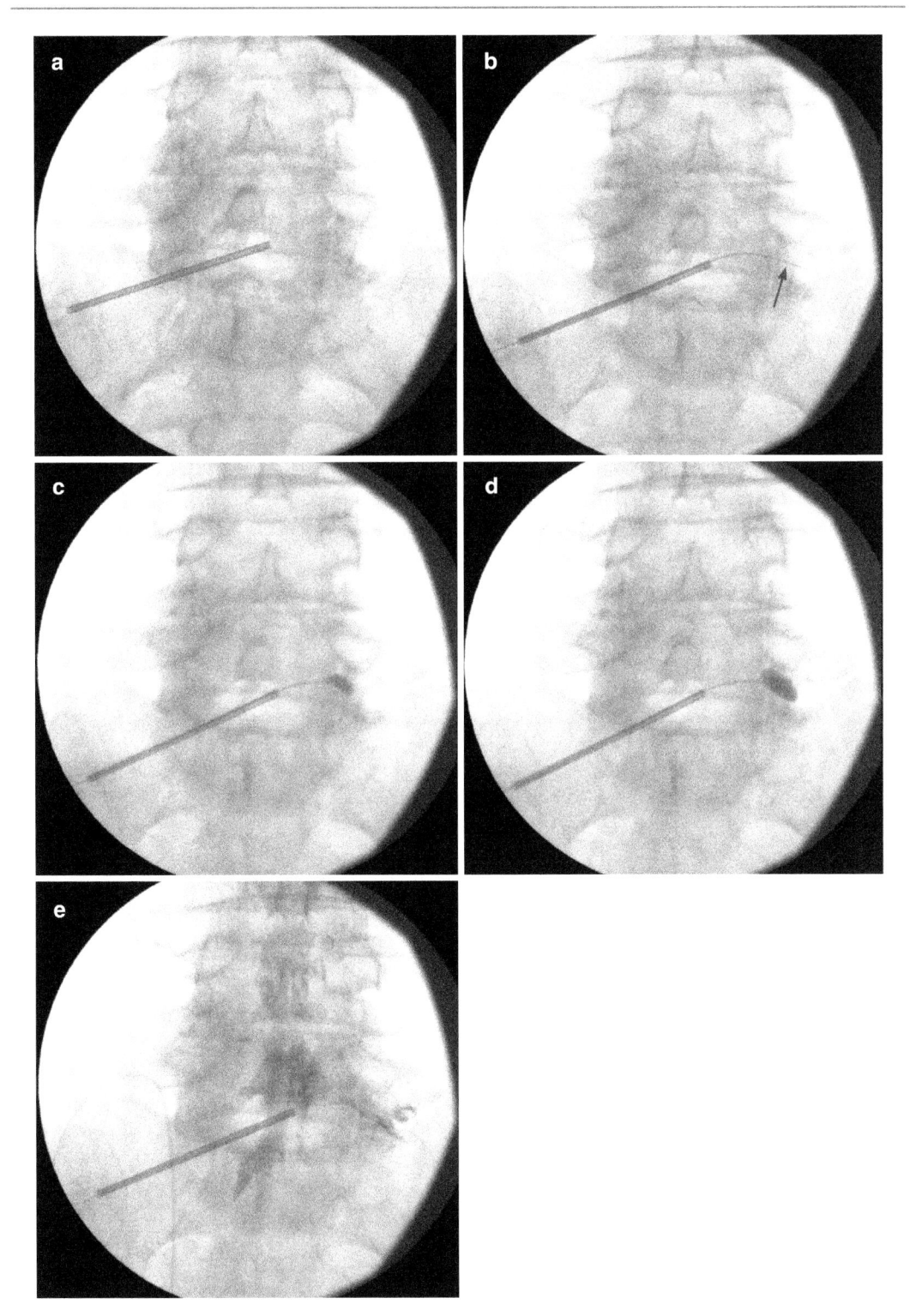

Fig. 5.45 The procedural order of the same level interlaminar ventral approach. (**a**) Insert the needle tip so that it will extend beyond the midline and reach the epidural space. (**b**) Insert the ZiNeuF03 catheter into the extraforaminal area. Arrow: ZiNeuF03 catheter. (**c, d**) Stepwise balloon inflation. (**e**) Inject the contrast dye with the ZiNeuF03 catheter

Choosing the easier one between accessing the L4–5 and L5–S1 interlaminar space in the same level interlaminar ventral approach should be considered. The width of the interlaminar space should also be considered; however, consideration of the site at which the interspinous gap is wider is more important. Choosing the site with a wider interspinous gap helps to prevent snagging when the needle is moved over to the opposite side (Fig. 5.47).

For the most part, the same level interlaminar ventral approach with the L5–S1 interlaminar approach is easier than the retrograde interlaminar ventral approach; however, while the former procedure may be easier, it cannot be performed on the preganglion area in many cases. As balloon decompression at all areas along the nerve path, including the preganglion, foraminal, and extraforaminal areas is recommended, the retrograde interlaminar ventral approach should be considered first. If this method is difficult, then the same level interlaminar ventral approach should be attempted (Fig. 5.48).

Case The patient had undergone a laminectomy 8 years prior. Bilateral L5 foraminal stenosis and adhesion at the surgical site prevented the ZiNeuS catheter's entry into the left and right intervertebral foramen through the caudal approach. Because of the history of laminectomy at the L5–S1 level, the interlaminar space in this area was wider; by contrast, the L4–5 interlaminar space

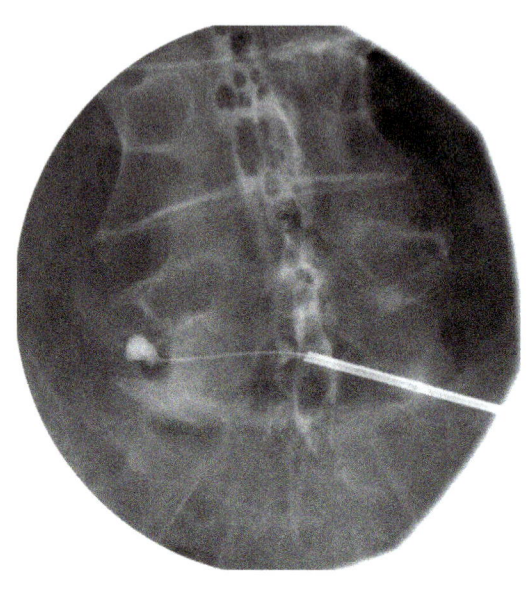

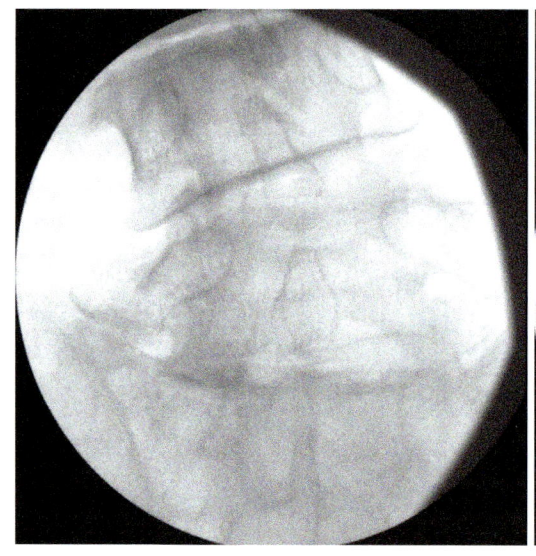

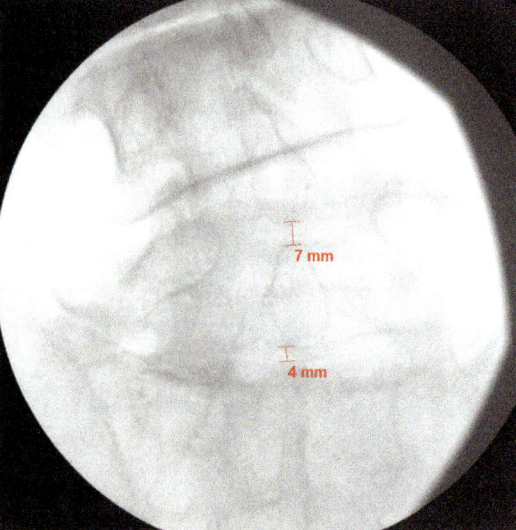

Fig. 5.46 Same level interlaminar ventral approach. The balloon is inflated after the ZiNeuF03 catheter has been inserted. Arrow: Filling defect is visible in the area of the balloon where the air has not been completely expelled

Fig. 5.47 Example of approaching the Lt. L5 intervertebral foramen. The L5–S1 interlaminar space is wider than the L4–5 interlaminar space, but the L5–S1 interspinous gap is narrower. Therefore, the retrograde interlaminar ventral approach in the L4–5 interlaminar space is easier for this case

5.3 Recommended Procedural Methods

was narrow. Accordingly, to enhance the convenience of performing the procedure, the same level interlaminar ventral approach was used to insert the ZiNeuF catheter into both sides and perform balloon decompression (Fig. 5.49).

The patient showed improvement in symptoms up to approximately 4 months after the procedure, but the procedure was subsequently repeated due to recurrence. Currently, the patient is in the 7th month of follow-up.

5.3.3 Cervical Interlaminar Approach

Balloon decompression in the cervical area requires special attention since it features a narrower epidural space and smaller intervertebral foramen than does the lumbar area. However, as long as the pain felt by the patient is monitored

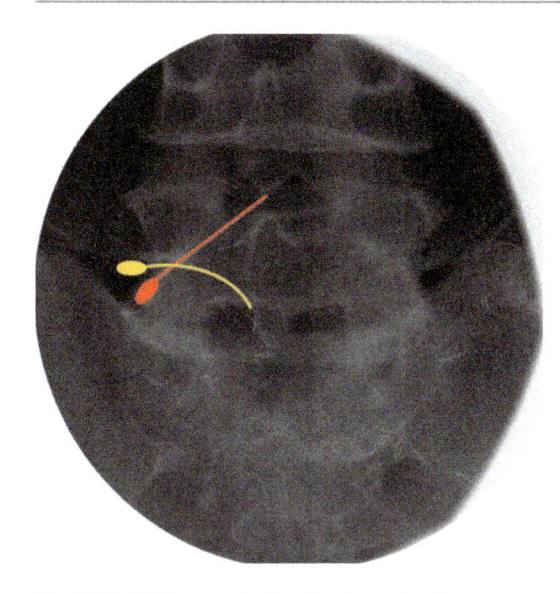

Fig. 5.48 Differences in the direction of catheter movement according to different interlaminar ventral approaches. Red catheter: Retrograde interlaminar ventral approach. Yellow catheter: Same level interlaminar ventral approach

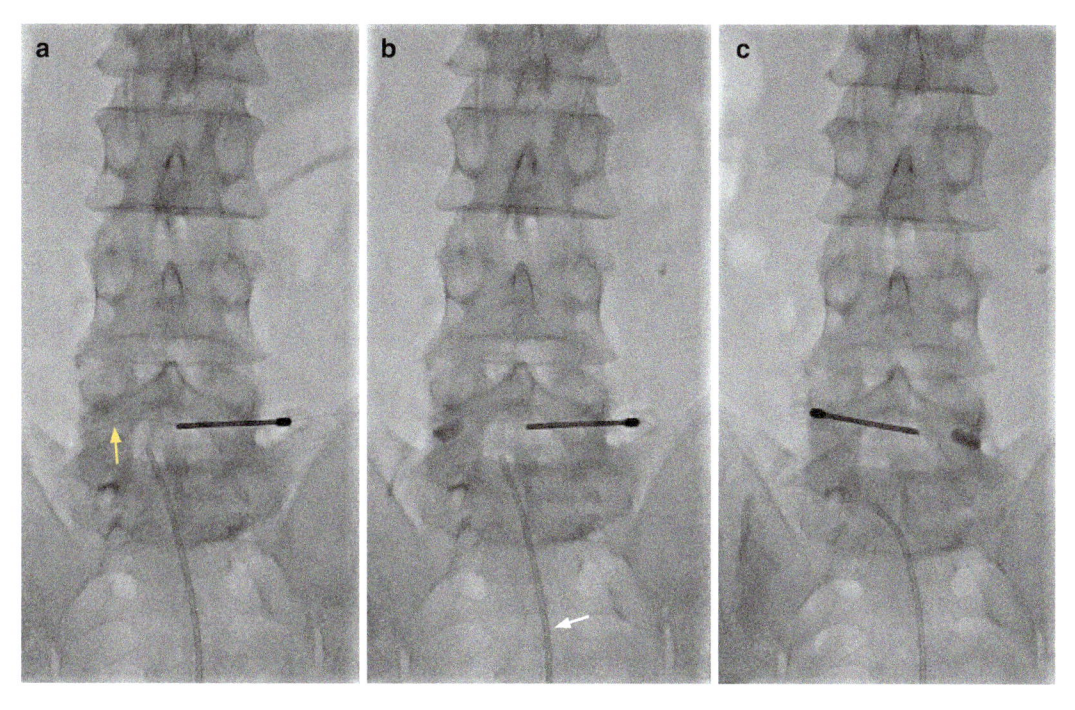

Fig. 5.49 (**a**, **b**) The performance of balloon decompression with the insertion of the guide needle into the same level interlaminar space, and the insertion of the ZiNeuF catheter into the Lt. L5 intervertebral foramen. (**c**) The performance of balloon decompression with the reinsertion of the guide needle in the opposite direction, and the insertion of the ZiNeuF catheter inserted into the Rt. L5 intervertebral foramen. Yellow arrow: ZiNeuF catheter. White arrow: ZiNeuS catheter

during balloon inflation, the procedure is no more dangerous than neuroplasty with the Racz catheter, which is commonly performed in the cervical area. The procedural methods are similar to those that employ the Racz catheter.

5.3.3.1 Procedural Methods

With the patient lying in a prone position on the operating table, a slightly elevated pillow should be placed in such a manner so as to support the chest of the patient and thereby create greater flexion in the cervical area. The endplate of cervical spine is aligned in the AP view with slight cephalad tilting of the C-arm. The entry point is set at the paramedian area at one or two levels below the interlaminar space, where the entry will be made (Fig. 5.50a), and the guide needle is inserted in the superomedial direction. From a three-dimensional perspective, the needle tip is inserted at an angle that allows it to be positioned on the midline when it reaches the epidural space (Fig. 5.50b). After switching the C-arm view to the contralateral oblique view by approximately 40–50°, the angle of the needle is adjusted under the C-arm view while the needle is inserted between the laminae in the target area (Fig. 5.50c).

The guide needle is inserted until its tip passes through the laminae and reaches the ligament flavum. The loss of resistance technique is unnecessary before the guide needle reaches the ligament flavum, and only the depth requires confirmation with the C-arm view (Fig. 5.50d). Whether the

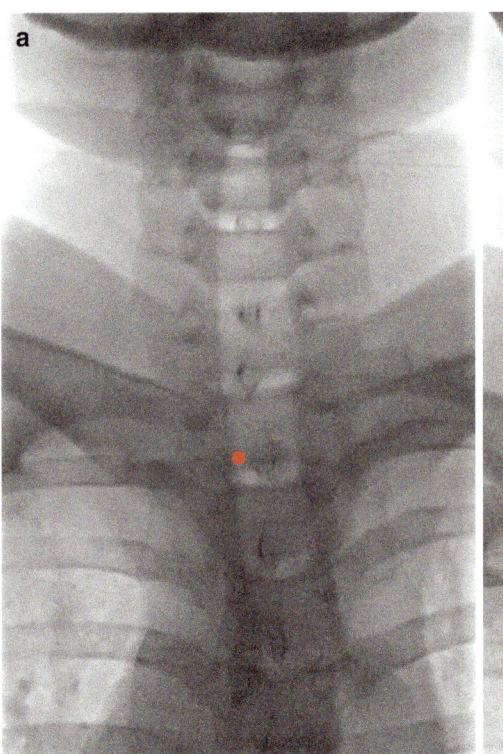

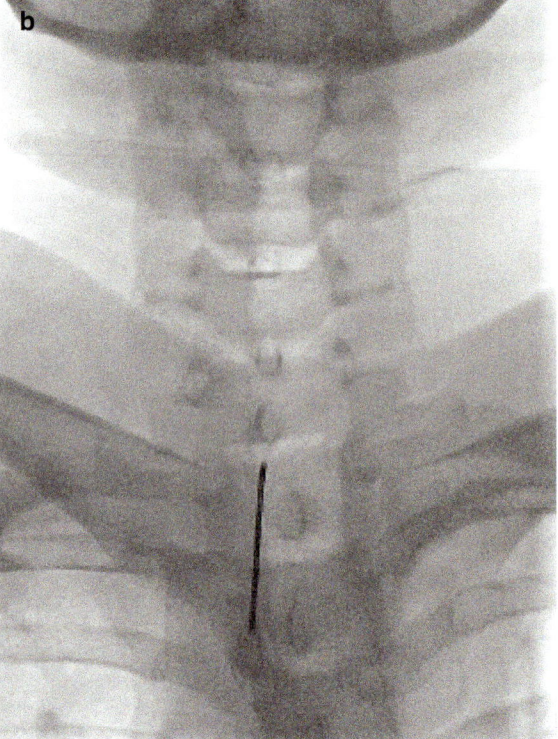

Fig. 5.50 The procedural order of cervical interlaminar approach. (**a**) The entry point is set to the paramedian area at one or two levels below the interlaminar space where the entry will be made. Red dot: Entry point. (**b**) The guide needle is inserted in a superomedial direction. (**c**) While referencing the 40–50° contralateral oblique view, the guide needle is adjusted to orient toward the area between the laminae in the target area. White arrow: Ligament flavum. (**d**) The guide needle is inserted at the point preceding the ligament flavum. (**e**) The positioning of the needle tip on the midline is checked in the AP view. (**f**) Finding the epidural space using the loss of resistance technique under the contralateral oblique view. (**g, h**) The ZiNeuF catheter is inserted up to the target area. Yellow arrow: ZiNeuF catheter. (**i, j**) The inflated balloon is gradually pulled down. Yellow circle: Inflated balloon

5.3 Recommended Procedural Methods 137

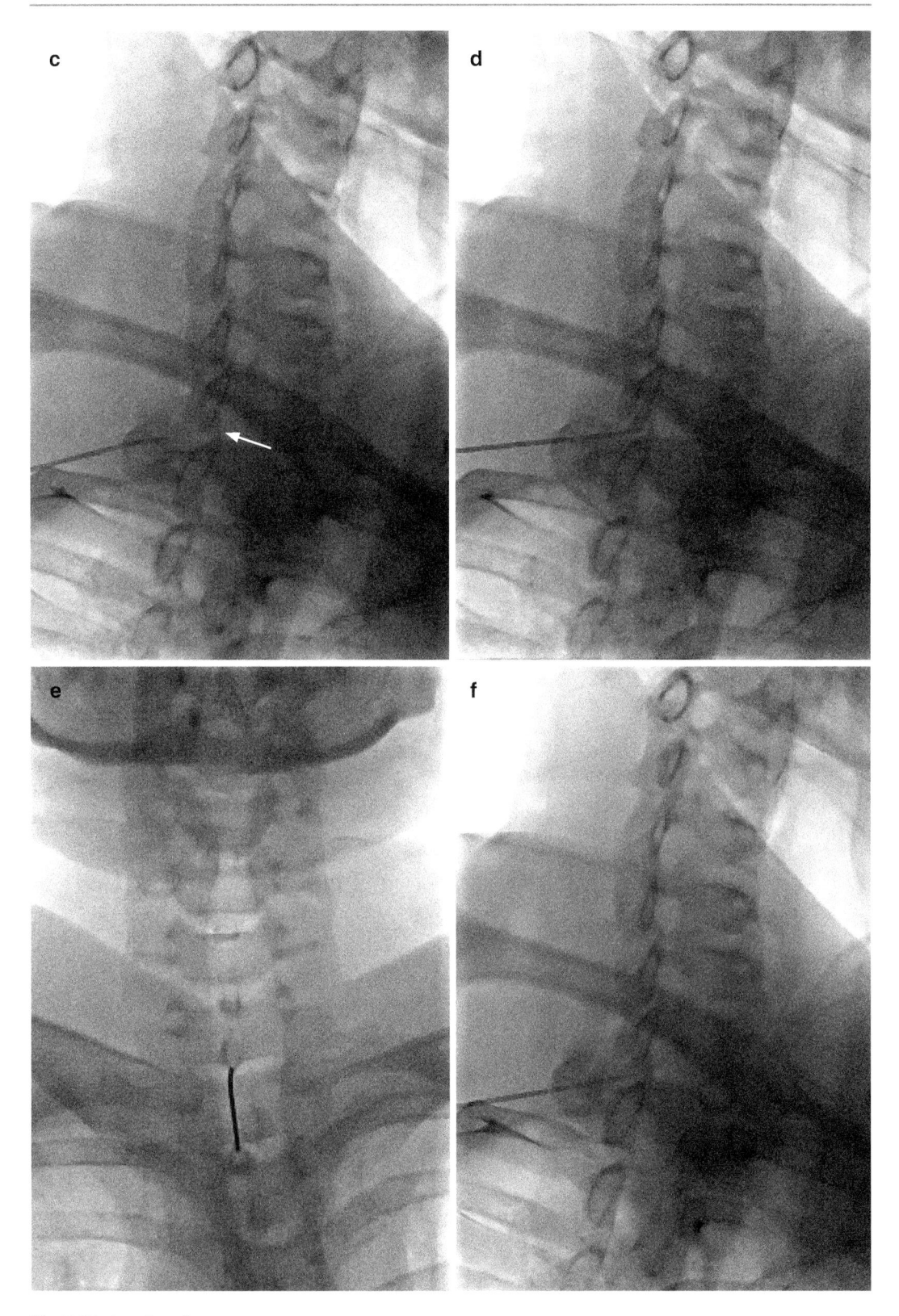

Fig. 5.50 (continued)

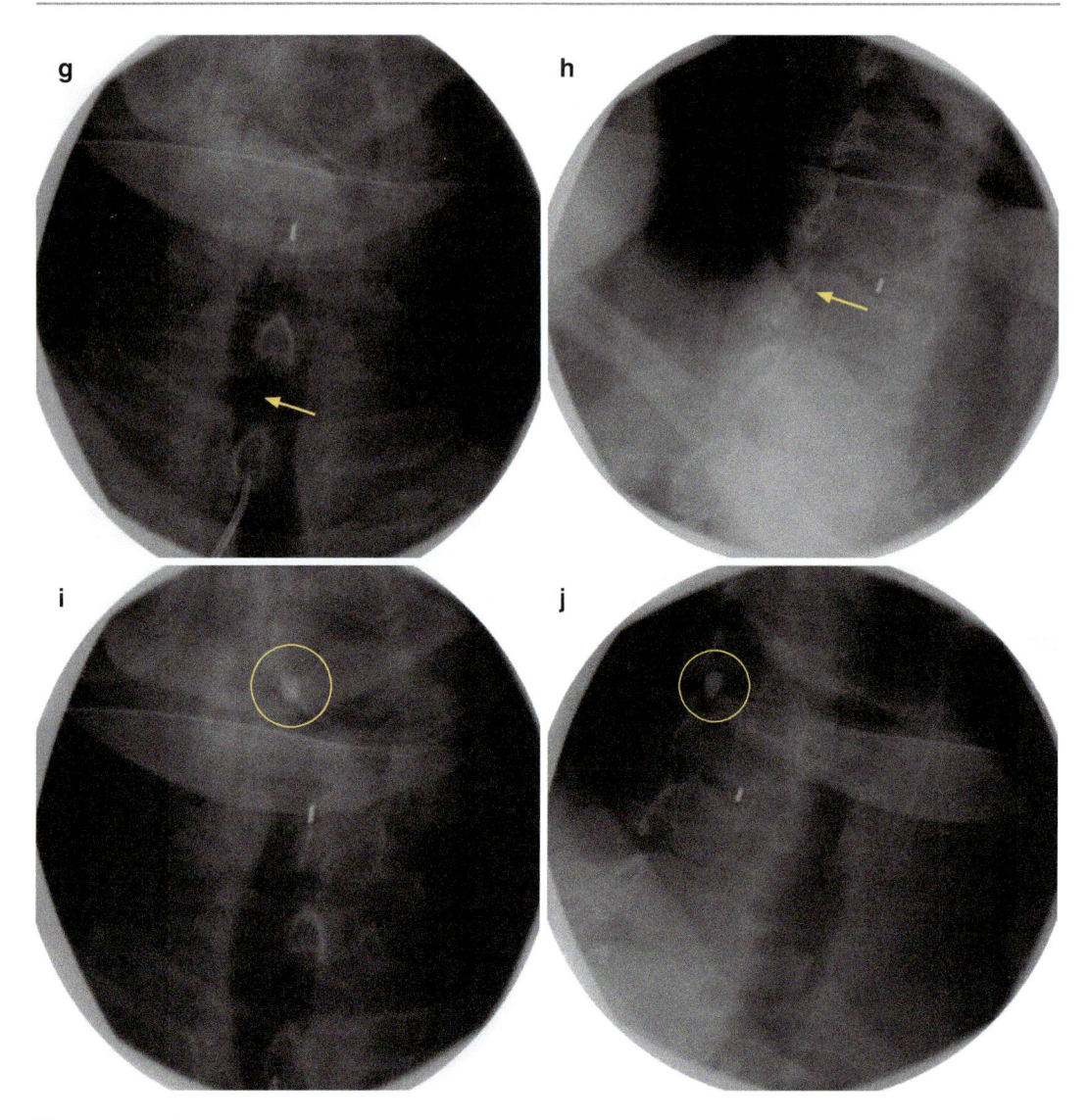

Fig. 5.50 (continued)

needle tip is positioned on the midline is checked again in the AP view (Fig. 5.50e). If the guide needle is positioned on the midline, the view is switched back to the contralateral oblique view. Under this state, the stylet is removed, and the needle is inserted to find the epidural space at a depth of 1–2 cm using the loss of resistance technique. Because the 40–50° contralateral oblique view is being used, the depth of the needle tip when the needle is placed in the epidural space will slightly pass the boundary of the ligament flavum (Fig. 5.50f).

To confirm whether the needle tip is positioned inside the epidural space, 1–2 cc of contrast dye is injected. If the tip is positioned inside the epidural space, the ZiNeuF catheter with a slightly bent tip for directional control is inserted. The catheter should be inserted as carefully as possible to prevent pain induced by dural irritation when the catheter is being inserted into the epidural space.

If the guide needle is positioned on the midline, the catheter may be advanced toward the head by following the midline of the posterior

5.3 Recommended Procedural Methods

epidural space. By gradually rotating the catheter itself to aim the catheter tip toward the target area and pushing slowly toward the head area, the catheter can approach the target area (Fig. 5.50g, h). Once the target area has been reached, the balloon should be inflated until the patient feels severe pain (within 0.1 cc of contrast dye), and the inflated balloon is carefully pulled down to reach the lower level and remove adhesion. If necessary, balloon decompression could be performed once more by reinserting it into the target area without the reinforcing wire (Fig. 5.50i, j).

When the guide needle reaches the epidural space, it may slip out to the intervertebral foramen or anterior epidural space on one side if the needle tip is not positioned on the midline. This may complicate ascendance to the upper level. Hence, if the operative plan requires upward movement, the needle tip must be positioned on the midline. However, if the goal is to enter the intervertebral foramen situated one or two levels above, then the needle tip could be tilted toward the affected area to allow it to reach the epidural space.

Balloon decompression in the cervical epidural space could be expected to provide alleviation of stenosis and adhesion in the posterior epidural space and area near spinal nerves. The injection of drugs after balloon decompression at the area near spinal nerves could spread into the anterior epidural space. All areas approachable by the Racz procedure could be approached with the ZiNeuF catheter. However, the method lacks the support of safety-related evidence; hence, more research may be required before adopting this attempt should be considered.

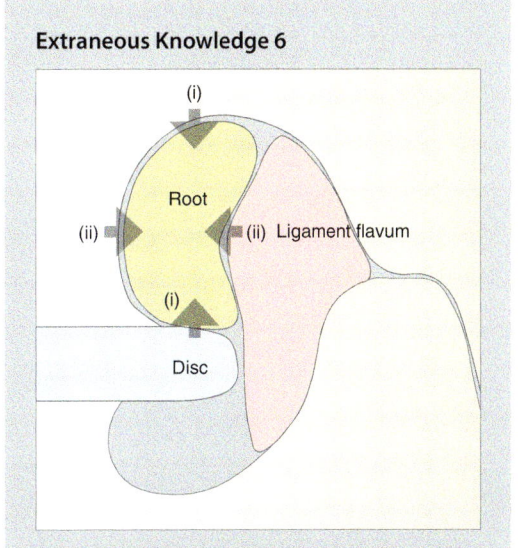

Extraneous Knowledge 6

Fig. E1 Mechanism of Foraminal Stenosis. (i) Stenosis caused by bony spurs or degenerative disc. (ii) Stenosis caused by hypertrophic ligament flavum or facet joint osteoarthritis. Stenosis could occur in two directions shown above

Methods for Executing the ZiNeuF03 Catheter Procedure

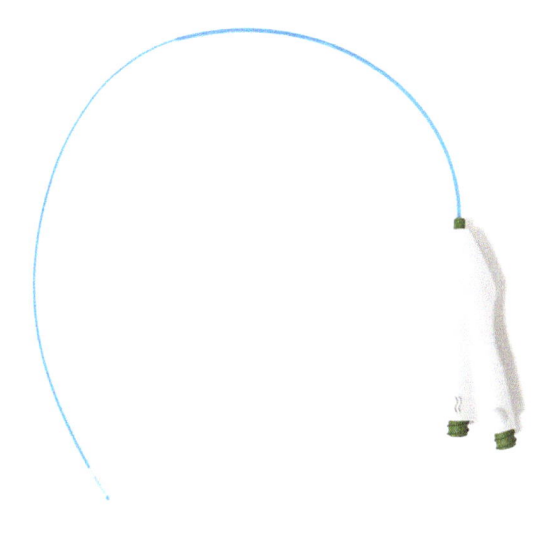

ZiNeuF03 catheter

6.1 Target Diseases

- Low back and leg pain caused by spinal stenosis
- Low back and leg pain caused by chronic disc herniation
- Low back and leg pain caused by epidural adhesion
- Post-spinal surgery pain syndrome

Electronic Supplementary Material The online version of this chapter (https://doi.org/10.1007/978-981-15-7265-4_6) contains supplementary material, which is available to authorized users.

6.1.1 Best Indications

Patients for whom conventional nerve block or neuroplasty achieved a short-lived therapeutic improvement.

Patients seeking the mitigation of their spinal stenosis-induced claudication.

: Among these patients, these indications apply to those in whom the lesion is localized to levels one or two.

While ZiNeuF03 features inferior lateral mobility and strength relative to the ZiNeu catheter, it is less expensive.

Since the catheter itself can be left in place for 2–3 days, it is useful for patients who require neuroplasty with hypertonic saline and balloon decompression together across several days.

Because it does not feature a lateral movement function, the use of this catheter is more appropriate for patients with lesions localized to levels one or two—especially lesions in the spinal canal—than for those with lesions in the intervertebral foramen. As will be explained later, it is also useful when employing the interlaminar approach.

6.2 Pre-Procedural Preparation

If the operative plan has scheduled the removal of the catheter and the patient's discharge on the same day as the procedure, prophylactic antibi-

© Springer Nature Singapore Pte Ltd. 2021
J. W. Shin, *Spinal Epidural Balloon Decompression and Adhesiolysis*,
https://doi.org/10.1007/978-981-15-7265-4_6

otic administration is unnecessary. However, if the operative plan mandates the continued administration of the drug by leaving the ZiNeuF03 catheter in place for 2–3 days, antibiotics should be intravenously administered before and after the procedure according to the methods prescribed for neuroplasty followed by treatment with anti-inflammatory analgesics and antibiotics for 3 days after the procedure; in the same manner as operations performed with the ZiNeu series, the patient is required to lay down such that his or her abdomen rests on top of the pillow and disinfection is conducted.

6.3 Recommended Procedural Methods

6.3.1 Insertion of the Guide Needle

Just as in procedures performed using the ZiNeu series catheters, two lines (one that connects the central area of the spine and another that connects the central point of the sacral hiatus) are drawn on the patient. A point slightly below the intersection between the two lines—i.e., the point at which the needle can be inserted parallel to the caudal epidural space in the lateral view—is set as the entry point (Fig. 6.1).

The guide needle should be inserted into the sacral hiatus in the lateral view, with the needle parallel to the caudal epidural space. The needle should be advanced along the midline drawn above the sacral hiatus of the patient to allow for the needle's placement on the spinal midline. After passing through the sacral hiatus, the needle is advanced 3–4 cm farther, and the stylet is removed.

When using the sheath-type needle, the sheath is advanced a slightly farther after stylet's removal. The excessive advancement of the sheath could compromise control of the catheter's direction. Hence, it should be advanced 3–4 cm past the sacral hiatus).

When inserting the guide needle, the C-arm images should be carefully monitored to control the direction or depth of the needle and ensure that bleeding does not occur when the needle tip injures the sacral bone. The direction of the guide needle bevel should be oriented such that it clearly enters the anterior epidural space as seen from the lateral view. The bevel should be directed toward the front of the patient to access the anterior epidural space (Fig. 6.2). Further details are provided in the subsection on guide needle insertion under the section on ZiNeu series procedural methods.

6.3.2 Epidurogram and Regional Anesthesia

Although an epidurogram is primarily performed to inform diagnosis along with the patient's symptoms, MRI findings, and response to nerve block, it can be administered prior to the procedure to

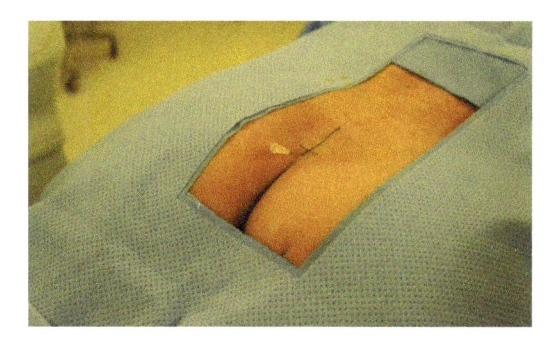

Fig. 6.1 The entry point is situated slightly below the intersection between the line connecting the central area of the spine and the line connecting the left and right cornu. The exact location is determined in the C-arm lateral view

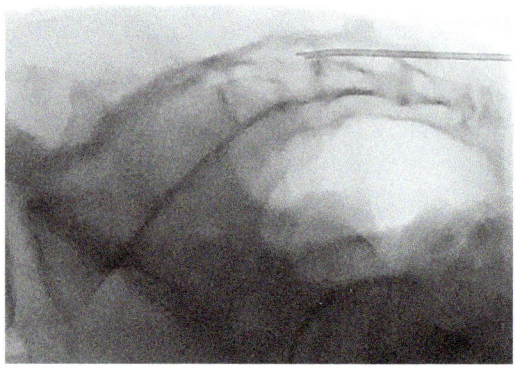

Fig. 6.2 Lateral view of the insertion of the guide needle into the epidural space

6.3 Recommended Procedural Methods

determine the site of operation. As with the procedures that use the ZiNeu series catheters, a mixture of contrast dye and 1% Lidocaine can be used for epidural anesthesia. This helps to achieve adequate pain reduction during the procedure and to prevent motor or sensory nerve paralysis, both of which are of clear utility to the patient and operator.

Prior to administering the local anesthetic mixture, it is paramount to check for abnormalities with 100% contrast dye. The procedure using the ZiNeuF03 catheter should have less pain that the procedures using the ZiNeu series catheters, and thus, the need for regional anesthesia is relatively lower.

6.3.3 Insertion of the ZiNeuF03 Catheter

When the catheter is inserted while its tip area slightly bent (Fig. 6.3a), there is a tendency to move toward the direction of the bend. When the bent tip is rotated to reduce the angle of bending or to make the tip area appear straight, the direction could be changed by an equivalent amount (Fig. 6.3b, c). In response to this tendency, if the syringe attachment port (catheter hub) is held and rotated gradually—in the same manner by which a steering while is turned—under C-arm view, the desired direction can be found, and the catheter can reach the target area (Fig. 6.4).

When rotating the catheter and changing its direction, it is important to use real-time C-arm view to find the moment when the orientation of the bent tip is similar to the direction intended by the operator. Once the operator becomes familiar with this directional control technique, the catheter can easily reach the desired area, as long as there is no severe adhesion or stenosis.

Because lesions are usually found in the retrodiscal area of the anterior epidural space, the catheter should be inserted into the anterior

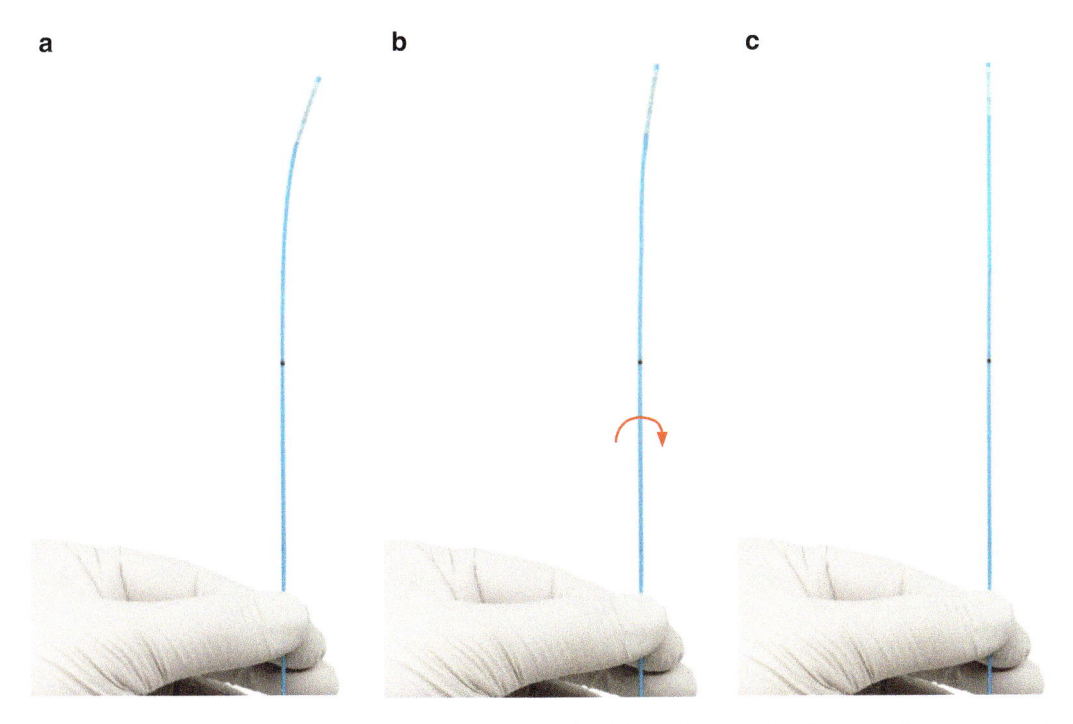

Fig. 6.3 (**a**) The catheter is bent to the right. (**b**) The catheter in **a** is rotated by 45°. (**c**) The catheter in **a** is rotated by 90°. Rotating the catheter from **a** to **c** decreases the angle of bending, while rotation by 90° makes the catheter appear as a straight line. (**a**, **b**) The catheter veers toward the right inside the epidural space to the same extent that the catheter tip is bent to the right. (**c**) The catheter tip does not sway to the left or right but advances in a straight line inside the epidural space

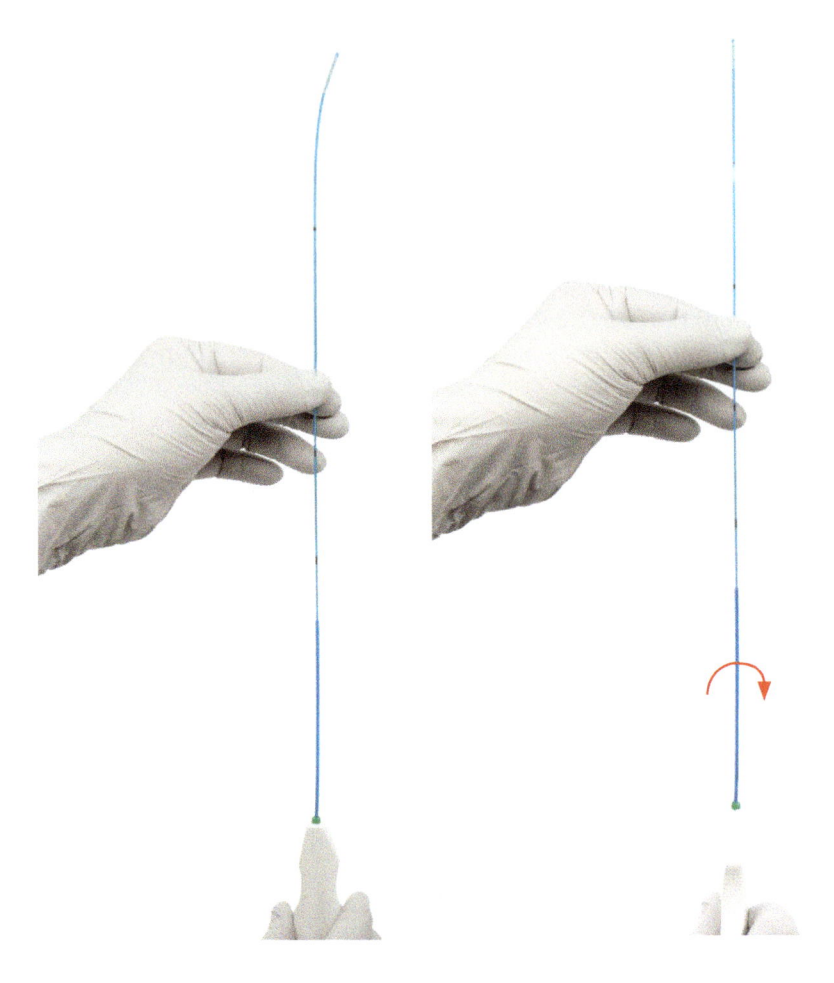

Fig. 6.4 Rotating the ZiNeuF03 catheter while holding its hub changes its angle of entry

epidural space when possible; hence, entry is initially made with the catheter bent toward the anterior of the patient (refer to Chap. 4 for details). However, unlike the ZiNeu series catheters, this catheter does not allow for lateral control; the catheter may therefore not allow entry into anterior epidural space. If the catheter must be placed inside the anterior epidural space, it is advisable to use the ZiNeu series catheters.

As explained earlier, entry into the intervertebral foramen should be completed by controlling the direction of the tip's bending when approaching the affected intervertebral foramen. If it is determined that entry cannot be made due to insufficient bending at the foraminal orifice, the reinforcing wire within the catheter must be removed and further bent before being reinserted into the catheter for another attempt at entry.

(Note that excessive bending could render reinsertion into the catheter difficult or damage the catheter as it is inserted.) In young patients with mild stenosis, entry into the intervertebral foramen should not be difficult. However, in patients with severe lesions or history of spinal surgery, it may be difficult to reach the affected area due to the catheter's thinness and lack of lateral control. In such cases, the use of the ZiNeu series catheters is advised. The most suitable equipment should be informed by the patient's medical history and MRI findings.

6.3.4 Balloon Decompression

Upon reaching the affected area, the reinforcing wire inside the catheter is removed, and a 5–10 cc

6.3 Recommended Procedural Methods

syringe half-filled with the contrast dye is connected to the catheter. The plunger is then forcefully pulled to remove the air. The plunger must be pulled and released with the syringe erect to ensure that the contrast dye inside the syringe flows into the catheter once the air is expelled. The syringe is subsequently removed, and a 1 cc Luer lock syringe filled with 0.1 cc of contrast dye is connected to the catheter (Fig. 6.5).

When the plunger is pulled to eliminate air, it is imperative to apply strong negative pressure; the air may not be completely expelled otherwise, causing air to remain inside the balloon when it is inflated with contrast dye. The retention of air inside the balloon could compromise the identification of the extent of balloon inflation in C-arm images and, in severe cases, could make the balloon appear ruptured. It is therefore important to apply strong negative pressure when expelling air (Fig. 6.6).

The following images depict balloon inflation with the ZiNeuF03 catheter (Figs. 6.7 and 6.8) (Video 6.1).

The level of pain felt by the patient should be monitored as 0.1 cc of contrast dye is gradually injected. If the pain is severe, the injection should

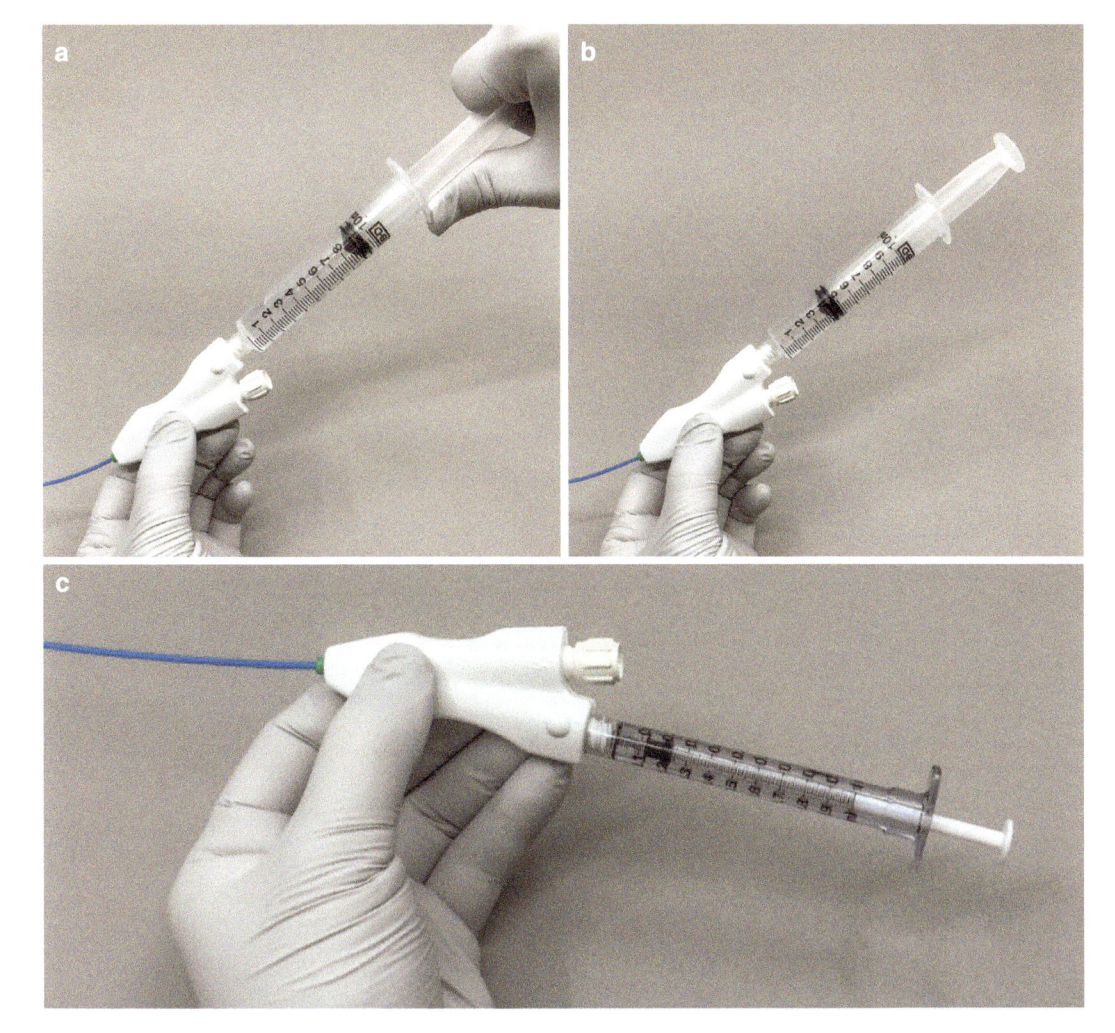

Fig. 6.5 (**a**) After connecting a 10 cc syringe filled with 3–4 cc of contrast dye to the balloon port, forcefully pulling the plunger expels any air remaining in the catheter. (**b**) The catheter fills with the contrast dye once the plunger is released. (**c**) The 1 cc Luer lock syringe filled with 0.1 cc of contrast dye is connected to the balloon port

Fig. 6.6 (**a**) Inflated balloon contains air that had remained in the catheter. (**b**) An inflated balloon without air

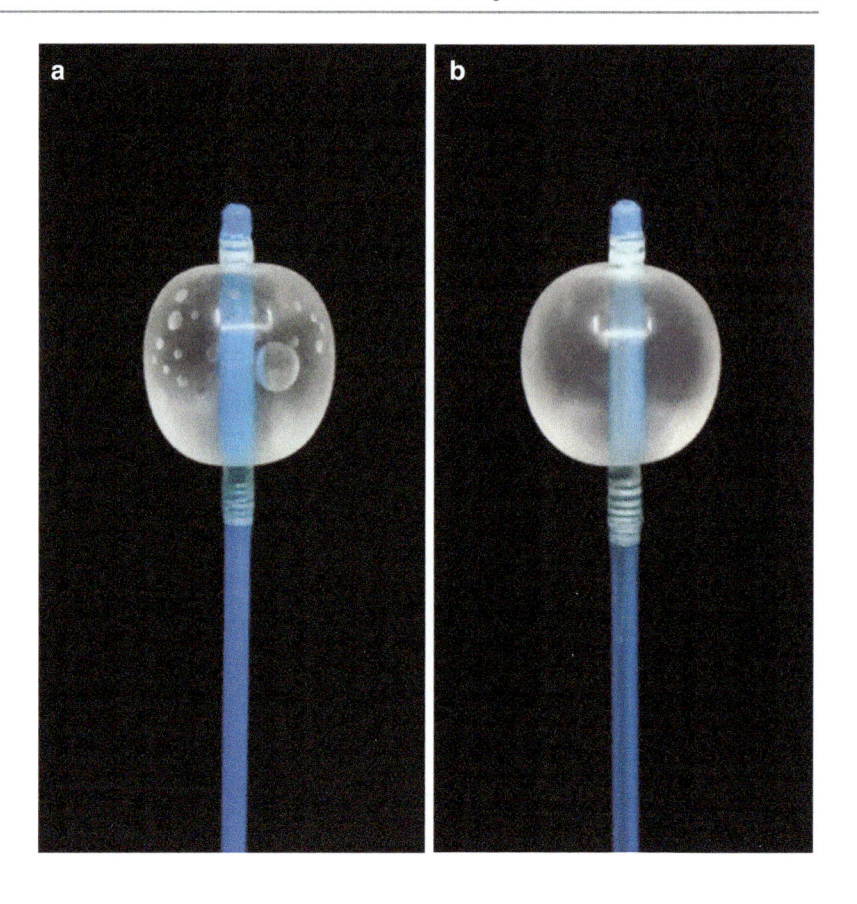

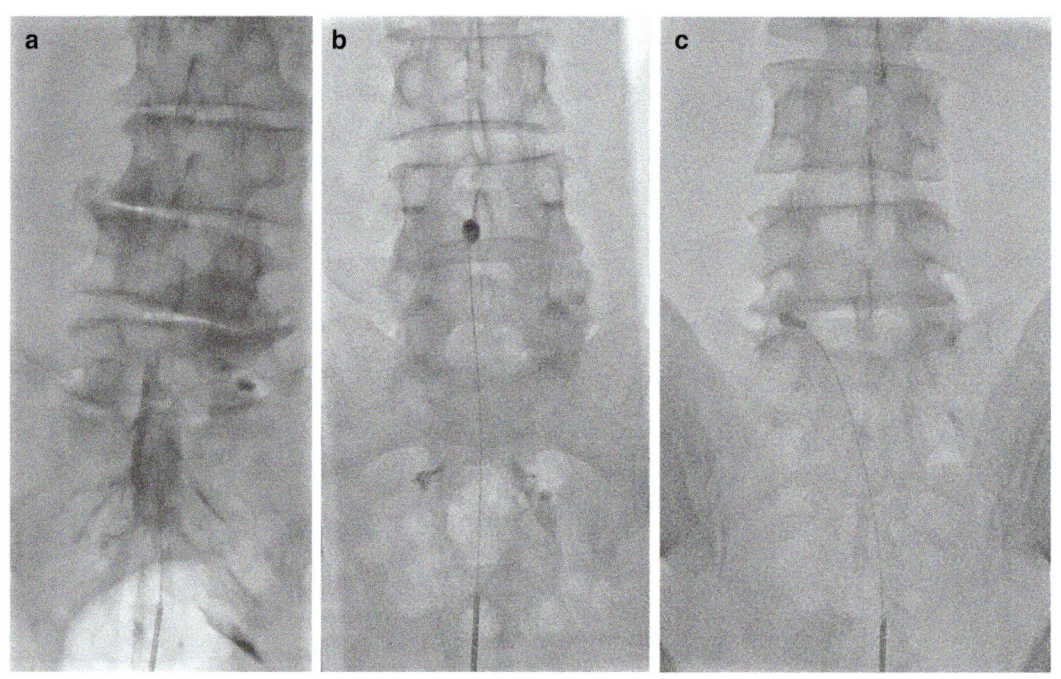

Fig. 6.7 (**a**) Inflation of the balloon in the right intervertebral foramen. (**b**) Inflation of the balloon in the L4–5 retrodiscal area. (**c**) Inflation of the balloon in the left L5–S1 retrodiscal area

6.3 Recommended Procedural Methods

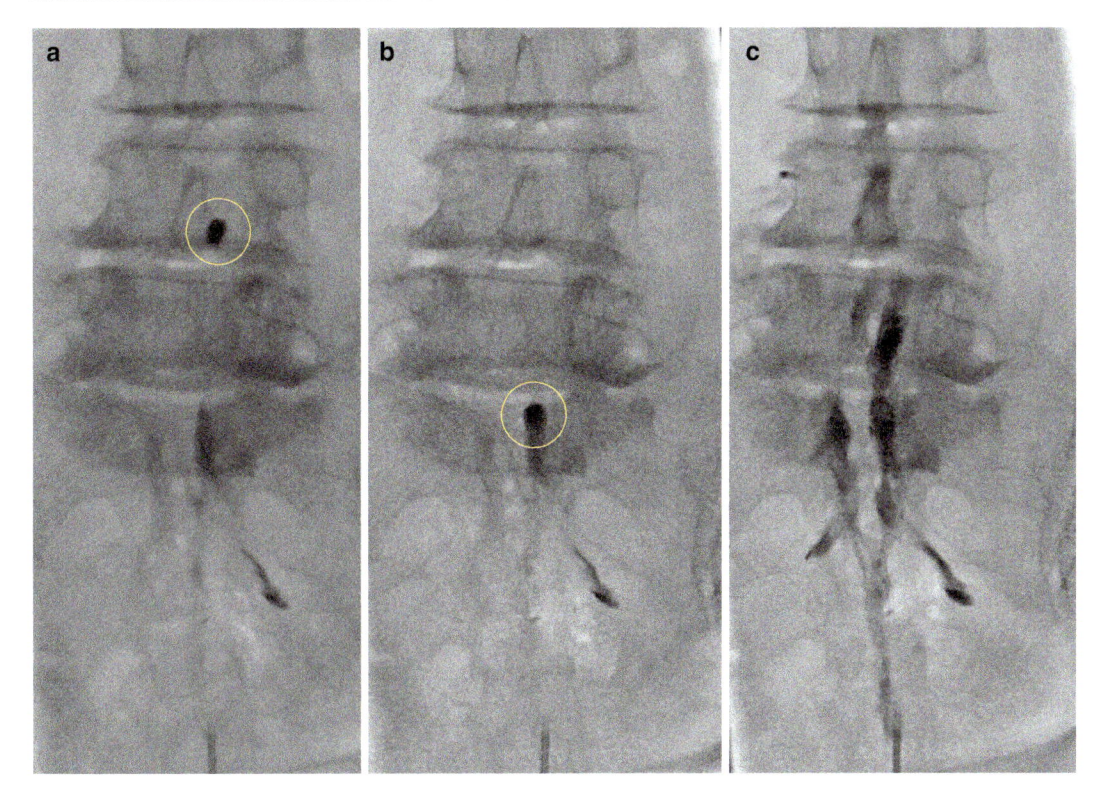

Fig. 6.8 (**a**) Inflation of the balloon at a site just above the L4–5 retrodiscal area. (**b**) Image of the inflated balloon being pulled down from the site shown in **a**. (**c**) Contrast images showing the spread of the dye into the area through which the inflated balloon had been pulled down. Circle: Inflated balloon

be terminated—even if all 0.1 cc had not been injected—and the balloon should be deflated after 2–3 s. Balloon inflation in a single spot should last no more than 5 s. After balloon inflation is completed in one area, the balloon is inflated according to the same method in other affected areas and their vicinities as the catheter is slowly withdrawn.

For procedures involving the intervertebral foramen, the author recommends that the balloon should be moved only when it is deflated; withdrawing an inflated balloon could induce pulling of the spinal nerves. However, when the procedure is performed in the central area, there is almost no risk of nerves being pulled. Therefore, pulling the balloon in an inflated state is acceptable when the operator attempts to complete the procedure across a wider area in less time. At this point, caution should be taken to ensure that the catheter is moved very slowly, and the procedure must not be performed in this manner if the patient feels any pain. If the patient feels pain when this method is employed, then the procedure must be performed by moving the catheter slowly while repeatedly inflating and deflating the balloon: for reemphasis, the balloon should never be quickly withdrawn when inflated (Fig. 6.8).

6.3.5 Contrast Dye Injection

Upon completion of balloon decompression, 100% contrast dye must be injected to check whether the contrast dye spread efficiently into the procedural site, whether dural puncture occurred during the procedure, and whether the drug is leaking into the blood vessels.

6.3.6 Irrigation

If the procedure yielded unsatisfactory results or the contrast images still indicate adhesion, irrigation with normal saline could be performed. Adequate saline irrigation in the areas with adhesion or stenosis could significantly help to improve symptoms. While there are some claims that more irrigation is more beneficial, the amount of irrigation performed should be determined in consideration of the patient's safety and other factors. Since using balloon decompression could yield good results with less irrigation volume, there is no need to be excessively aggressive when conducting irrigation.

6.3.7 Therapeutic Drug Injection

After irrigation with normal saline and waiting for 2–3 min to reduce the possibility of dilution, a local anesthetic/steroid mixture is injected (2–4 cc per site). If necessary, the site of operation can be moved to allow for the performance of the procedure according to the same method as that adopted to treat other affected areas.

6.3.8 Removal of the Needle or Sheath

If the resistance is felt at the guide needle tip when the catheter is removed, the needle and catheter should be adjusted slightly before the removal of the catheter is reattempted. If that still does not work, then they are removed together. If possible, it is better to remove the guide needle and catheter together. This almost never happens when a sheath is used. If the treatment plan involves leaving the ZiNeuF03 catheter in place for 2–3 days, then a tearable sheath must be used. Upon completion of the procedure, the sheath is removed by pulling it laterally to tear it; only the catheter, which is secured to the skin, is left in place (Fig. 6.9).

6.3.9 Drug Administration After Admission

If balloon decompression did not yield satisfactory results or the patient's symptoms include neuropathic pain, the administration of hypertonic saline for 1–2 days is advised. Some may receive inpatient treatment, while others may receive drug administration on the following day during their outpatient visits.

The method of administration first prescribes the injection of 4 cc of 1% Lidocaine, waiting 2–3 min, and then slowly injecting 3 cc of 5% hypertonic saline solution; the drug is to be administered up to three times a day at intervals of 1–3 h. On the following day, the drug is administered again up to three times.

In patients who do not have diabetes, 5 mg of dexamethasone can be administered at once during or after the procedure. Alternatively, it can be mixed with hypertonic saline solution and administered portion-wise. The total amount should not exceed 5 mg.

If the catheter has been accurately placed in the affected area, balloon decompression can be performed two to three additional times per day. The drug could be administered while the balloon is inflated when necessary.

6.3 Recommended Procedural Methods

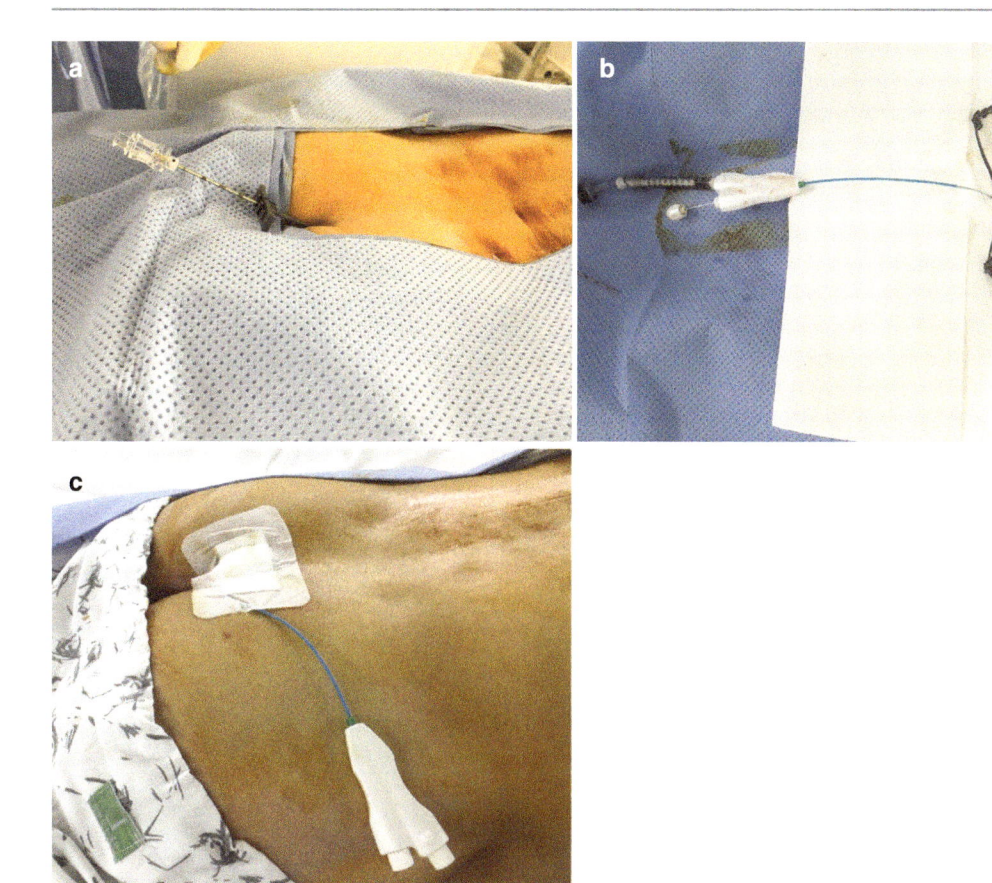

Fig. 6.9 (**a**) After inserting the guide needle containing the sheath into the caudal epidural space, only the sheath is pushed farther inside. (**b**) To leave the catheter in place for 2–3 days after the procedure, the sheath is removed by pulling it laterally to tear it. (**c**) After removing the sheath, the catheter is secured to the skin

Extraneous Knowledge 7

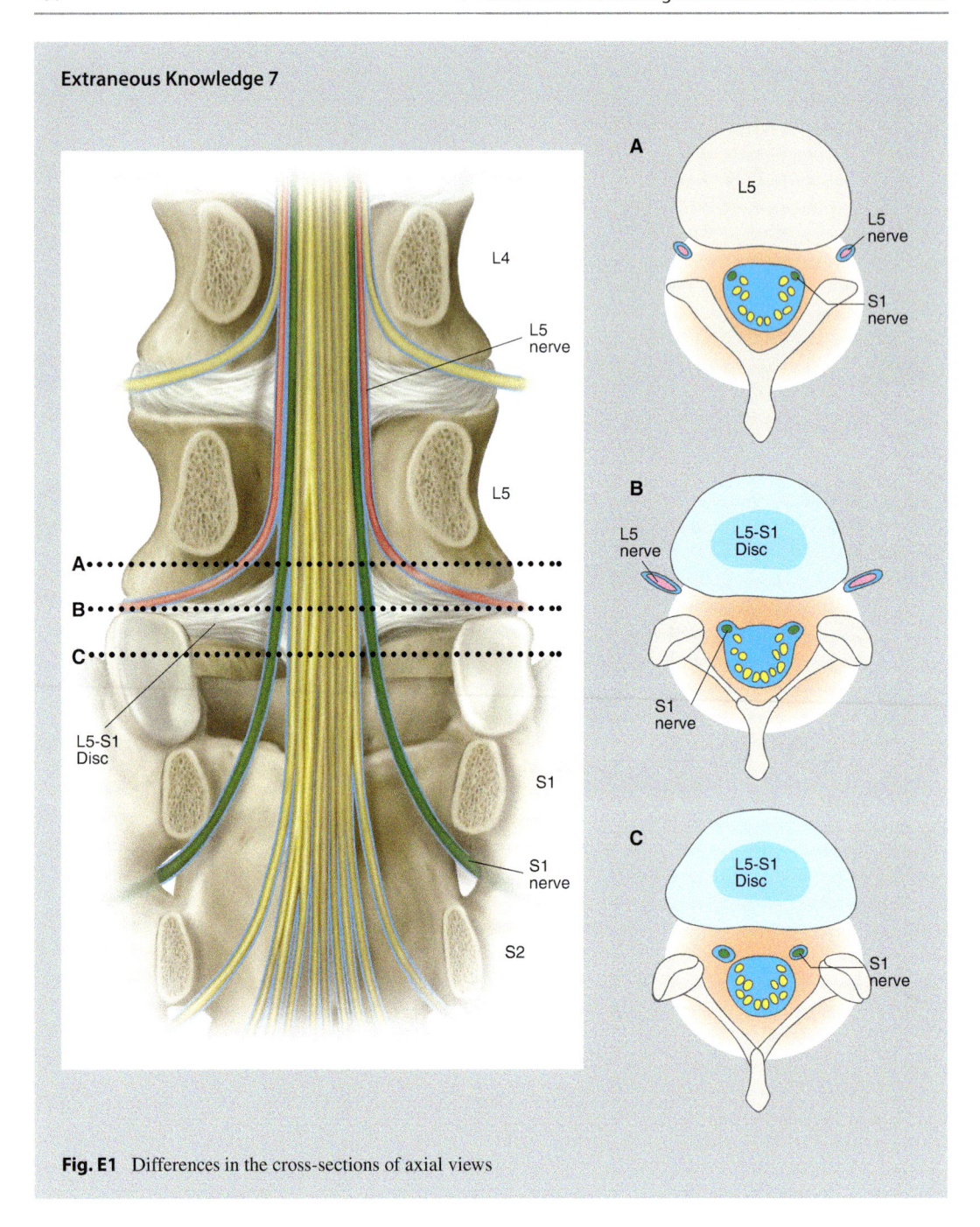

Fig. E1 Differences in the cross-sections of axial views

Dural Puncture

7

Dural puncture is a common occurrence in the nonsurgical treatment in the epidural space, but the operator should always exercise caution: not adopting the proper response measures could cause serious sequelae.

7.1 Problems That Could Arise from a Dural Puncture

7.1.1 Post-Dural Puncture Headache (PDPH)

Continued cerebrospinal fluid (CSF) drainage due to dural puncture decreases intracranial pressure to below normal levels of pressure, which can cause headache. In other words, when the volume of the CSF decreases, brain tissue inside the cranium descends when the affected person stands or sits, further increasing tension in structures sensitive to pain. This could cause orthostatic headache and various clinical symptoms, including neck pain, nausea, vomiting, diplopia, blurred vision, photophobia, hearing impairment, and tinnitus. Such headache and clinical symptoms tend to disappear while the affected individual is lying down but worsen when he or she stands up or sits down.

PDPH tends to occur more commonly among young individual than older adults and among women than men—i.e., more common among people with more abdominal fat. It is also observed to occur more often when a thick needle is used. PDPH usually presents immediately after the procedure ends but tends to disappear after 2–3 days. However, if the pain is too severe or there is no improvement after 3–4 days, an epidural blood patch procedure should be performed; this operation draws approximately 10–15 cc of blood from the patient and injects it into the suspected site of epidural puncture.

Due to the nature of the procedure, balloon decompression or neuroplasty may often result in puncture of the area with stenosis or adhesion. However, when the catheter is removed, the punctured area has the tendency to close immediately due to stenosis or adhesion. Hence, patients that actually require the blood patch procedure are fortunately rare. In particular, while dural puncture during the procedure occurs more commonly in patients who have undergone spinal fusion and have extensive and very severe adhesion, PDPH is very rare. The author has yet to observe the presentation of PDPH among such patients.

7.1.2 Drug Injection into the Punctured Area

If a local anesthetic is administered in the presence of dural puncture, total spinal anesthesia could occur, inducing symptoms such as the loss of consciousness, hypotension, cardiac arrest,

© Springer Nature Singapore Pte Ltd. 2021
J. W. Shin, *Spinal Epidural Balloon Decompression and Adhesiolysis*,
https://doi.org/10.1007/978-981-15-7265-4_7

and apnea. Among the cases that have been referred to the author for legal consultation, two involved serious sequelae-related disability caused by the lack of timely recognition of apnea and loss of consciousness in the patient during neuroplasty. Because it is a very dangerous complication, the drug injection must be injected after the dural puncture during the procedure is confirmed to be absent. Operators must perform the procedure while checking the patient's condition.

7.2 Tips Concerning Dural Puncture

1. When performing the pre-procedural epidurogram, it is advisable to perform epidural anesthesia using a mixture of contrast dye and Lidocaine. Before injecting this drug mixture, 3–5 cc of 100% contrast dye must be injected to confirm that the drug is being injected into the epidural space. The purpose of this is mostly to check whether the drug is being injected into a blood vessel but it to assess the possibility of dural puncture that may occur during the process of inserting the guide needle through the sacral hiatus if the thecal sac has descended abnormally.
2. If the drug containing the local anesthetic will be administered during the procedure after the catheter or guide needle has been administered, the drug must be injected after the 100% contrast dye has been used to confirm that the drug will be administered to the epidural space.
3. To reduce dural puncture when advancing the site of adhesion or stenosis with a catheter, the procedure should be performed by moving the catheter slightly to the left and right (swing) rather than stabbing the catheter toward the head (Fig. 7.1).
4. When dural puncture is suspected, or the contrast dye has been injected into a blood vessel, particulated steroids, including triamcinolone, must not be used. This is because the inflow of particulated steroids into the dural space could

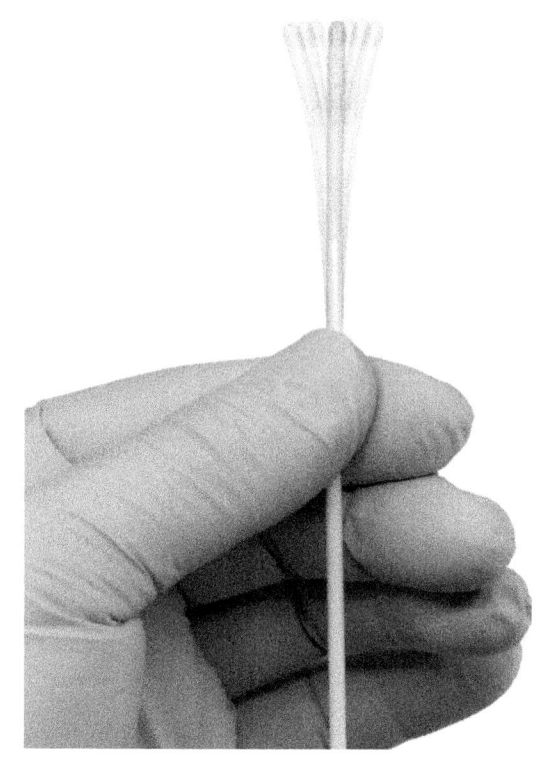

Fig. 7.1 The gradual movement of the catheter tip from right to left (swing) when advancing the catheter toward the head

cause arachnoiditis, while inflow into a blood vessel could cause embolization.

By strictly adhering to these four tips, dangerous complications can be avoided.

7.3 Findings Indicative of Dural Puncture

The task of suspecting and discriminating the presence of dural puncture is paramount to the safety of the procedure. The findings indicative of dural puncture during the procedure are as follows; in such cases, contrast dye must be used for confirmation.

1. The epidural space houses nerves, blood vessels, fat, and fibrotic substances. Accordingly, slight resistance may be felt when a catheter is being inserted therein. In particular, because

7.3 Findings Indicative of Dural Puncture

the patient is lying in a prone position during the procedure, the anterior epidural space becomes narrower—i.e., greater resistance may be felt when inserting the catheter into the anterior epidural space than into the posterior epidural space. However, if at some point the catheter is able to move laterally without impediment while inside the spinal canal and there is almost no resistance when the catheter is advanced toward the head of the patient, dural puncture should be suspected. In some cases, when the catheter punctures the dura, the operator may actually feel some sense of penetration. Whether such a sensation can be attributed to the removal of adhesion or dural puncture should be checked immediately with the contrast dye.

Figure 7.2 shows endoscopic images of normal epidural space, the site of dural puncture, and the intradural space when dural puncture is present. CSF and nerve bundles are usually present in the intradural space; hence, there is almost no resistance when the catheter moves through this space. However,

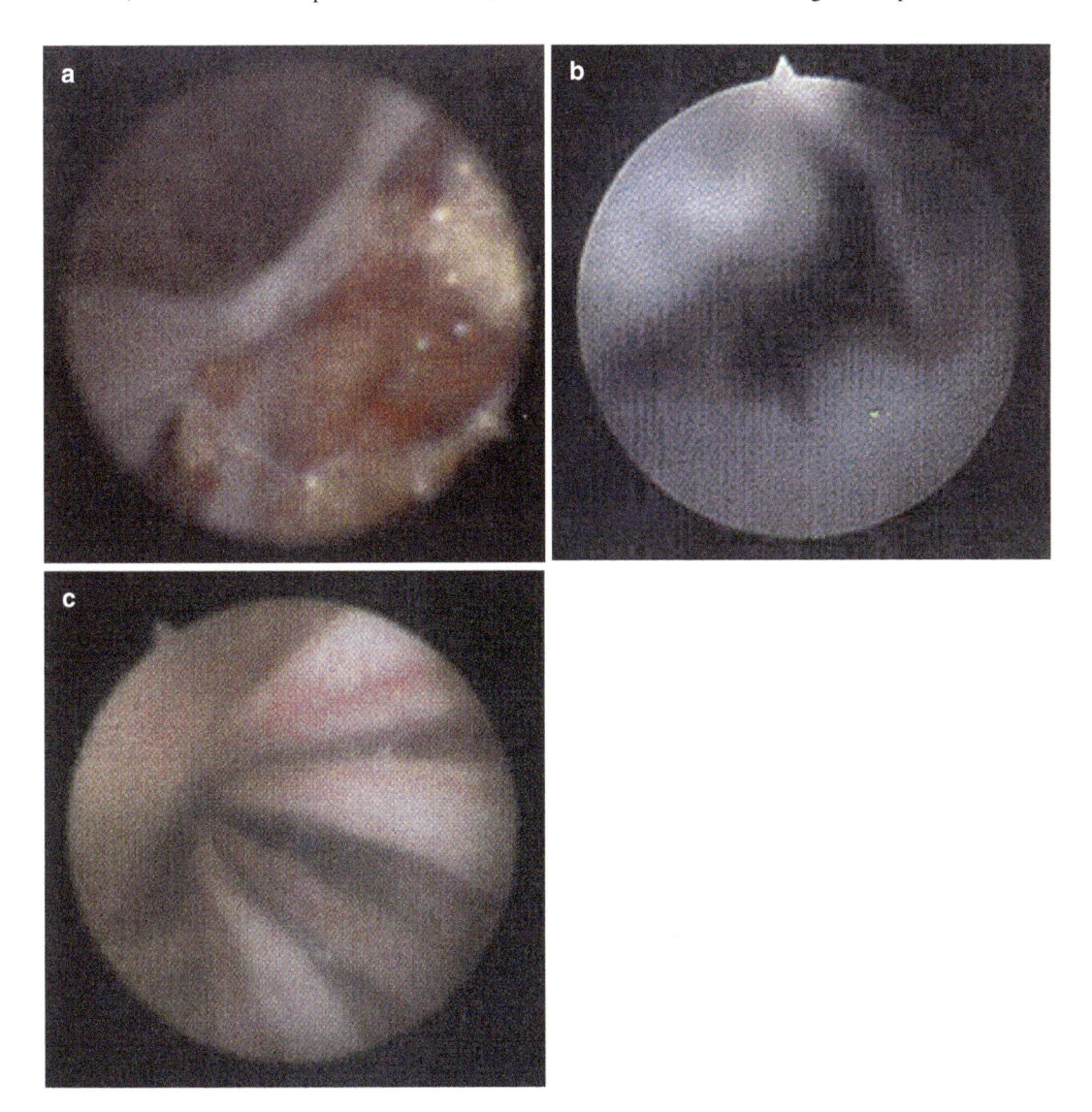

Fig. 7.2 Epiduroscopic findings. (**a**) Normal epidural space: The dura, fat tissues, and blood vessels are observed. (**b**) The punctured dura. (**c**) Presence of CSF and nerve bundles inside the dura

such catheter movement often causes abnormal nerve irritation or pain. In such cases, as the pain is not excessively severe, the level of pain cannot be used as an indicator for discriminating whether the operator has accessed the intradural space.
2. If the insertion of the catheter from the spinal canal into the intervertebral foramen cannot be achieved despite the absence of severe stenosis or adhesion, the catheter may be inside the dural space. As shown in the figure below, the dura mater wraps around nerve roots and forms the dural sleeve—i.e., the catheter cannot exit the intervertebral foramen and pass through this narrow space (Fig. 7.3).

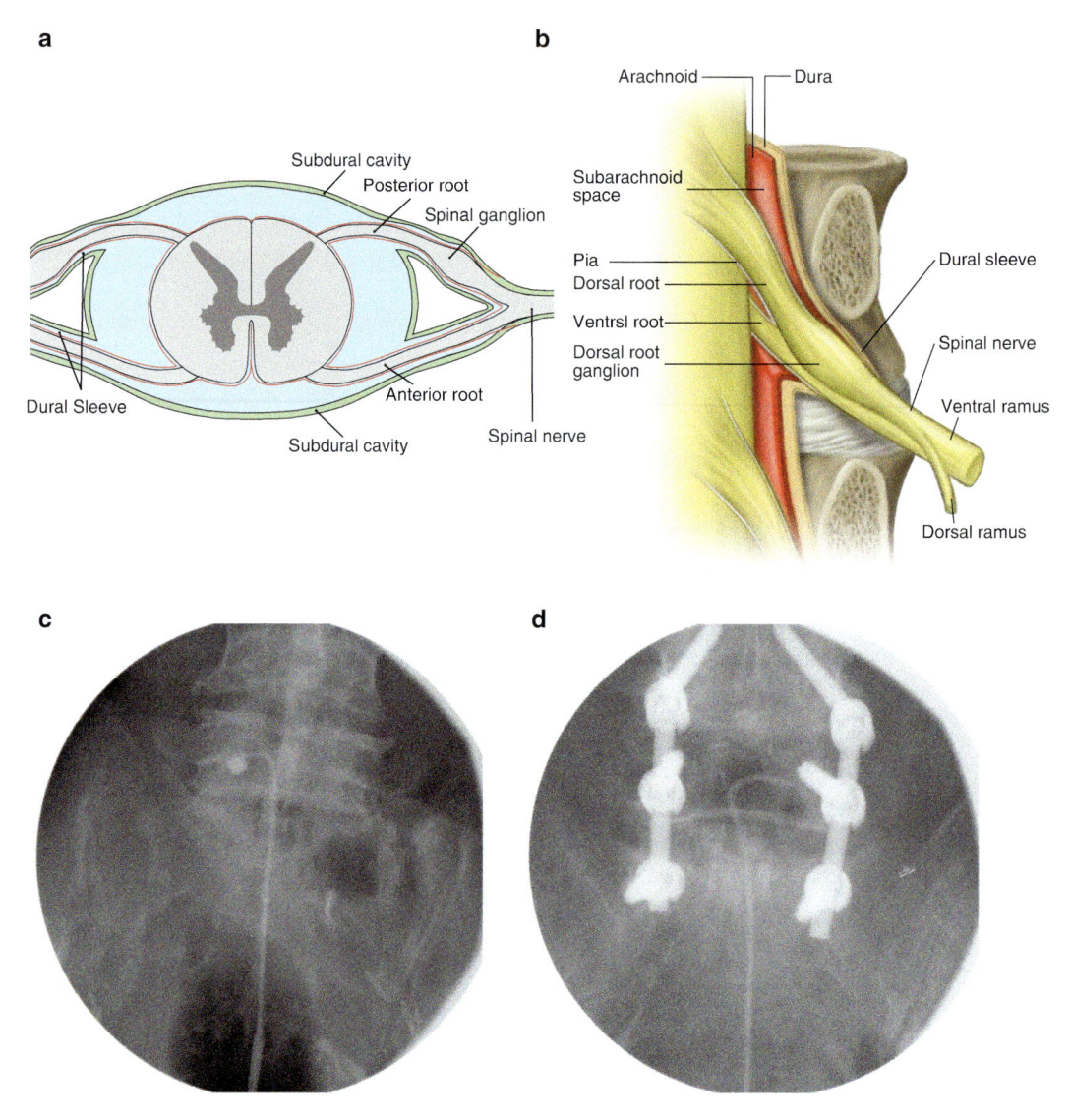

Fig. 7.3 (**a**, **b**) The dura mater forms the dural sleeve and connects to the intervertebral foramen. It is impossible for the catheter to enter the intervertebral foramen through this narrow space. (**c**, **d**) Because the catheter is in the intradural space, it cannot advance from the foraminal orifice into the intervertebral foramen

7.4 Characteristic Contrast Image Findings Indicative of Dural Puncture

Without endoscopy, the presence of dural puncture must be determined by referencing contrast images. Hence, familiarity with the features of the epidural and intradural spaces as seen on contrast images and the ability to differentiate such findings is important. The following helps to provide this knowledge by comparing characteristics of epidurography and myelography findings indicative of dural puncture (Figs. 7.4, 7.5, 7.6, 7.7, 7.8, 7.9, 7.10, 7.11 and 7.12).

1. AP myelography findings are symmetrical. Multiple strands of lines can be observed inside due to the cauda equina fibers. By contrast, an epidurogram does not show any fibers. It presents a disorganized appearance with the holes scattered sporadically throughout; these holes represent fat within the epidural space characteristic to epidurograms (Figs. 7.4, 7.5 and 7.6).
2. Myelograms feature distinct and smooth margins that spread, while epidurograms have indistinct margins.
3. Lateral findings of myelograms reveal the contrast dye ascending from the anterior of the spinal canal as a half-moon shape resembling a cup being filled with wine. This phenomenon is due to the fact that the patient was in a prone position when the myelogram was obtained and that the contrast dye is heavier than the CSF (Fig. 7.6b). In the myelograms of patients with severe spinal stenosis, the contrast dye may not appear to fill the stenosed area or might be cut off due to a lack of

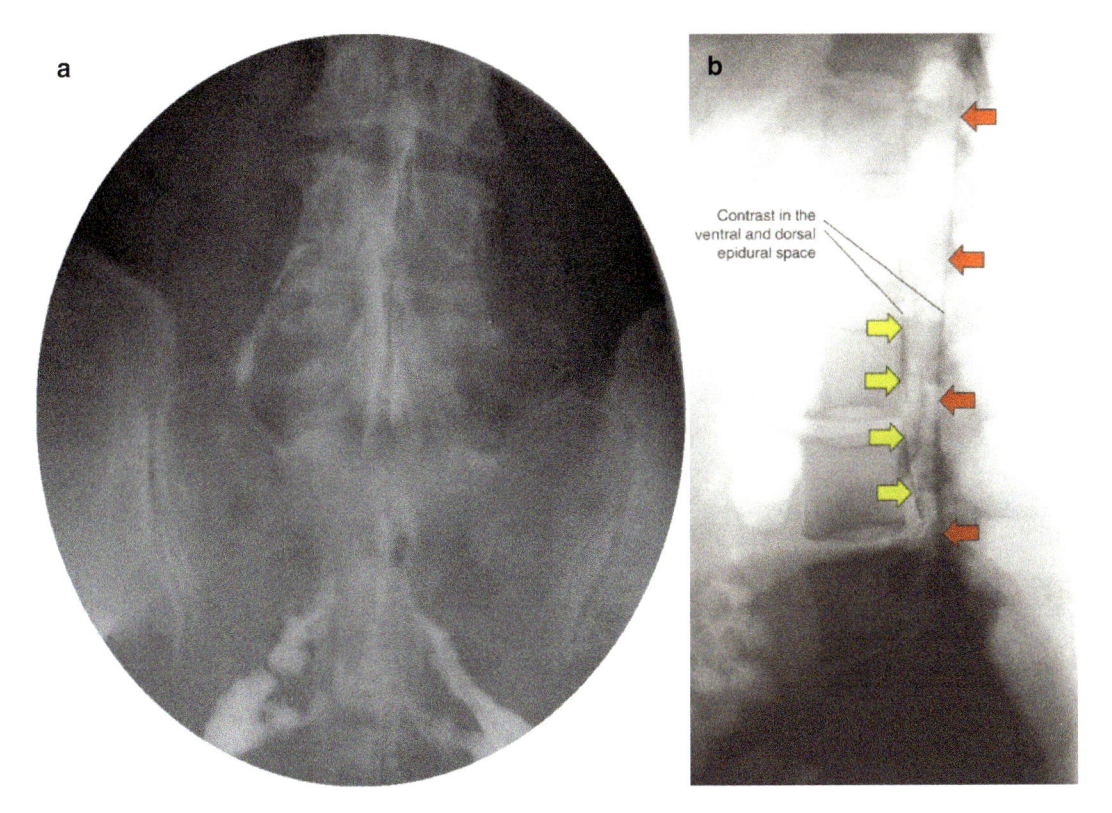

Fig. 7.4 Normal epidurogram findings. (**a**) Christmas-tree-like spreading with rough margins and an irregular, disorderly appearance due to the sporadic distribution of adhesion and fat tissue. Contrast image findings do not show equina fibers. (**b**) The lack of severe adhesion allows the contrast dye to spread well into the anterior and posterior epidural spaces. In the anterior epidural space, the contrast dye spreads close to the posterior surface of the vertebral body. Yellow arrow: Anterior epidural space. Red arrow: Posterior epidural space

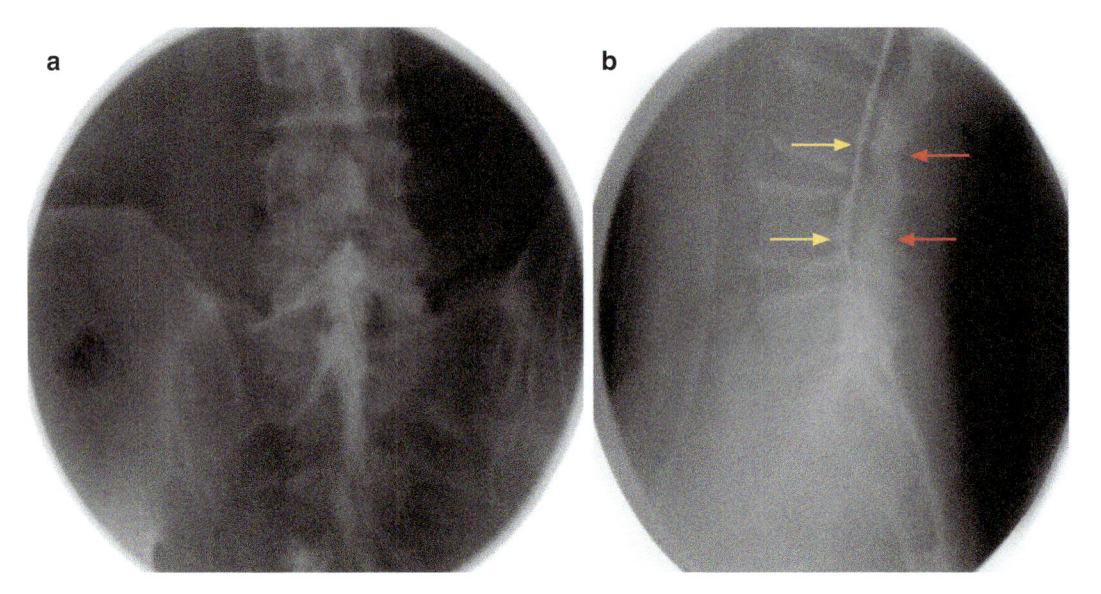

Fig. 7.5 Normal epidurogram findings. (**a**) Christmas-tree-like spreading with a disorderly appearance. (**b**) Both the anterior and posterior epidural spaces are contrast-enhanced. The dye spreads with no space between the anterior epidural space and the posterior surface of the vertebral body. Yellow arrow: Anterior epidural space. Red arrow: Posterior epidural space

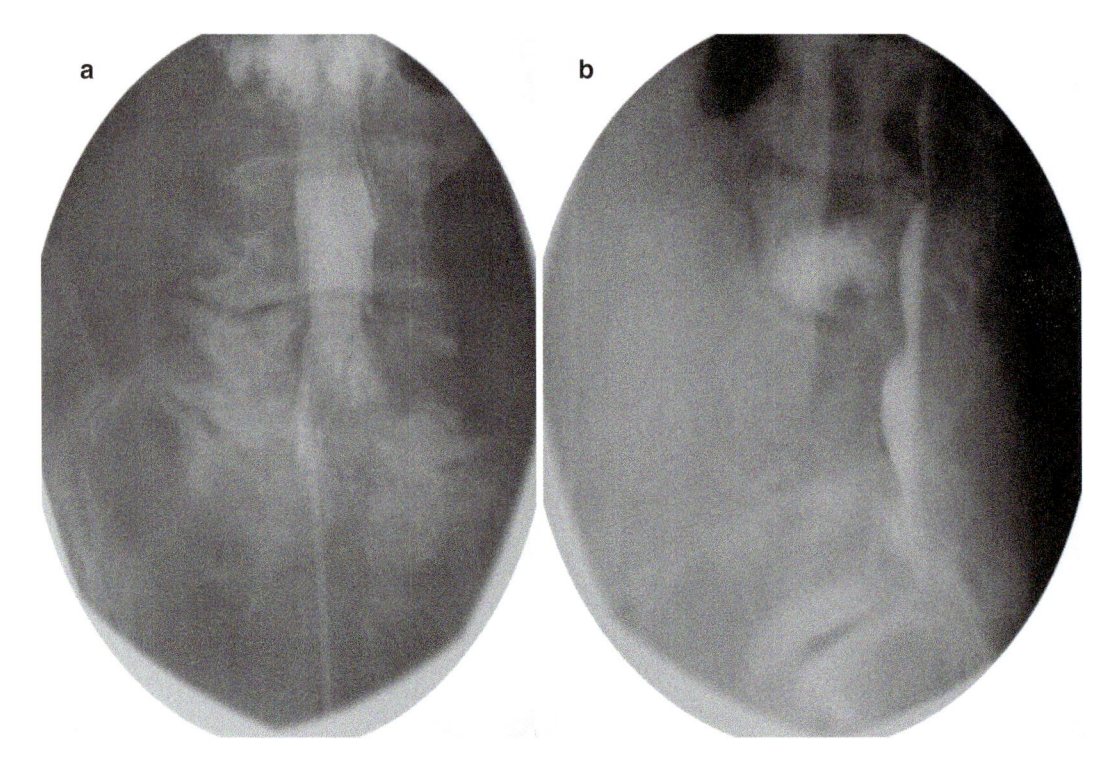

Fig. 7.6 Myelogram findings with dural puncture. (**a**) Contrast image findings are symmetrical, the margins are distinct, and the cauda equina fibers are visible inside. The contrast dye ascends from the catheter tip to the head with more efficacy than can be reasonably expected. (**b**) The contrast dye ascends and spreads evenly, similar to the half-moon shape observed when wine is poured into a cup

7.4 Characteristic Contrast Image Findings Indicative of Dural Puncture

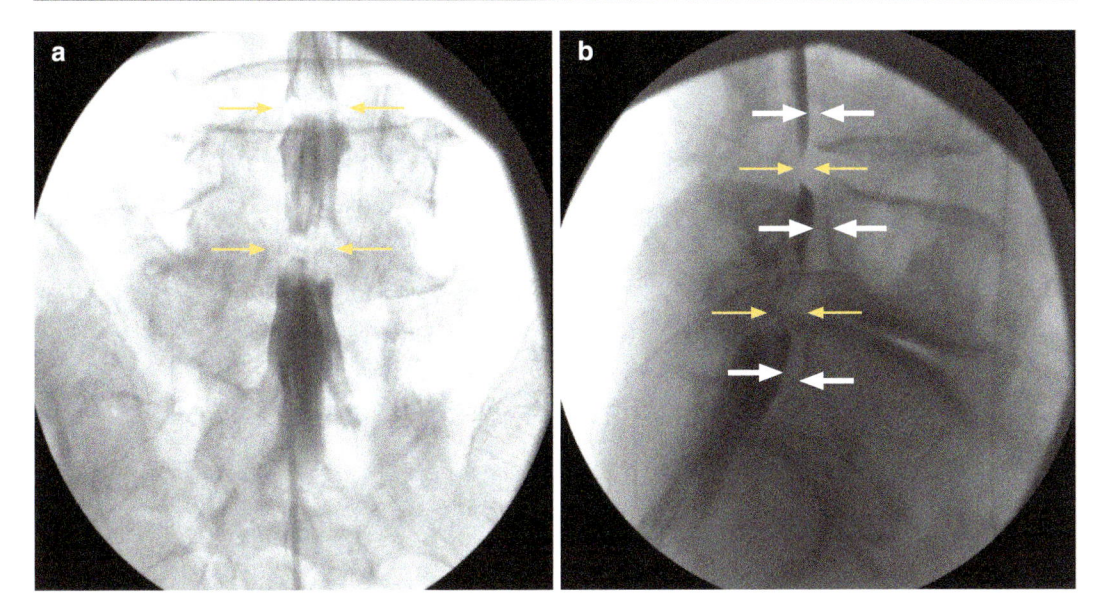

Fig. 7.7 Myelogram findings in a patient with severe stenosis. (**a**) Severe stenosis results in the appearance of filling defects, as the contrast dye cannot fill the retrodiscal area of the stenosed area. (**b**) The empty space between the posterior surface of the vertebral body and dura to where the contrast dye does not spread is the anterior epidural space. Yellow arrow: Filling defect. Between the white arrows: Anterior epidural space

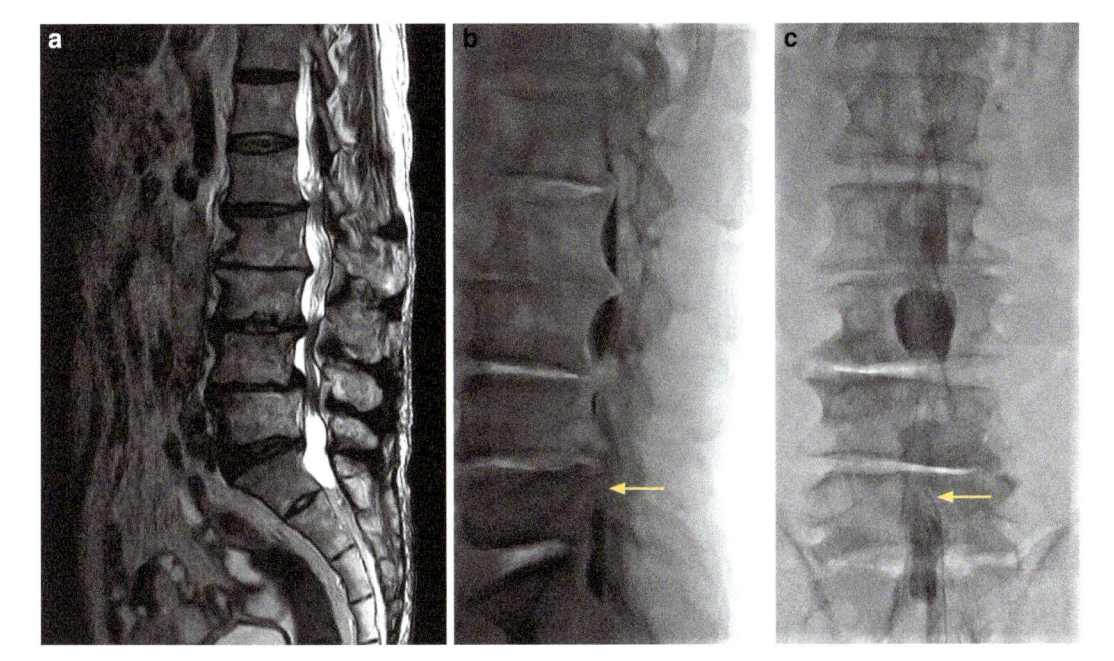

Fig. 7.8 Dural puncture during an operation performed with the Racz catheter. (**a**) MRI findings. Multilevel central stenosis. (**b**, **c**) Contrast image findings after dural puncture. Puncture occurred when passing through the Rt. L5–S1 central area. The contrast dye spreads easily toward the head relative to the catheter. The filling defect is seen in the stenosed area, along with distinct margins and nerve fibers. Arrow: Racz catheter tip

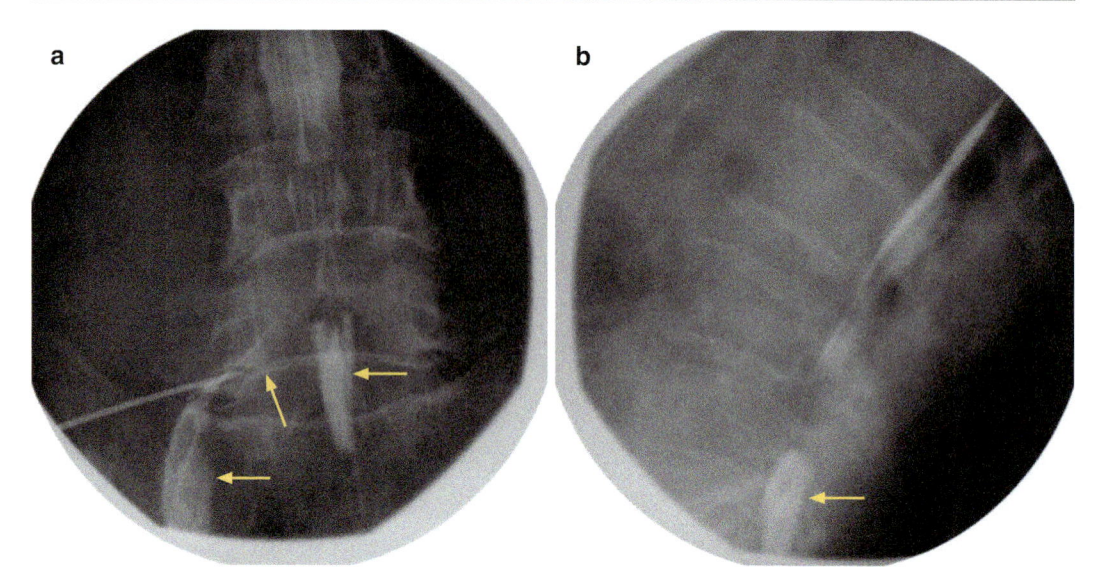

Fig. 7.9 Lt. L5 transforaminal block performed after dural puncture during the caudal approach. The upper and lower representations of contrast spread correspond to the myelogram and epidurogram, respectively. In the latter, the cauda equina fibers are contrast-enhanced. Arrows: Epidurogram

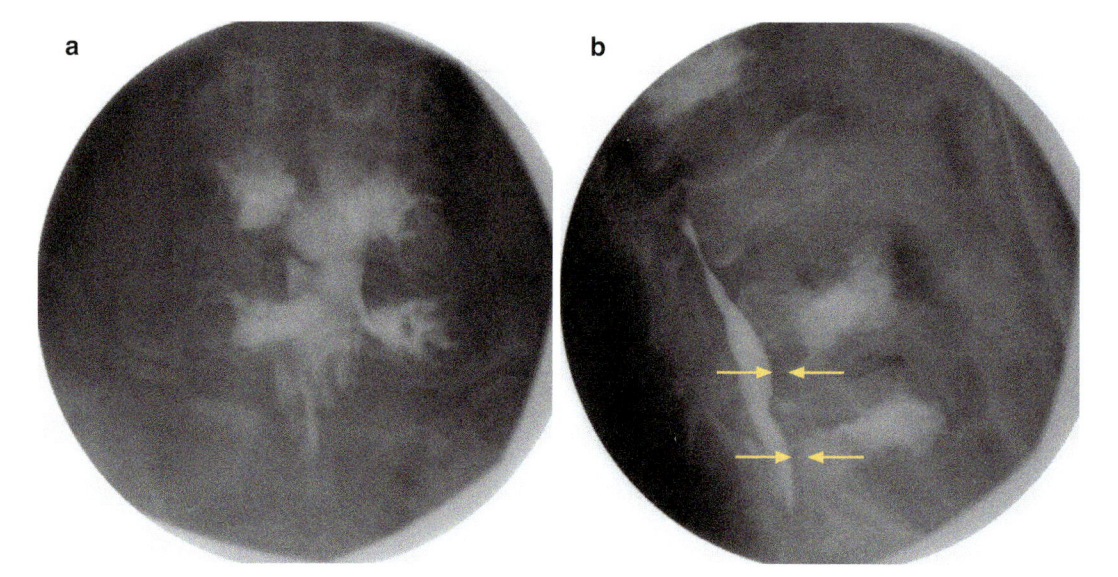

Fig. 7.10 Myelogram findings obtained during balloon decompression in a patient who had undergone multilevel vertebroplasty. (**a**) The AP findings show no fat density and distinct margin contrast despite unclear findings concerning the cauda equine fibers. (**b**) In the lateral findings, the fluid level in the intradural space was visible, resembling the filling of a cup with wine, and the anterior epidural space, into which the contrast dye did not spread, was also visible. Between arrows: Anterior epidural space

volume; the latter is indicative of a filling defect (Fig. 7.7).

From such findings, the clinician should discriminate the spread of the contrast dye spreading into the anterior epidural space: the narrow area situated between the posterior longitudinal ligament and the dura. The pattern of contrast dye spread in this area can thus

7.4 Characteristic Contrast Image Findings Indicative of Dural Puncture

Fig. 7.11 Contrast image of only the anterior epidural space. Findings show filling defects in the posterior epidural space as well as all other areas. (**a**) The AP findings feature irregular margins and fail to indicate any cauda equina fibers. (**b**) In the lateral findings, thin and irregular spreading is observable. The resemblance between the fluid level and the pouring of wine into a cup is absent. The dye spreads close to the posterior surface of the vertebral body. The findings shown in (**a**) and (**b**) provide evidence for the absence of dural puncture and the exclusive spread of the contrast dye into the anterior epidural space

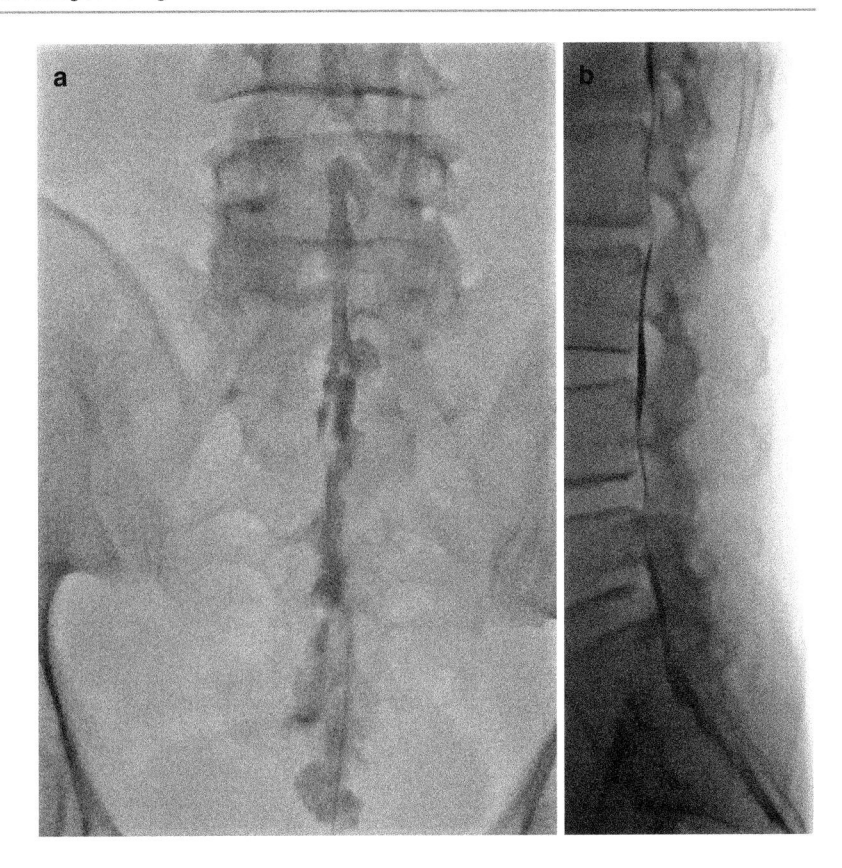

appear similar to the myelogram findings indicative of dural puncture. Because the anterior epidural space is located anterior to the dura, the contrast dye spreads close to the posterior surface of the vertebral body; however, if dural puncture is present, the thin anterior epidural space anterior to the spread of the contrast dye may appear as empty space. This point should be kept in mind as comparisons and are made between findings from the AP and lateral views (Figs. 7.6, 7.7, 7.8, 7.9, 7.10 and 7.11).
4. The contrast dye spreads easily toward the head in myelograms. As this balloon procedure is performed with patients who have stenosis or adhesion, filling defects may appear in the tip of the catheter or the drug may not ascend well. If the drug spread with unexpected efficiency toward the head, myelogram should be suspected (Figs. 7.6 and 7.8).
5. When a small amount of contrast dye is used when the myelogram is obtained, the contrast images may become blurry or even completely disappear within a few seconds. This is because the dye becomes diluted in the CSF as it spreads into the wide intradural space. During epidurography, the contrast dye is absorbed without being diluted; the contrast image findings are thus retained for relatively longer periods.

In rare cases, the contrast dye may spread into the subdural space situated between the dura and arachnoid, suggesting that the dural layers have split. In such cases, if local anesthetic is administered, symptoms may appear more quickly than when it is administered into the epidural space—although slower than when it is administered in the same dose into the intrathecal space—and may anesthetize upper levels. Hence, the operator must exercise caution. Contrast image findings characteristically show very clean margins, no features attributable to fat or cauda equina fibers, and the spread of the contrast dye in pocket form

Fig. 7.12 Myelogram was observed due to dural puncture during the performance of an interlaminar epidural block. Consequently, the needle was withdrawn slightly and adjusted to enable the contrast dye to spread into the posterior epidural space. (**a**) AP myelogram findings show distinct margins and cauda equina, while the epidurogram features holes attributable to fat tissues. (**b**) Upper and lower panels correspond to the simultaneous viewing of the myelogram and epidurogram, respectively, in the lateral view. Yellow arrow: Myelogram. White arrow: Epidurogram. Purple arrow: Myelogram and epidurogram mixed together

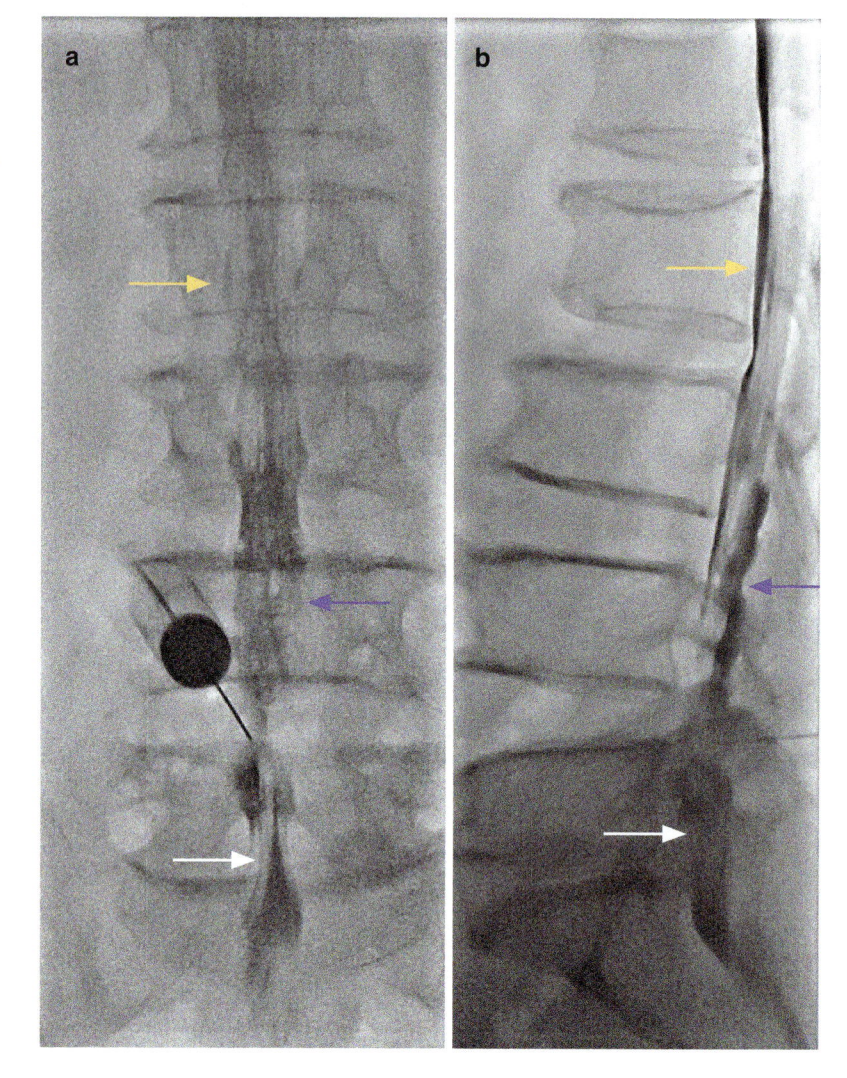

as the dye spreads and the dural space is extending. Just as with the intradural space, the drug should not be injected into the subdural space, and the procedure should be performed by using a different approach (Figs. 7.13, 7.14 and 7.15).

The following examples will help to improve the discrimination and interpretation of contrast image findings of the epidural space: specifically, discerning the findings indicative of dural puncture.

7.5 Coping Strategies for Dural Puncture

Before administering drugs during the procedure, including local anesthetic, contrast dye must be injected to confirm that the epidural space has been reached. Injection of local anesthetic into the intradural or subdural space could cause total spinal anesthesia and thereby cause fatal complications such as a sudden drop in blood pressure,

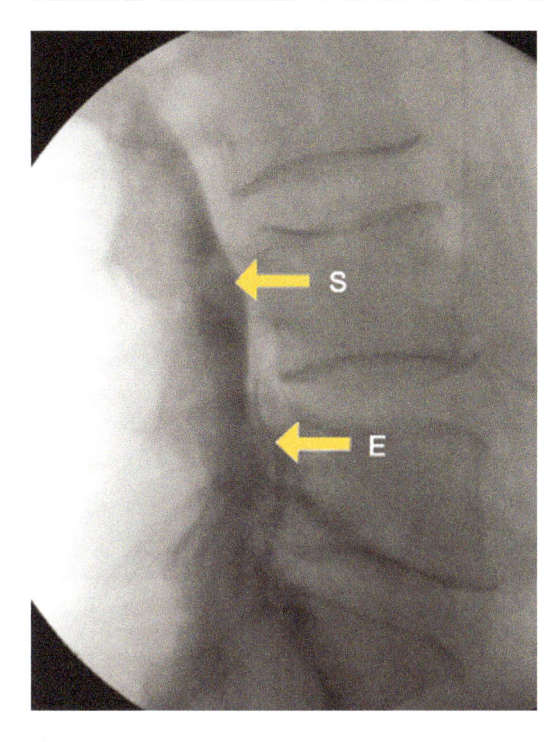

7.5 Coping Strategies for Dural Puncture

cardiac arrest, and the loss of consciousness. However, terminating the procedure due to dural puncture could raise the level of dissatisfaction in the patient due to low improvement relative to the expended cost. The following methods help to progress the procedure after dural puncture is discovered and provide strategies for coping with a sudden drop in blood pressure and/or loss of consciousness.

7.5.1 Performing the Procedure by a Different Path After Discovering Dural Puncture

Case 1 A 61-year-old male patient complained of being unable to walk for more than 10 min due to low back pain and bilateral S1 radiculopathy (Fig. 7.16). His leg pain was more severe in the left leg than in the right leg. His MRI findings indicated L4–5 central stenosis. Despite three rounds of epidural block, improvement in his symptoms lasted only 3–4 days. Accordingly, balloon decompression using the ZiNeu catheter was performed.

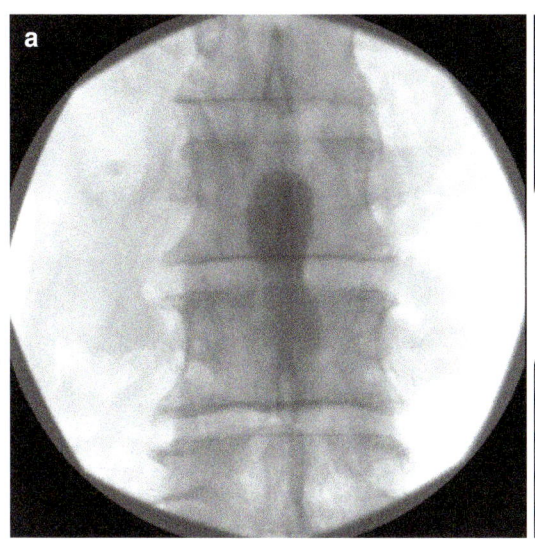

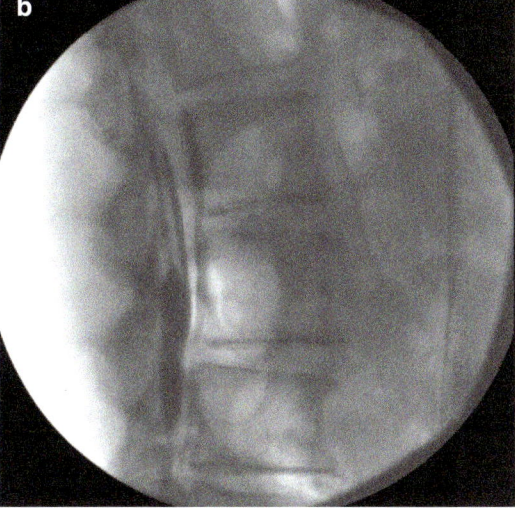

Fig. 7.13 Contrast images of the subdural space. Spread is localized to the posterior dural space and the margins are very distinct, while the contrast images do not reveal any equina fibers or fat tissues. Arrow S: Subdural, E: Anterior epidurogram

Fig. 7.14 Subdural contrast image findings. The dye spreads like a water sac. (**a**) The margins are very distinct, while the contrast images do not reveal the equina fibers or fat tissues. (**b**) The spread of the dye is localized to the posterior dural space

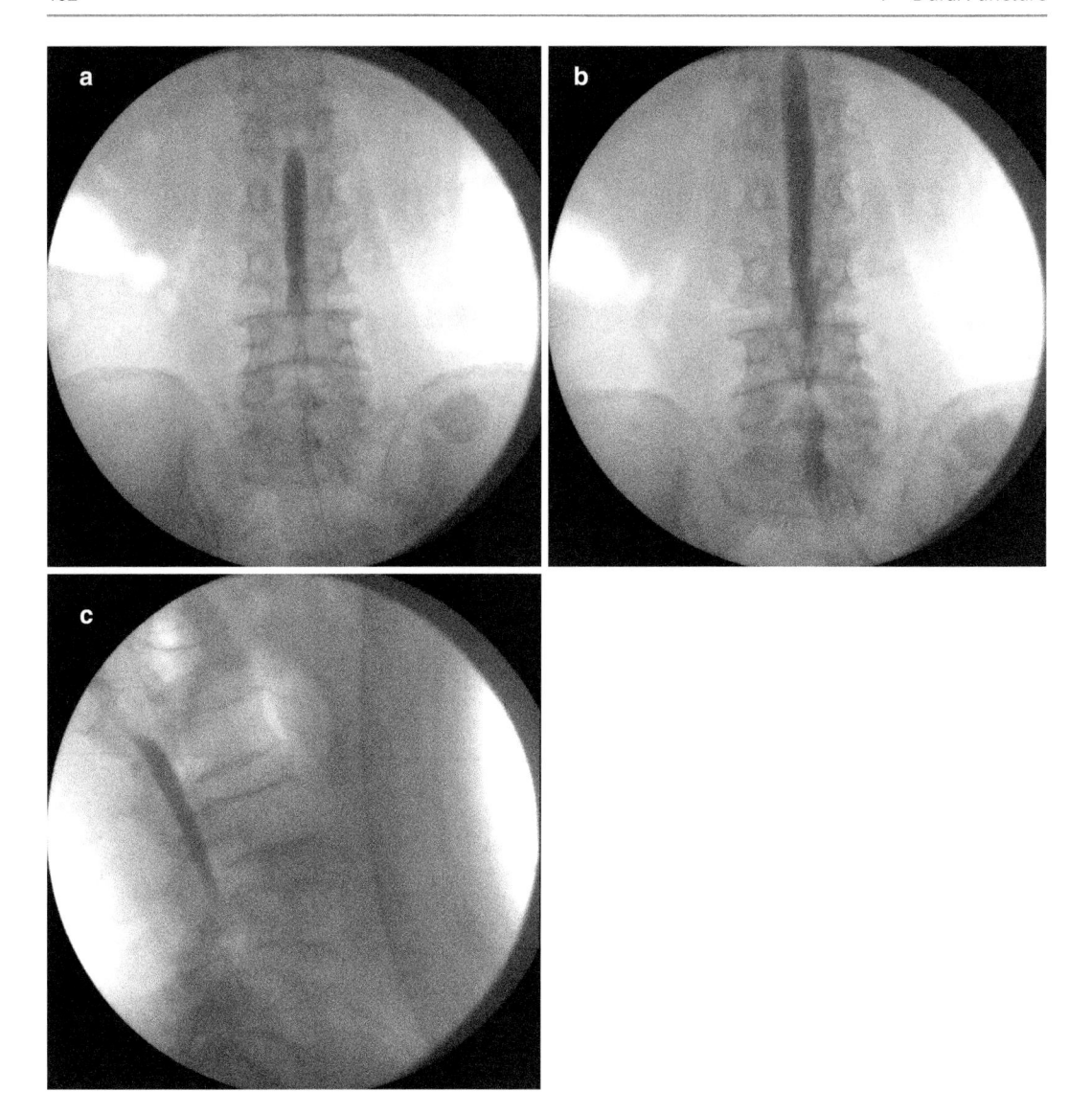

Fig. 7.15 Subdural contrast image findings. (**a**) The margins are very distinct, while the contrast images do not reveal any equina fibers or fat tissues. (**b**) When more contrast dye was injected, the dye spread more toward the head. (**c**) The dye spread like water in a sac and was localized to the posterior dural space

This patient suddenly complained of severe pain when the area near the L4–5 level was approached in an attempt to enter the left epidural space. Consequently, 3 cc of contrast dye was injected, revealing dural puncture (Fig. 7.17a, b). Accordingly, the catheter was withdrawn to the S3–4 level, and the L4–5 retrodiscal area was reached by a different path to the right of the originally selected approach. Balloon decompression was performed after confirming the epidural space with the contrast dye (Fig. 7.17c, d).

If the site of dural puncture is known, the procedure can be reattempted through the side opposite to the site of puncture (i.e., a different path). Once a path is created inside the epidural space with the movement of the catheter, the catheter has the tendency to advance through the

7.5 Coping Strategies for Dural Puncture

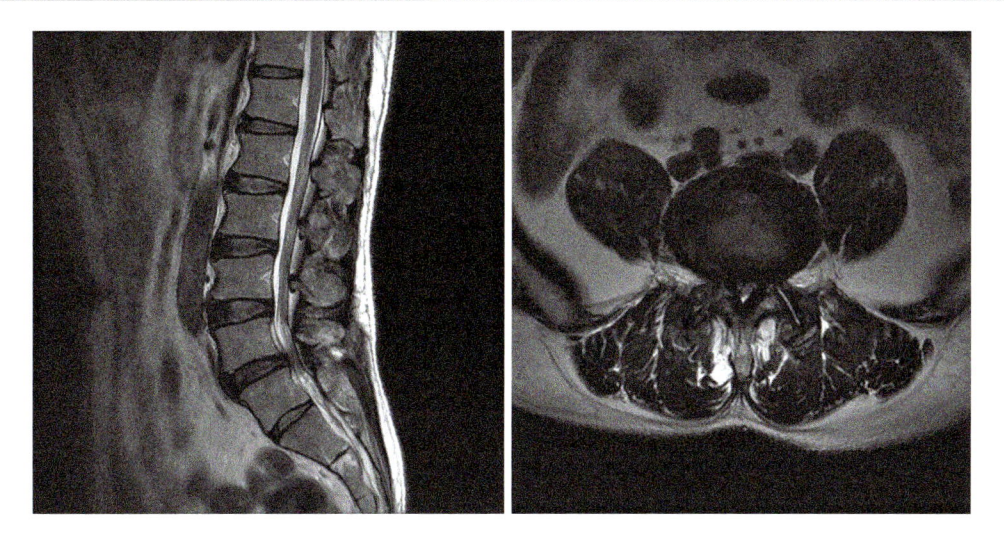

Fig. 7.16 MRI findings. L4–5 central stenosis

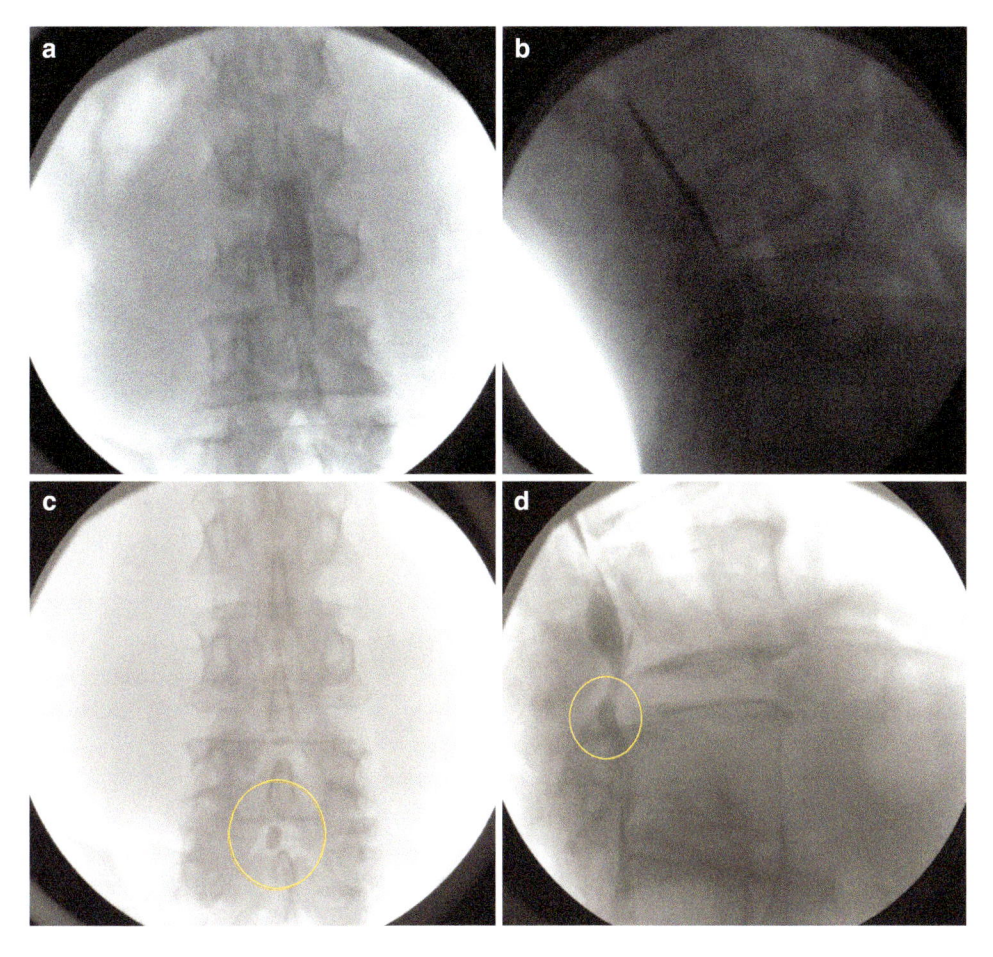

Fig. 7.17 (**a**, **b**) Myelogram due to dural puncture. (**c**, **d**) The balloon inflated in the L4–5 retrodiscal area, which was accessed by a different path. Circle: Inflated balloon

same path when the procedure is repeated. Hence, the catheter should be sufficiently withdrawn toward the coccygeal area before a new path is sought.

Case 2 A 63-year-old male patient had 20-min claudication due to low back pain and radiating pain in the left leg that began 8 years prior. Dural puncture occurred during entry into the central area of the spinal canal. Consequently, the catheter was withdrawn toward the coccygeal area and reinserted slightly to the left by a different path. The Lt. L5 intervertebral foramen was thus successfully accessed.

If the catheter was in the intradural space, the entry of the catheter into the intervertebral foramen would have been impossible. The inflation of the balloon in the anterior epidural space was confirmed (Fig. 7.18).

As in this case, if a dural puncture occurs, the procedure can be performed on the target intervertebral foramen by gaining entry through a different path.

7.5.2 The Performance of an Alternative Procedure Following Dural Puncture

Case A 66-year-old male patient had undergone spinal fusion surgery 5 years prior. On account of pain in the lower back and both legs that became severe during the 4 months prior to his clinical presentation, he underwent several rounds of epidural block at another hospital. However, the improvement in his symptoms did not last very long. Accordingly, balloon decompression in the spinal canal and both L5 intervertebral foramen was indicated. However, the original procedure was ceased due to a dural puncture that occurred while approaching the L5–S1 central area. Instead, only the bilateral L5 transforaminal epidural block was performed (Fig. 7.19).

When dural puncture occurs in the spinal canal during the procedure—as in this case—the procedure can be completed by gaining entry through a different path. However, if the procedure is difficult and the expected effect of the procedure is low, then the procedure could be completed by safely performing only the transforaminal block and not being overly aggressive.

Local anesthetic should be administered with extreme caution—even in cases in which the catheter was reinserted through a different path or another procedure was performed after the dural puncture had occurred—because the previous site of dural puncture may still be exposed, and the drug may partially flow into that site. Before administering the therapeutic drug, the contrast dye must be used to ensure that the drug will not be injected into the intradural space. Once dural puncture occurs, the approach should be made by a different path, or a different procedure should be performed. Moreover, the dose of the drug being injected should be reduced from the normal level, and any administered steroids should be confirmed as non-particulated (e.g., dexamethasone).

7.5.3 Coping Strategies for When the Drug Is Administered to the Punctured Site

Continued monitoring of the patient's condition during the procedure is paramount to the safety of the procedure. For this same reason, regional or local anesthesia is recommended over general anesthesia.

The procedure must be performed while continuing to monitor the patient's state of consciousness and vital signs. If any abnormalities are detected, the catheter and guide needle should be removed immediately, and emergency measures should be prepared after placing the patient in a supine position. Any delays in determination and decision by the operator may lead to irreversible complications.

Emergency precautions to be taken when the drug is administered to the punctured site are the same as those performed in response to deleterious vital signs. While ensuring that the patient's aspiration is maintained, the patient's airway is secured, and adequate oxygen is supplied. If there is a drop in blood pressure or heart rate, 5–10 mg of ephedrine is repeatedly administered

7.5 Coping Strategies for Dural Puncture

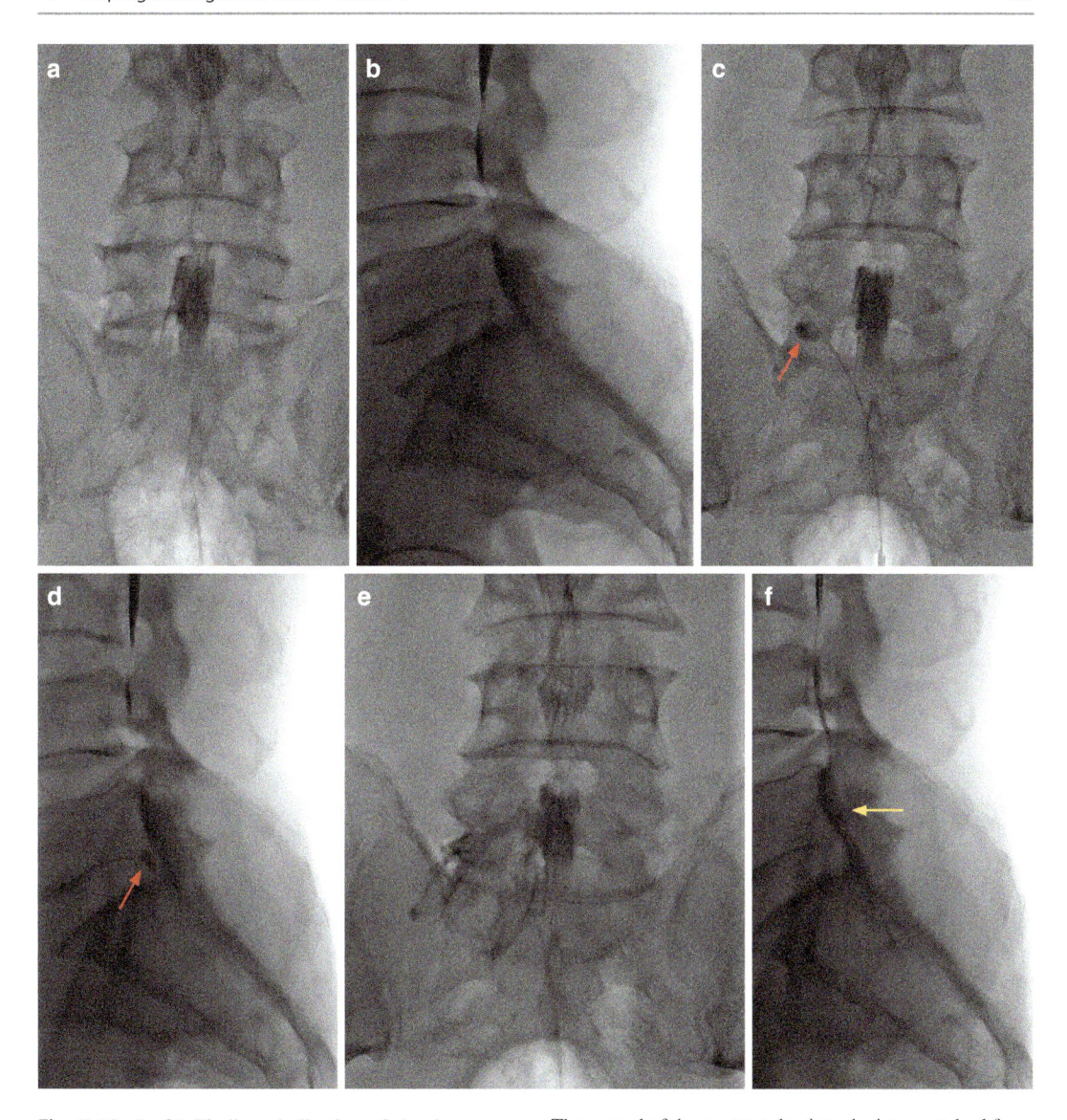

Fig. 7.18 (**a**, **b**) Findings indicative of dural puncture during entry into the spinal canal. The filling defect is seen in the area with L4–5 stenosis, and the cauda equina fibers are visible. (**c**) The inflation of the balloon after entry into the Lt. L5 intervertebral foramen was attained by a different path, and the site of dural puncture was avoided. (**d**) Lateral view of the inflation of the balloon in the anterior epidural space. The contrast dye did not spread there. (**e**) The spread of the contrast dye into the intervertebral foramen after balloon decompression. (**f**) In contrast to Figure (**b**), the contrast dye spreads into the anterior epidural space. A myelogram and epidurogram obtained after dural puncture and the completion of the foraminal procedure, respectively, can be seen simultaneously. Red arrow: Inflated balloon. Yellow arrow: Myelogram and epidurogram findings are shown together

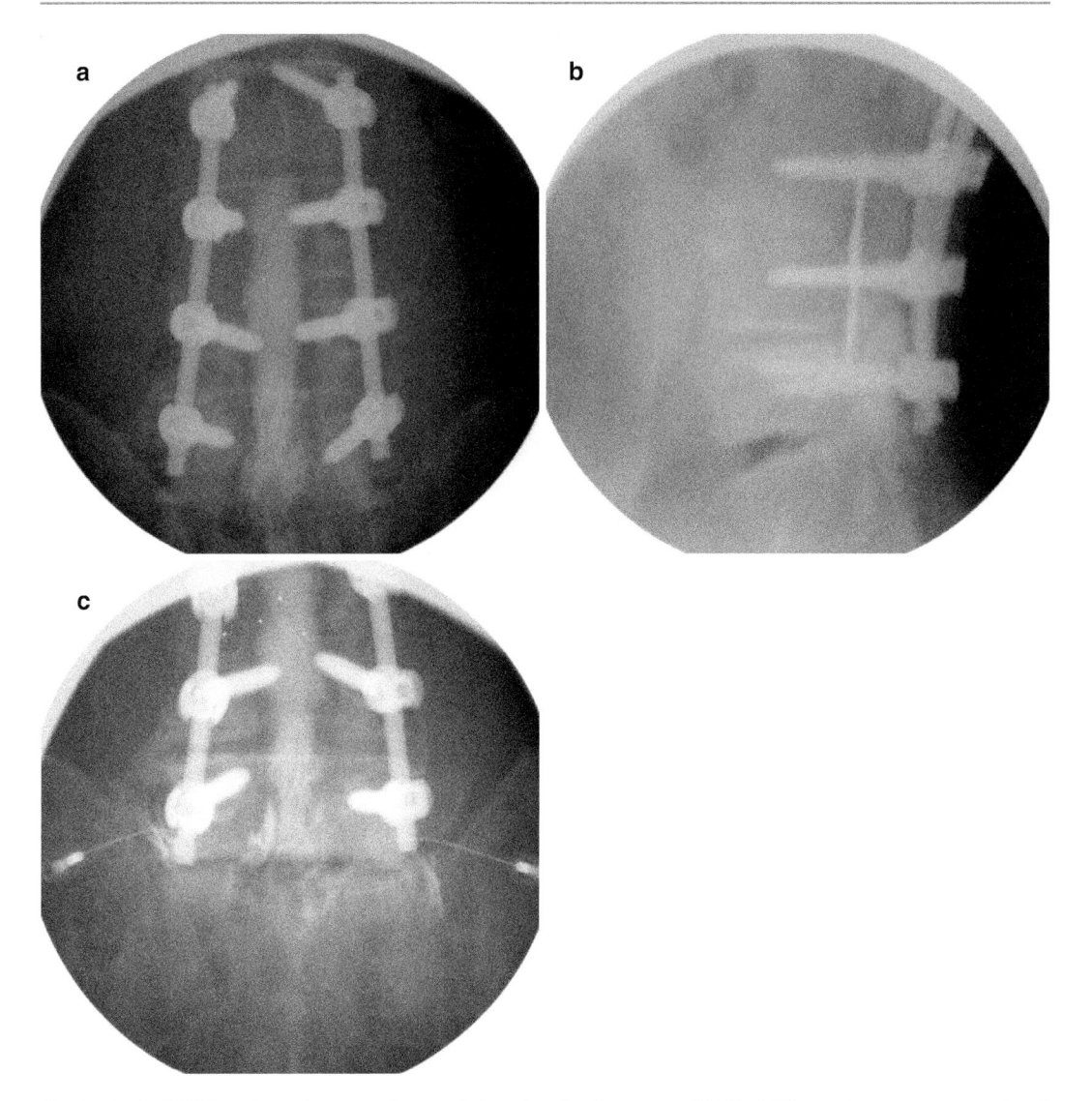

Fig. 7.19 (**a**, **b**) When 4 cc of contrast dye was injected after the catheter tip had reached up to the L5–S1 level, the dye spread up to the L3 level. There was evidence of dural puncture. (**c**) The ZiNeu catheter was removed, and a bilateral L5 transforaminal epidural block was performed

to stabilize the patient's vital signs. The patient is then closely monitored, and his or her vital signs are carefully maintained until he or she recovers.

If a local anesthetic is injected into the intradural space or a blood vessel, timely response could assure recovery without any sequelae. In particular, the injection of local anesthetic into the intradural space causes spinal anesthesia, where the level of anesthesia increases in proportion to the administered concentration. In such cases, the patient's vital signs should be attended until the patient's level of anesthesia gradually decreases, and consciousness as well as motor and sensory nerve functions have been recovered.

The injection of local anesthetic into the intradural space or a blood vessel could occur anytime during the procedure; hence, preparation should be made for early detection and timely response. In the meantime, the patient's condition must be continuously monitored during the procedure.

Extraneous Knowledge 8

Femoral head osteonecrosis (avascular necrosis: AVN) must be differentiated from degenerative spinal diseases

A 57-year-old male patient visited the pain clinic at our hospital due to left sacral and leg tingling sensation (L5 dermatome) and inguinal pain that had presented 5 months earlier. The patient stated that his pain in the sacral area as well as lower back felt like an electric shock when his left foot hit the ground and when sitting for 20–30 min, respectively. He also mentioned that the regular consumption of analgesics did not improve his condition. During the physical examination performed at our hospital, the patient complained of slight pain during Patrick's test, and tenderness on the gluteus medius muscle and posterior sacroiliac joint area was found. The electromyogram performed at an outside hospital was normal. The patient reported that a single round of epidural steroid injection and two rounds of trigger point injection received at an outside hospital produced only temporary improvement.

While the sacral and leg pain felt by the patient may have been caused by degenerative spinal disease, sacroiliac joint syndrome and related pain was suspected as a more substantiated diagnosis because of the mild pain experienced during Patrick's test and the tenderness found in the gluteus medius muscle and posterior sacroiliac joint area. As hip joint disorder was also considered as a differential diagnosis, a bone scan and hip MRI were performed.

Since both tests revealed bilateral femoral head osteonecrosis, the department of orthopedic surgery was consulted. When sacral and leg pain or tingling occurs, a lumbar MRI is usually performed to rule out degenerative spinal disease, which is found in most elderly patients with such symptoms. Treatment for this condition usually targets the spine. However, femoral head osteonecrosis could be mistaken for spinal disease, and the patient's condition may therefore not be treated properly.

The author has found several cases of femoral head osteonecrosis; in every instance, the satisfaction of identifying the patient's condition was overshadowed by the concern about possible misdiagnosis.

The method for identifying femoral head osteonecrosis is rather simple. In patients with sacral and leg pain, whether the results from Patrick's test are positive should be checked. The patient should further be asked if he or she experiences inguinal pain when walking. If femoral head osteonecrosis is thus suspected, translateral and frog-leg view, bone scan, and hip MRI must be performed. It is advisable to always perform Patrick's test when conducting physical examinations of outpatients.

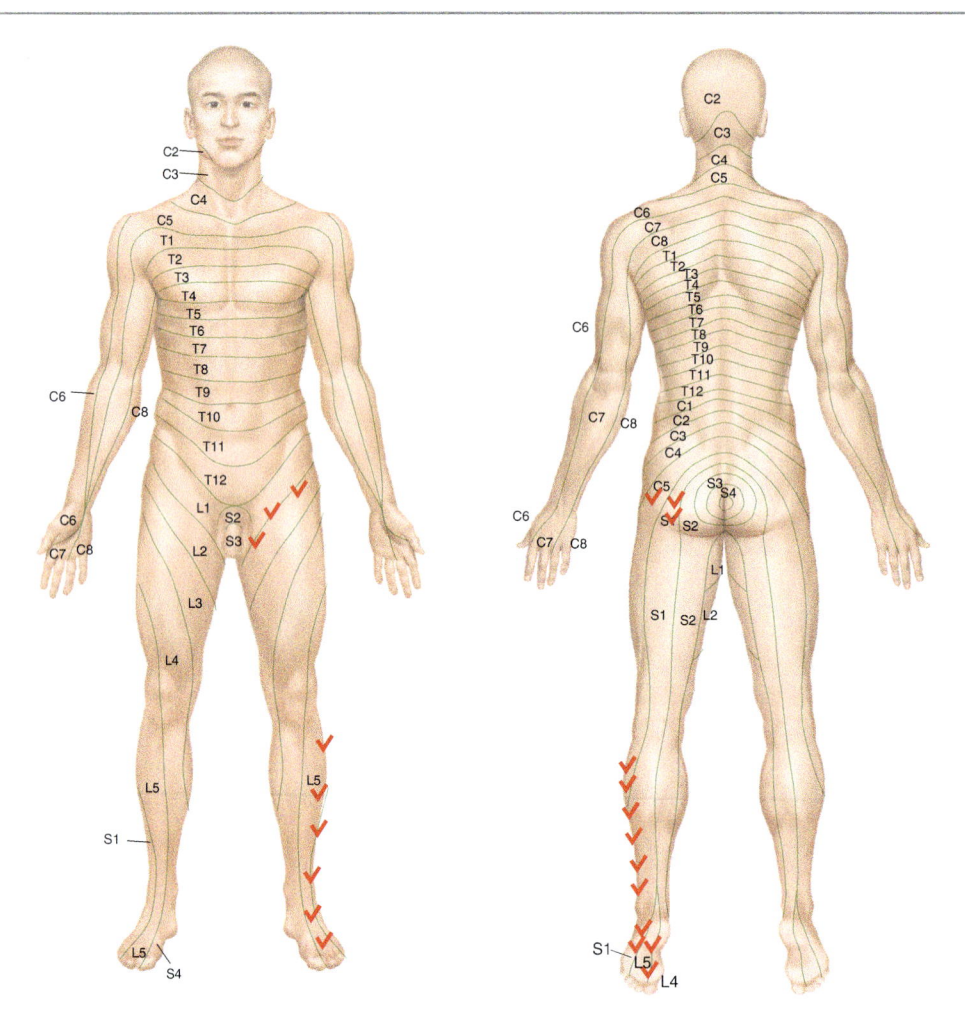

Fig. E1 Red: sites of pain

7.5 Coping Strategies for Dural Puncture

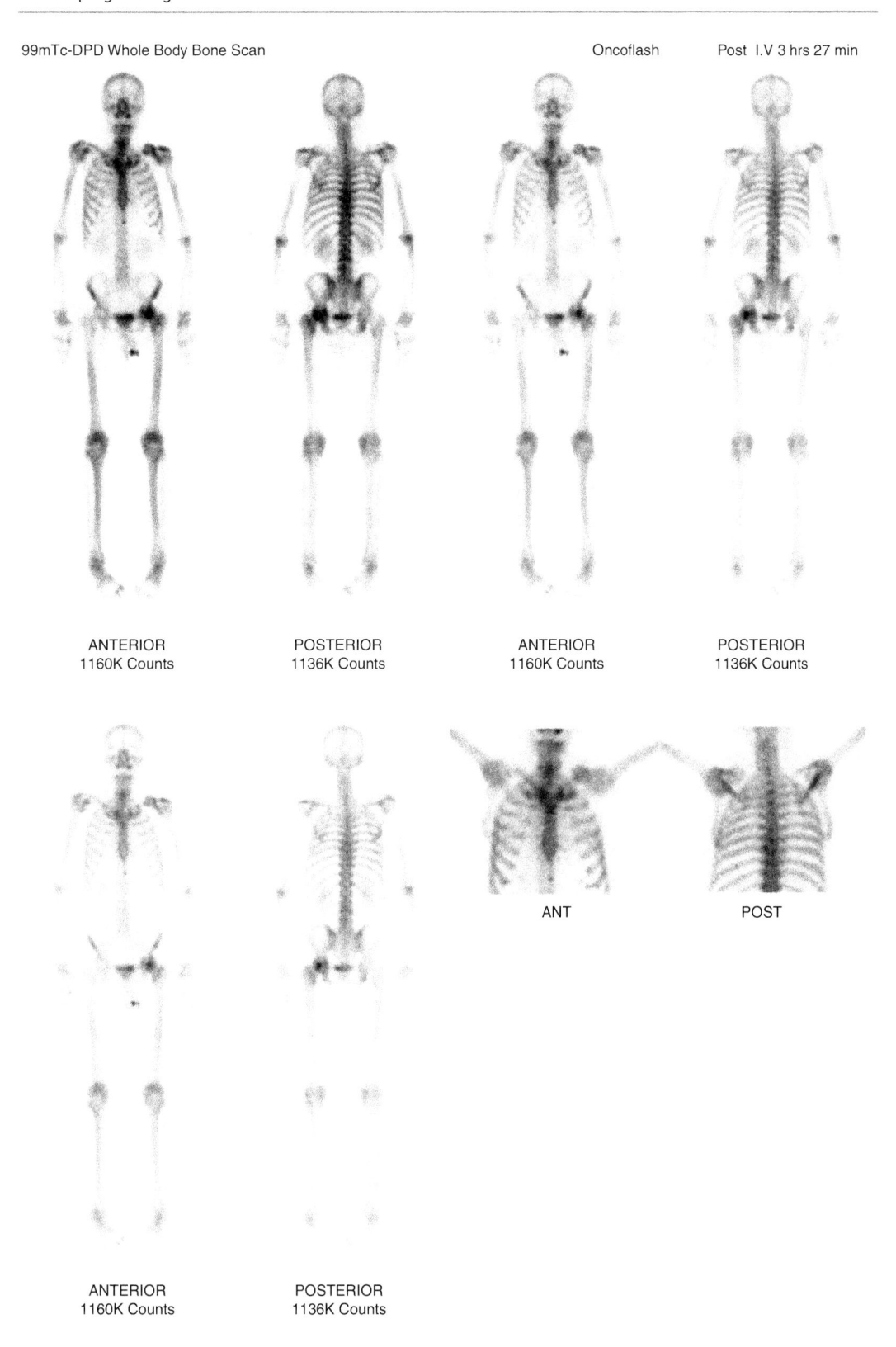

99mTc-DPD Whole Body Bone Scan Oncoflash Post I.V 3 hrs 27 min

ANTERIOR 1160K Counts POSTERIOR 1136K Counts ANTERIOR 1160K Counts POSTERIOR 1136K Counts

ANT POST

ANTERIOR 1160K Counts POSTERIOR 1136K Counts

Fig. E2 Bone scan findings. Bilateral femoral head osteonecrosis

Bibliography

1. Schutze G. Epiduroscopy, spinal endoscopy. Berlin: Springer. pp. 23, 88, 120.

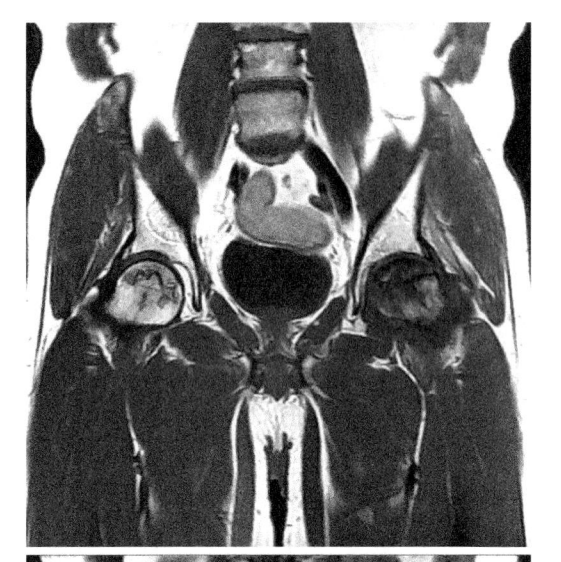

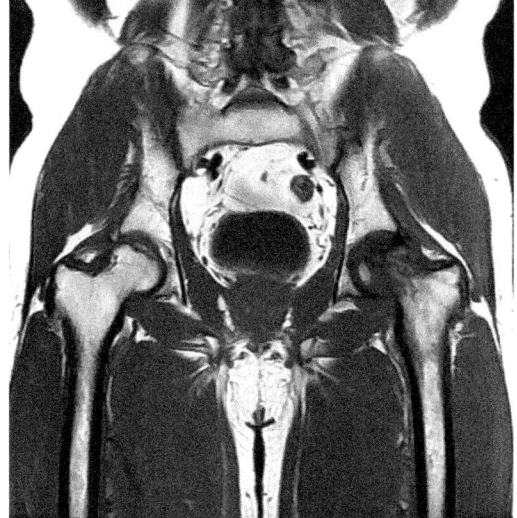

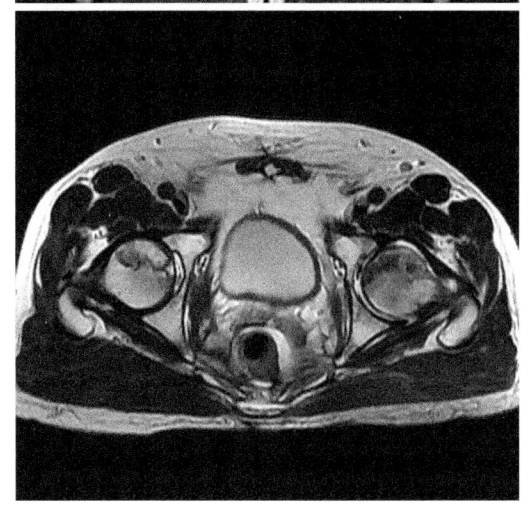

Fig. E3 MRI findings. Bilateral femoral head osteonecrosis

Method for Catheter Selection

The location and severity of lesions, as well as the extent of degenerative progression, vary much between patients. Accordingly, selecting the catheter that is best suited to address each patient's case becomes an important part of the treatment process, as catheter selection has a significant impact on the success of the procedure.

For example, the ZiNeu02 catheter may be selected when adhesion is not very severe, as it is relatively inexpensive and less irritating to the patient. However, if the unexpectedly strong adhesion renders compromises the use of the ZiNeu02 catheter, the operator may wish he or she had selected the ZiNeu01 or ZiNeuS catheter instead; and realizing this during the procedure may place the operator in a difficult situation. Therefore, in tandem with the analysis of the patient's condition and MRI findings, an accurate understanding of the characteristics and features of the different types of catheters must inform the selection of equipment.

While informed by the experiences of the author, the method of catheter selection explained below is only a recommendation; other choices are available depending on the tendencies and preferences of the operator.

8.1 Catheter Selection Recommendations According to Case

8.1.1 Selecting Between the ZiNeu01 and ZiNeuS Catheters

While the ZiNeu01 and ZiNeuS catheters both have the same outer diameter (2.3 mm), they also feature some key differences. The ZiNeuS catheter can be used together with an endoscope, and its tip area bends easily to form an articulation. By contrast, the ZiNeu01 catheter cannot be paired with an endoscope, and its tip cannot be articulated; the entire catheter bends when it is pulled laterally (Fig. 8.1).

It is easier to approach the foraminal orifice with the ZiNeuS catheter, as its tip area bends easily. Moreover, this catheter causes less pain since it can enter the intervertebral foramen parallel to the spinal nerves. However, due to the nature of the articulation, the tip area of this catheter is inevitably weaker than those of catheters incapable of articulation. In patients with severe foraminal stenosis or adhesion, the ZiNeuS catheter equipped with an articulated tip may therefore be used to approach the foraminal orifice more easily but may fail to penetrate into the intervertebral foramen. This same problem is inherent to all articulated catheters used to approach the caudal epidural space. By contrast,

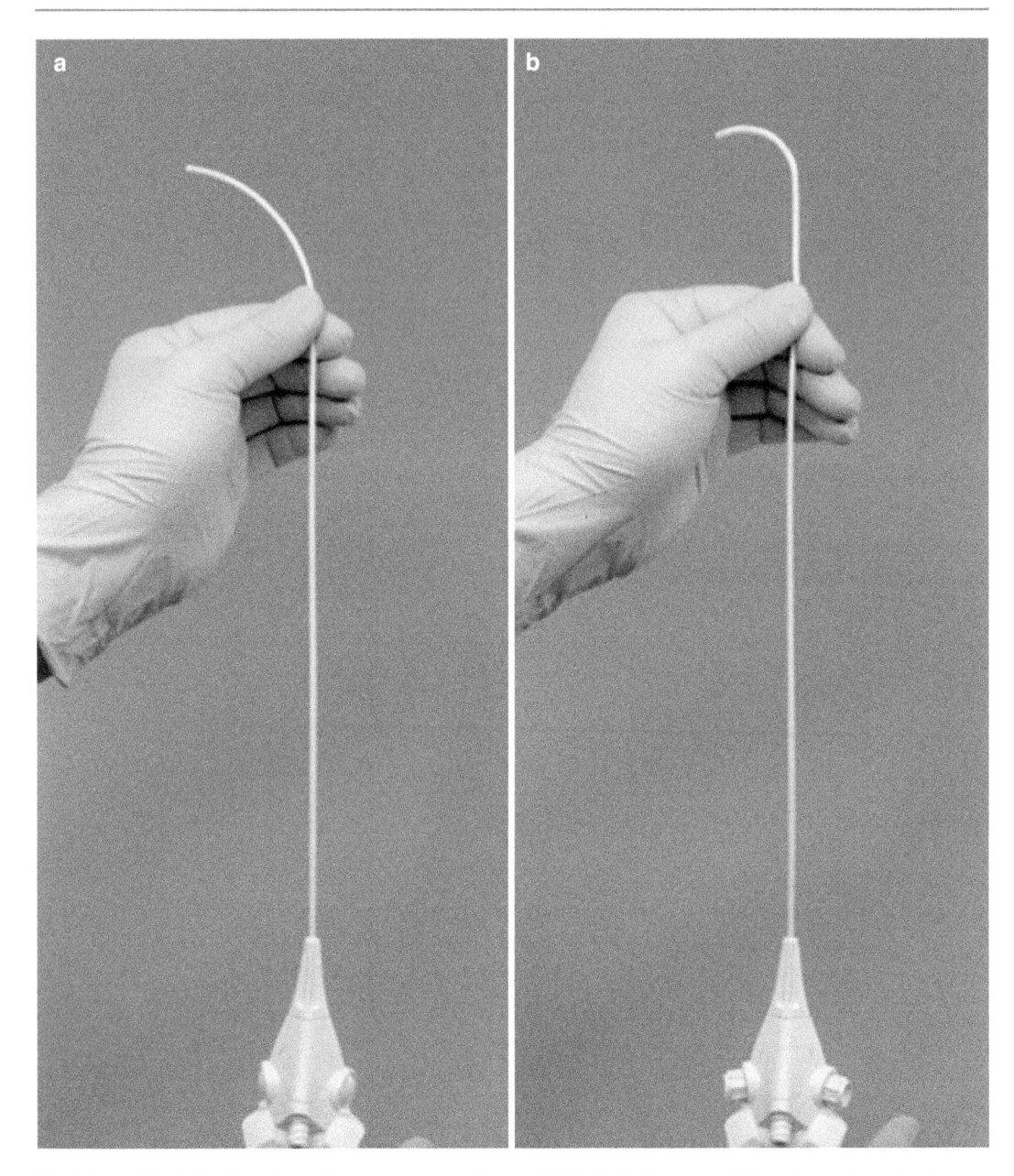

Fig. 8.1 (**a**) The ZiNeu01 catheter. The entire catheter bends. (**b**) The ZiNeuS catheter. The articulated part bends more

while using the ZiNeu01 catheter without an articulated tip may complicate the approach to the foraminal orifice, it is strong enough to penetrate into the intervertebral foramen, increasing the likelihood of a successful procedure across the entire intervertebral foramen (Figs. 8.2, 8.3 and 8.4). Since it is difficult for novice operators to use the ZiNeu01 catheter to approach the foraminal orifice, they should first familiarize themselves with the employment of the ZiNeuS catheter before trying to use the ZiNeu01 catheter.

When the ZiNeu01 catheter is used, its tip often slips after reaching the subpedicular area and enters the intervertebral foramen, which could irritate the spinal nerves located

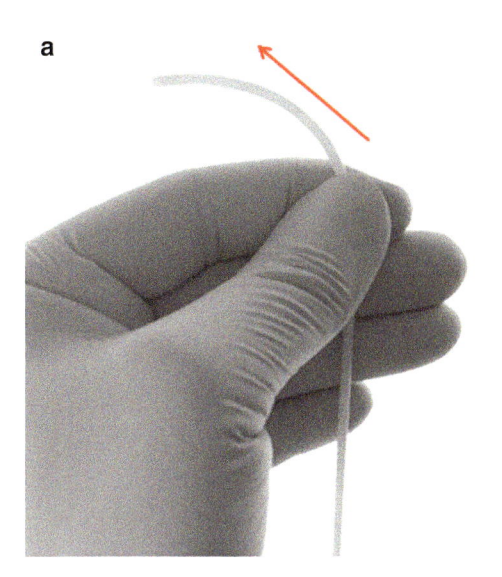

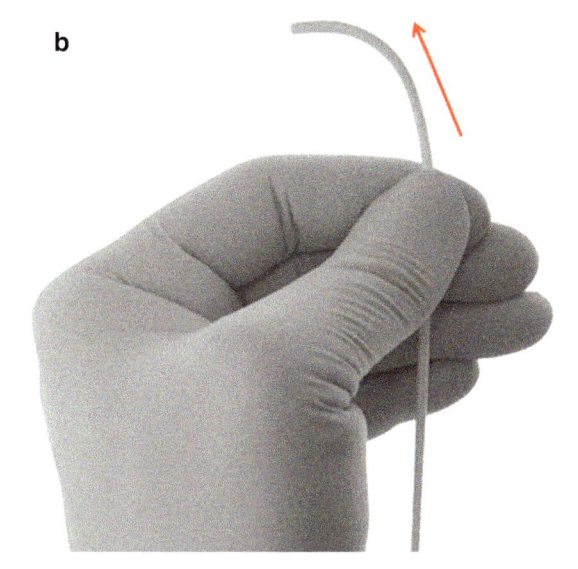

Fig. 8.2 Differences between the ZiNeu01 and ZiNeuS catheters based on the articulation of their respective tips. (**a**) The bending of the unarticulated tip of the ZiNeu01 catheter. If the catheter is inserted in this state, the force advances the catheter toward the intervertebral foramen, which increases the success rate of entry into the intervertebral foramen. (**b**) The bending of the articulated tip of the ZiNeuS catheter. The tip bends more easily, but if the catheter is inserted in this state, the force tends to advance the catheter more toward the head than the intervertebral foramen, which weakens the entry force and compromised access into the intervertebral foramen

immediately below the pedicle. This outcome eventually causes more severe pain than do eventualities resultant of using the ZiNeuS catheter.

These properties account for the variance among the preferences of operators. The author's own recommendations are as follows:

1. The ZiNeu01 catheter is selected for cases in which the intervertebral foramen or several levels of the spinal canal are the site of operation, those in which balloon decompression must be performed inside the intervertebral foramen, and those in which entry may be complicated by severe stenosis or adhesion. The ZiNeuS catheter is selected for cases in which entry appears to be easy due to the lack of severe foraminal stenosis or adhesion and for those in which the procedure itself is suspected to be easy and feature a limited possibility of inducing pain.

2. The ZiNeu01 catheter is selected for cases in which the procedure is performed only on the spinal canal with no need to enter the intervertebral foramen due to the site of the lesion; this catheter's strength achieves excellent adhesion removal.
3. The ZiNeu01 catheter is selected for cases in which the patient has previously undergone spinal surgery, as most of these cases exhibit severe adhesion.
4. The ZiNeuS catheter is selected for cases in which an endoscope must be used.

8.1.2 Selecting the ZiNeu02 Catheter

The ZiNeu02 catheter has an outer diameter of 1.55 mm and is thus recommended for operators who feel that catheters with outer diameters of 2.3 mm to be too thick. Because the catheter is

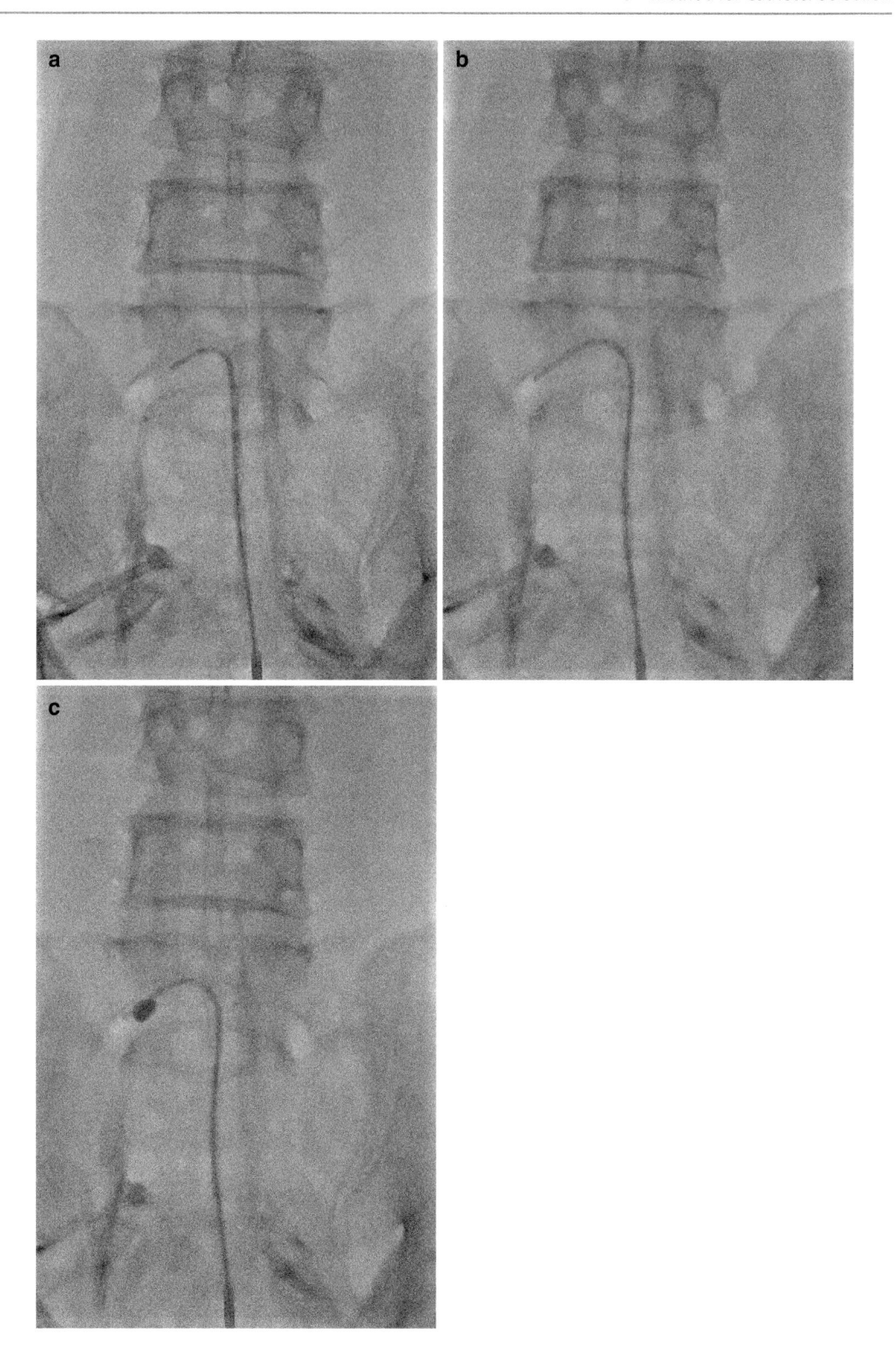

Fig. 8.3 (**a**) A case in which entry with the ZiNeuS catheter was precluded by severe foraminal adhesion. (**b**, **c**) When the ZiNeu01 catheter was used in the same patient, entry into the intervertebral foramen was successful, and balloon inflation at the exact location was completed

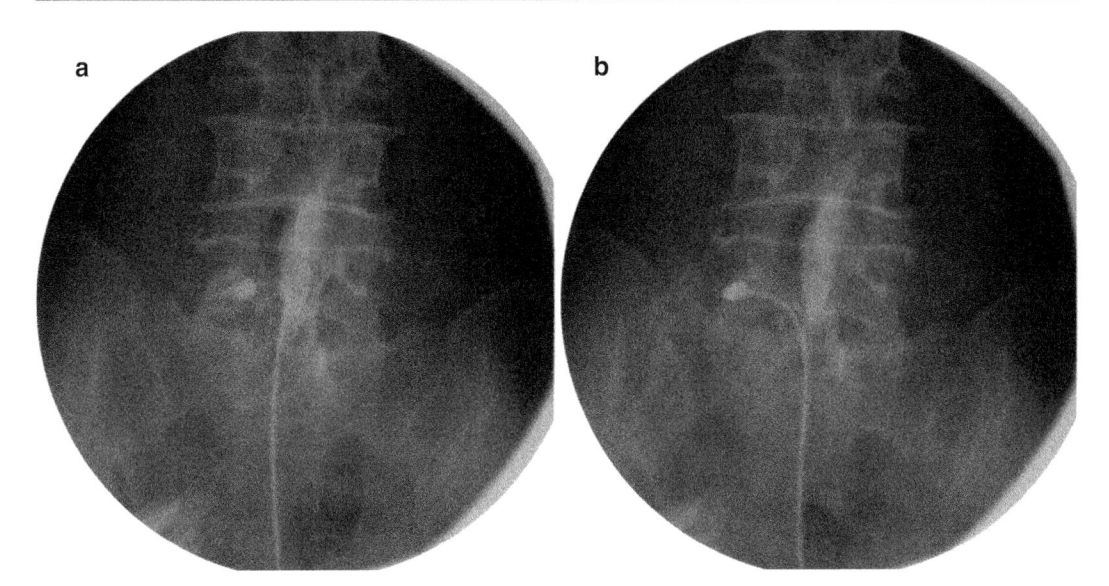

8.1 Catheter Selection Recommendations According to Case

Fig. 8.4 (**a**) A case in which the ZiNeuS catheter could not be advanced due to foraminal adhesion. (**b**) When the ZiNeu01 catheter was used in the same patient, entry into the intervertebral foramen was successful, and balloon inflation at the exact location was accomplished

thin, it facilitates the insertion of the guide needle, causes less pain, and is associated with a lower complication rate than are catheters with diameters of 2.3 mm. However, the success rate of the procedure may be low because the catheter enables the exertion of relatively low force. The author typically uses this catheter in cases of non-severe stenosis or of lesions situated at multiple levels of the spinal canal or intervertebral foramen. In particular, younger pains are more sensitive to pain; hence, the ZiNeu02 catheter should be selected for such patients whenever possible.

Although the ZiNeu02 catheter contains a guidewire, it has little impact on increasing the strength of the catheter. Accordingly, the guidewire is not used in many cases; the contrast dye is passed through the catheter instead to make the catheter more readily visible in C-arm images. The author typically uses the guidewire to facilitate drug delivery by passing the wire through the intervertebral foramen and creating a path by which entry into the intervertebral foramen is facilitated—not for reinforcing strength. A more thorough description of this is included in the section on the procedural methods used for the ZiNeu catheter.

The ZiNeu02 catheter has a relatively high satisfaction rating since it features higher strength than expected—despite being thin. However, as mentioned earlier, if the ZiNeu02 catheter was selected because the procedure was suspected to be easy, and is in fact complicated by severe adhesion or stenosis, the selection of the 2.3-mm catheter would have likely been more prudent. Therefore, a 2.3-mm catheter should always be used unless the patient is young or there are specific indications to the contrary.

8.1.3 Selecting Between the ZiNeuF and ZiNeuF03 Catheters

Unlike the ZiNeu series catheters, ZiNeuF and ZiNeuF03 have limited lateral mobility and weak strength due to their thinness. However, they offer the advantage of being less costly. The ZiNeuF catheter is a 2F balloon catheter with a reinforcing wire, whereas the ZiNeuF03 catheter is a 3F balloon catheter with reinforcing wire, which also allows concurrent balloon decompression and drug administration.

If the lesion is localized inside the intervertebral foramen, using the transforaminal or interlaminar approach could provide high success rate than the caudal approach. The reason is, because of the short distance from the needle tip to the lesion, the force used to penetrate into the lesion becomes stronger. In other words, when attempting to enter the intervertebral foramen by the caudal approach, the distance from the sacral hiatus to the intervertebral foramen is farther, causing the penetrating force to be weaker than the transforaminal or interlaminar approach. Therefore, the ZiNeu series catheter could be used with the caudal approach in cases with lesions in multiple sites, but when the lesion is localized in the intervertebral foramen, it is better to use the ZiNeuF series catheter with the transforaminal or interlaminar approach.

8.2 Catheter Selection Recommendations According to the Procedural Approach

8.2.1 Transforaminal Approach

Thinner catheters, such as the ZiNeuF catheter, cause less pain and facilitate access into small, narrow areas. In the intervertebral foramen, because the needle tip and the target area come into close contact with each other, the drug must be injected through the needle to ensure that the drug spreads efficiently into the target area. When the ZiNeuF03 catheter is inserted, and the drug is injected through the catheter, the drug may leak through the needle (backflow). Therefore, the ZiNeuF catheter is recommended for the transforaminal approach rather than the ZiNeu03 catheter.

8.2.2 Interlaminar Approach

When injecting the drug through the needle upon completion of the procedure, the drug may not always spread efficiently into the intervertebral foramen; as this complication requires drug injection through the catheter, the ZiNeuF03 catheter is well-suited to this procedure. However, operators who prefer thinner catheters may use the ZiNeuF catheter to perform balloon decompression and subsequently inject the drug after rupturing the balloon in the target area by overinflating it. Alternatively, they can rupture the balloon after completely withdrawing the ZiNeuF catheter from the body, reinsert a catheter that includes a reinforcing wire, and inject the drug.

8.2.3 Caudal Approach

The ZiNeu Series catheter is undoubtedly superior to the ZiNeuF03 catheter with respect to the convenience of use and associated operative success rates. However, in the cases listed below, using the ZiNeuF03 catheter to perform the procedure in a manner similar to the use of the Racz catheter and injecting hypertonic saline for 2–3 days should be considered. This strategy features the particular advantage of allowing for the repeated performances of balloon decompression with the catheter left in the target area across several days.

> Cases in which injecting hypertonic saline after placing the ZiNeuF03 catheter should be considered:
>
> - In patients with lesions localized to one or two sites and mild cases in which entry with the ZiNeuF03 catheter may be possible—i.e., cases in which the procedure appears to be easy and performed with this much strength.
> - Patients with lesions in the spinal canal than that are less severe than those in the intervertebral foramen.
> - Patients who, on account of exhibiting neuropathic pain, are associated with a high risk of failing to respond to treatment. Balloon decompression and the administration of hypertonic saline for 2–3 days could help to alleviate neuropathic pain.
> - Severe cases in which the use of ZiNue series catheters is not expected to yield much improvement due to overly extensive/severe stenosis or adhesion. The cost-effectiveness of the ZiNeuF03 renders it superior in this case.

8.2 Catheter Selection Recommendations According to the Procedural Approach

- Patients for whom the use of the ZiNeu series catheter would incur an excessive financial burden.

8.2.4 Simultaneous Application of Two Approaches

When lesions present in multiple levels of the spinal canal or intervertebral foramen, the ZiNeu series catheter should be used. However, as aforementioned, this catheter is deficient in some cases: it may not allow for the exertion of enough strength to penetrate the intervertebral foramen when there is severe stenosis or adhesion. The ZiNeuS catheter is more susceptible to this shortcoming than is the ZiNeu01 catheter without articulation. Indeed, the weakness of the catheter may also preclude the performance of balloon decompression at the site of the major lesion. In such cases, the employment of the ZiNeu series catheter in all areas, except the intervertebral foramen, is recommended. The ZiNeuF series catheter can then be additionally inserted into the intervertebral foramen via the transforaminal or interlaminar approach to complete the procedure. In other words, the procedure can be performed with the ZiNeu series catheter when lesions present in several levels of the spinal canal or intervertebral foramen; if entry into the intervertebral foramen is impossible, the ZiNeuF series catheter could be subsequently inserted into the intervertebral foramen via the transforaminal or interlaminar approaches to complete the procedure (Figs. 8.5 and 8.6).

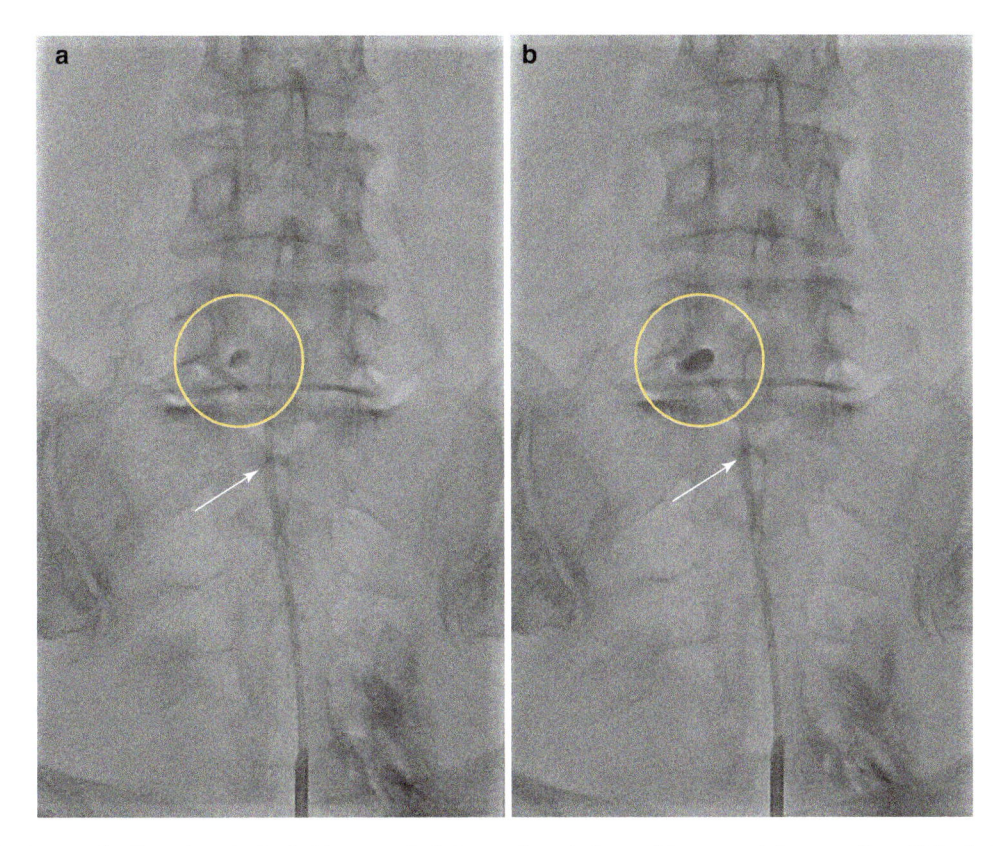

Fig. 8.5 (**a**, **b**) Entry into the Lt. L5 intervertebral foramen with the ZiNeuS catheter could not be achieved. As a result, the ZiNeuF catheter was inserted into the Lt. L5 intervertebral foramen via the transforaminal approach and was used to inflate the balloon. (**c**) The AP and (**d**) lateral views of the contrast dye spreading efficiently into the expanded area after the procedure. Circle: The inflated balloon of the ZiNeuF catheter that was inserted into the intervertebral foramen. Arrow: The ZiNeuS catheter inserted into the caudal space

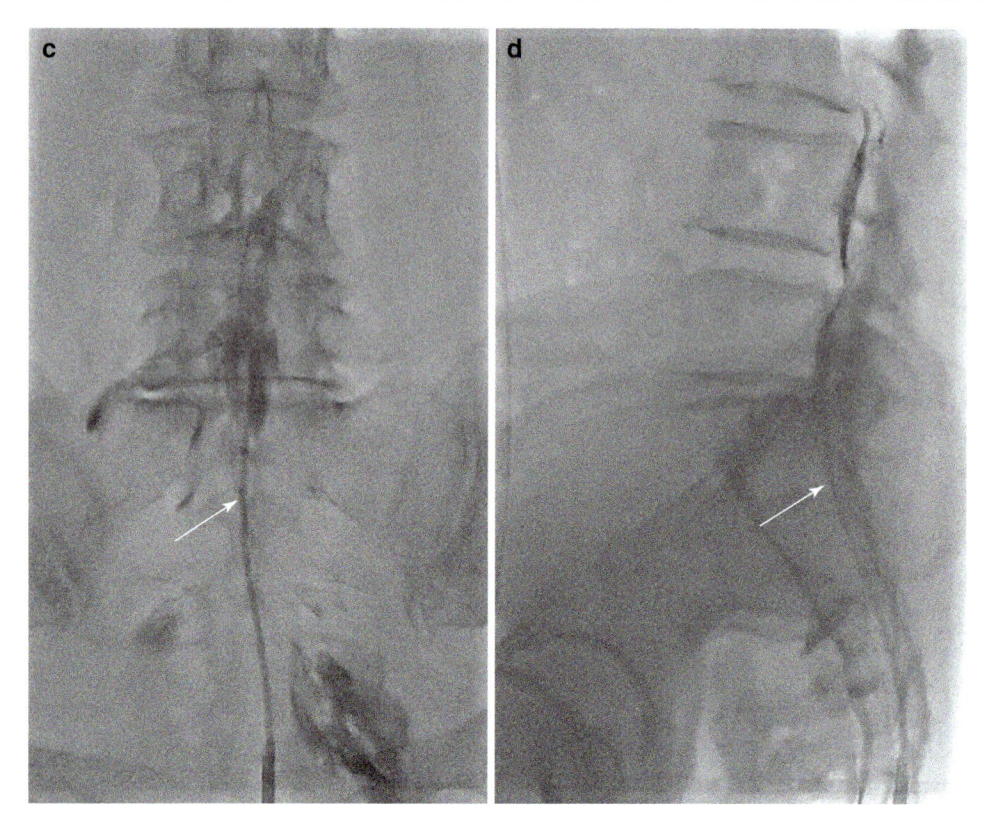

Fig. 8.5 (continued)

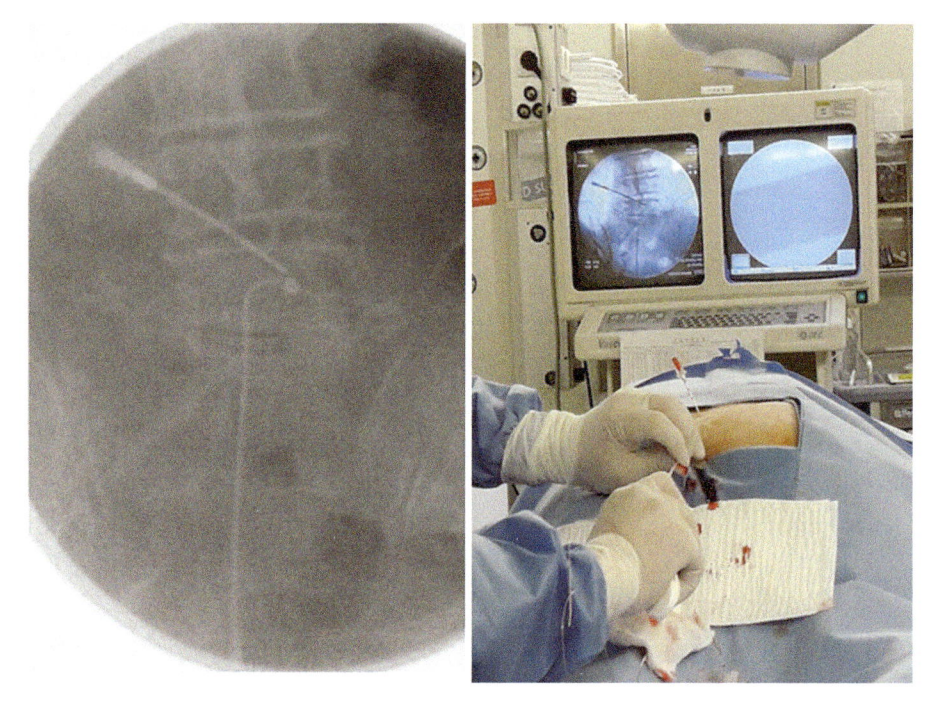

Fig. 8.6 A case in which entry into the Rt. L5 intervertebral foramen using the ZiNeuS catheter could not be achieved, and the transforaminal approach was rendered difficult by the high iliac crest. The ZiNeuF catheter was subsequently inserted into the Rt. L5 intervertebral foramen via the interlaminar approach

8.2 Catheter Selection Recommendations According to the Procedural Approach

Generally, there are only one or two types of medical devices available. From the operator's perspective, this limitation of options may facilitate selection; however, procedures may fail due to the unavailability of appropriate devices. Hence, employing devices that can adapt to a variety of cases—as in the case of the ZiNeu catheters—could be useful when considering the resultant increases in the success rate of procedures and their cost-effectiveness.

Extraneous Knowledge 9

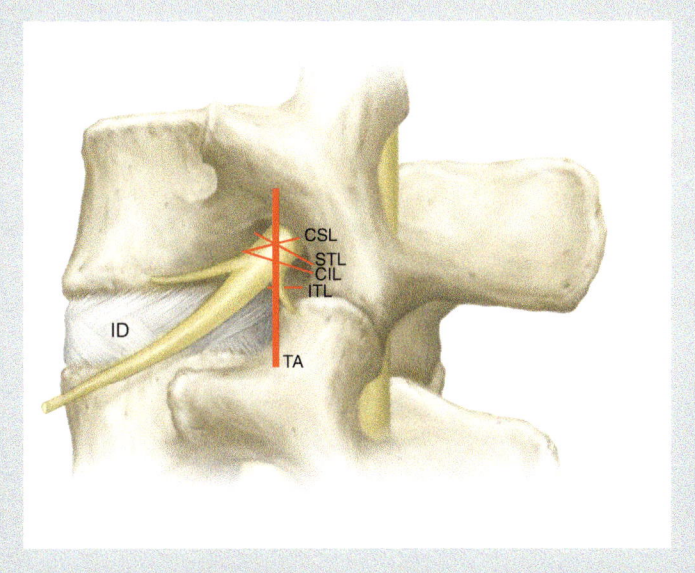

CSL : corporotransverse superior ligament
CIL : corporotransverse inferior ligament
STL : superior transforaminal ligament
ITL : inferior transforaminal ligament
TA : tendinous arcus of intertransverse ligament

Fig. E1 Types and functions of the transforaminal ligament

The ligaments shown in the figure are commonly observed transforaminal ligaments. Their key functions include partitioning blood vessels, nerves, and lymphatic vessels to prevent them from interfering with or compressing each other, as well as preventing nerve traction and reducing stenosis.

The superior aspect of the intervertebral foramen is wide, forming an inverted triangular structure. If the inferior transforaminal ligament (ITL) that supports the spinal nerves from beneath were not present, the spinal nerves would descend into the narrow area of the inferior aspect of the intervertebral foramen, causing stenosis or compressing blood vessels thereat band impairing circulation. Hence, intentional injury to this ligament is not desirable.

Some theories claim that transforaminal ligaments could actually exacerbate cases of foraminal stenosis and thus argue for the cutting or removal of these ligaments. While most of the ligaments are observable up to the L1–L3 intervertebral foramen, the number of observable ligaments decrease in the L4–L5 intervertebral foramen—i.e., the lower level of the intervertebral foramen—where foraminal stenosis usually occurs. However, as this area features relatively fewer ligaments, removing the ligaments may contribute significantly to the resolution of stenosis. In fact, injury to the inferior transforaminal ligament may actually exacerbate stenosis. Therefore, whether resecting the transforaminal is therapeutically beneficial requires further research.

9

Methods for Determining the Site of Procedure According to Case

Just as with any procedure, many factors can influence the outcome of balloon decompression, including whether the right patients were selected, whether the diagnosis and areas targeted by the procedure were correct, whether the operator performed the procedure on all areas that required treatment, and the drugs administered during the procedure as well as their manner of delivery.

While developing the ZiNeu catheters and promoting balloon decompression, the author has trained many physicians and observed the performance of numerous procedures by other doctors. It thus became clear that an excessive number of procedures were completed in haste due to limited time, too many patients were misdiagnosed, and errors were made concerning the areas requiring treatment. In particular, in many cases involving patients with foraminal lesions, the operator performed one or two rounds of balloon decompression and injected the drug after haphazardly inserting the catheter into the spinal canal rather than expending the necessary effort to insert the catheter into the intervertebral foramen. Performing the procedure in such a manner compromises the benefits of balloon decompression, and the operation consequently differs very little from an epidural block. Needless to say, the outcome of such instances would be unsatisfactory. While the lack of improvement in the patient's symptoms may be ascribed to misdiagnosis or an inappropriately performed procedure, the operator and patient may instead consider balloon decompression itself to have been ineffective.

This chapter will provide detailed explanations of actual cases that illustrate the type of procedure to be performed for various patients. It is hoped that this chapter will facilitate referencing the patient's specific condition to select the area(s) to target during the procedure. Briefly, when determining these area(s), the patient's symptoms, MRI findings, and epidurogram findings should be assessed comprehensively. Moreover, the procedure should not be performed in areas unrelated to the symptoms.

9.1 Cases Involving Procedures in the Retrodiscal Area at the Level Immediately Above the Intervertebral Foramen

Case 1 A 72-year-old man complained of low back, Rt. L5 radiculopathy and claudication after 20 min of walking. Although low back pain was reduced slightly after neuroplasty was performed with the Racz catheter 2 years previously, the patient's leg pain did not improve. A few subsequent rounds of epidural block showed improvement that lasted only 1 week. MRI findings showed Rt. L5 foraminal stenosis and L4–5 central stenosis, whereas the epidurogram findings showed fill-

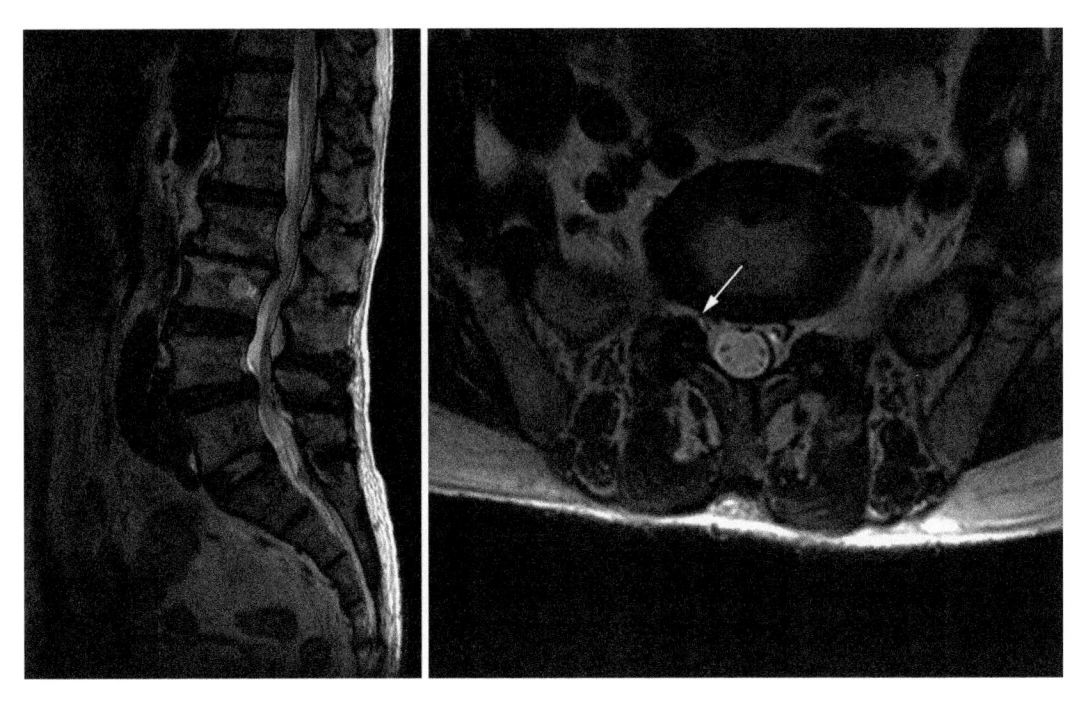

Fig. 9.1 MRI findings. Central L4–5 stenosis with Rt. L5 foraminal stenosis. Arrow: Rt. L5 foraminal stenosis

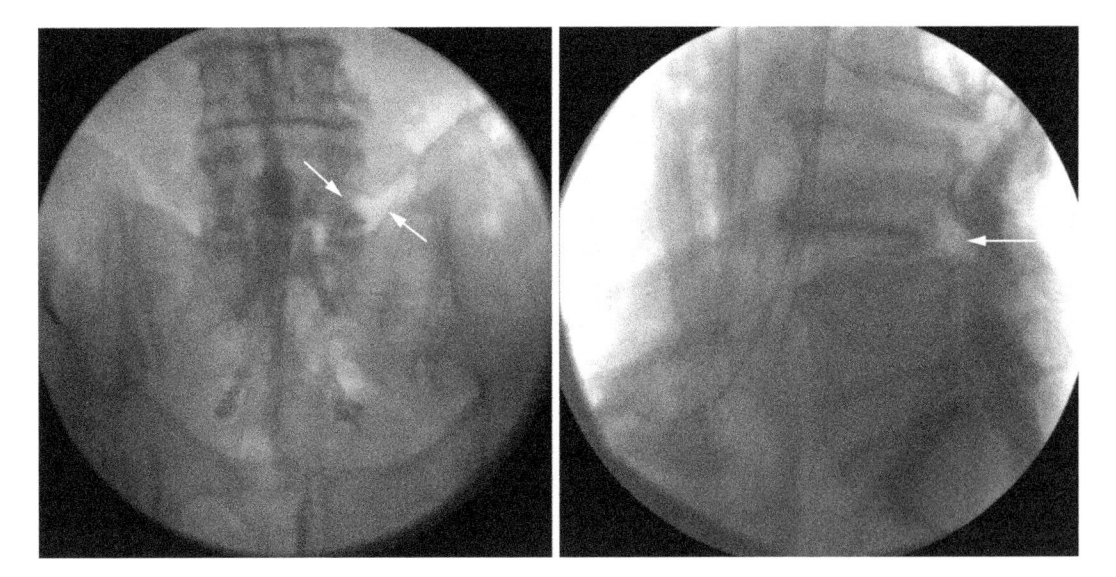

Fig. 9.2 Epidurogram findings. Observations of filling defects in the superior aspect of the Rt. L5 foramen and L4–5 retrodiscal area are consistent with the patient's symptoms. Arrow: Filling defect areas

ing defects in the superior aspect of the Rt. L5 foramen, i.e., around the root, and L4–5 retrodiscal area (Figs. 9.1 and 9.2). Based on these findings, it was determined that the procedure should be performed on the Rt. L4–5 retrodiscal area, superior aspect of the Rt. L5 foramen, and Rt. L5 preganglion area. Balloon decompression was performed accordingly. After the procedure, all filling defects were resolved, and the patient maintained a good condition up to the 9-month follow-up with an NRS of 2 points and experienced no difficulty in walking (Figs. 9.3 and 9.4).

9.1 Cases Involving Procedures in the Retrodiscal Area at the Level Immediately Above...

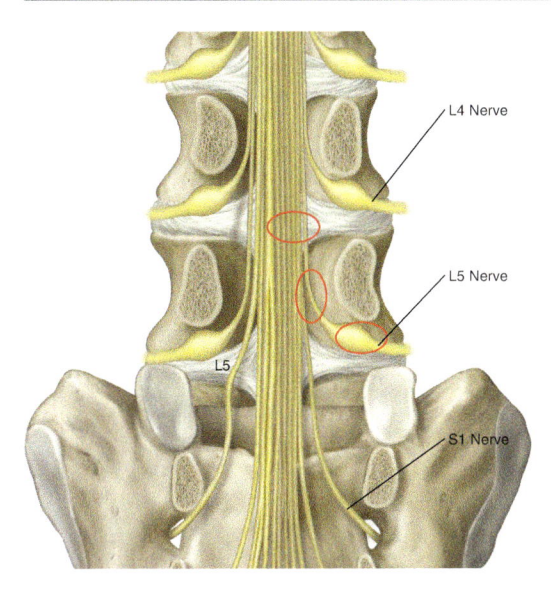

Fig. 9.3 Circle: Areas where the procedure was performed. After conducting the procedure through the anterior epidural space, it was also performed in the central area of the posterior epidural space

As illustrated by the case presented above, if L4–5 central stenosis is present and the patient's symptoms include Rt. L5 radiculopathy, filling defects in the superior aspect of the Rt. L5 foramen, preganglion, and L4–5 retrodiscal area should be checked and the procedure should specifically target those areas. Rt. L5 radiculopathy or claudication occurs when a lesion presents in at least one of these three areas. Because there were no symptoms on the patient's left side, the procedure in the retrodiscal area targeted only the right side. Adhesion in the posterior epidural space is highly associated with low back pain, but the patient evinced almost no filling defects in the posterior epidural space and his low back pain was not severe. Accordingly, the procedure was not performed in the posterior epidural space; however, time permitting, conducting the procedure therein would be prudent. As the success of procedure in the Rt. L5 foramen was important for the treatment of this patient, the procedure was performed with the ZiNeu01 catheter.

If the patient exhibits L4 radiculopathy and an L3–4 central lesion or stenosis, balloon decompression should be performed in the L3–4 retrodiscal area, L4 preganglion, and L4 foramen. In such cases, the catheter must always be inserted into the superior aspect of the foramen adjacent

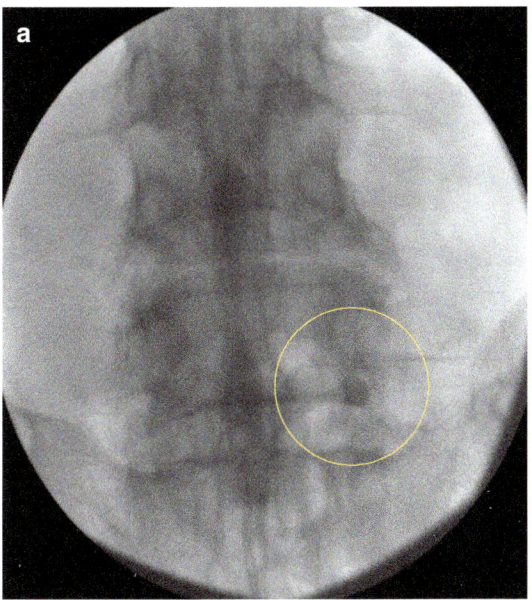

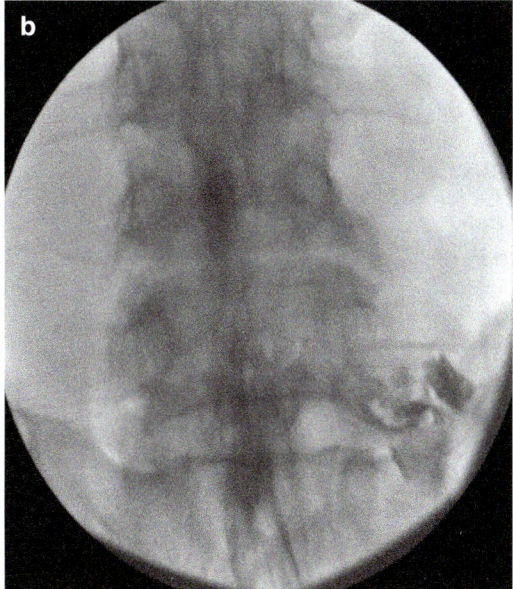

Fig. 9.4 (**a**) Image of balloon decompression performed in the Rt. L5 foramen. (**b**) Image of filling defects resolved after balloon decompression in the Rt. L5 foramen. (**c**) Image of balloon decompression performed in the Rt. L4–5 retrodiscal area. (**d**) Epidurogram image of filling defects in the retrodiscal area before the procedure. (**e**) Image of filling defects resolved after the procedure and the spread of the contrast dye spreading into the anterior epidural space. Yellow circle: Inflated balloon. Arrow: Anterior epidural space

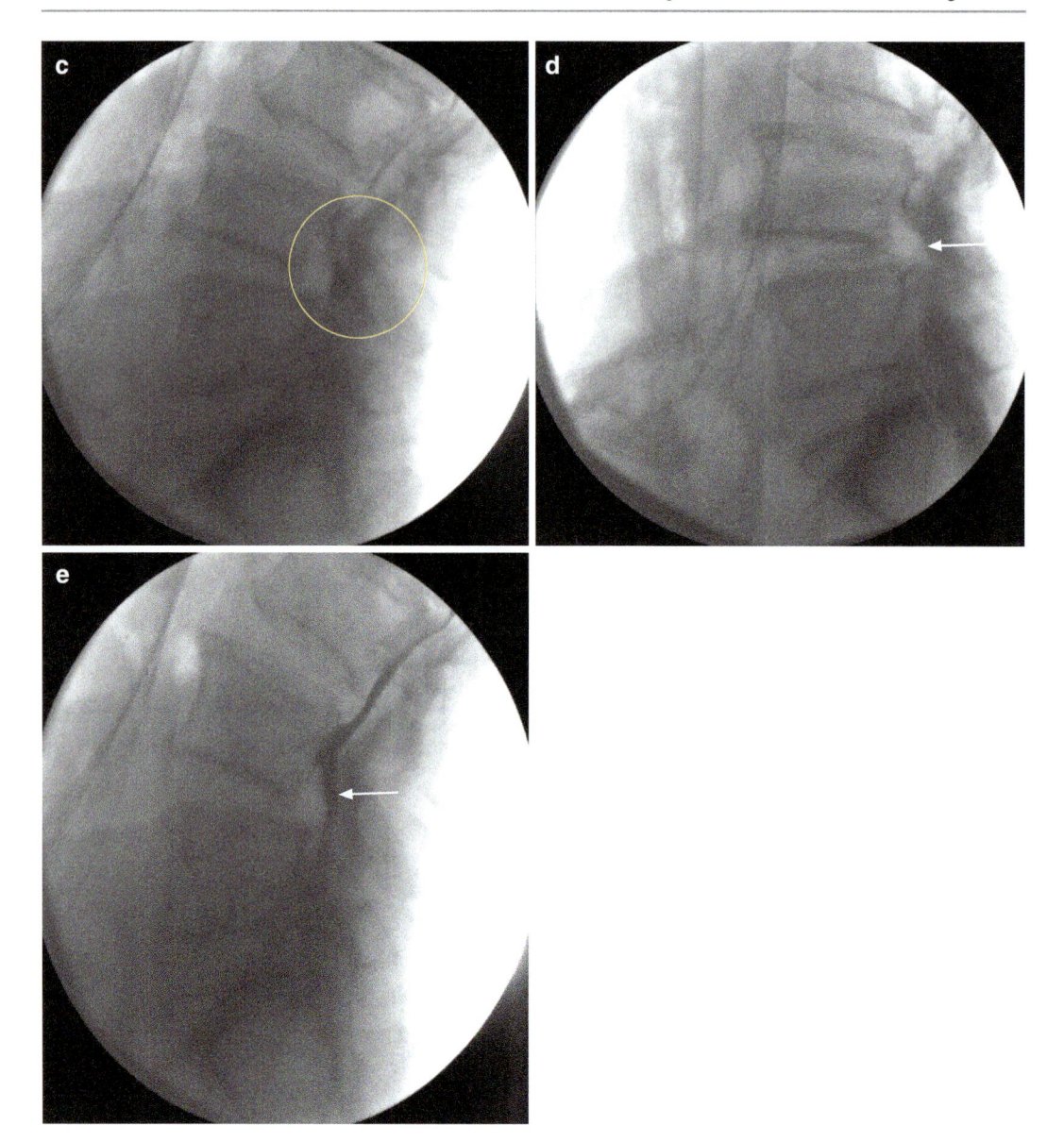

Fig. 9.4 (continued)

to the nerve's trajectory—there is a high likelihood of adhesion being present near this area.

Case 2 A 74-year-old man who had undergone L4–5 PLIF surgery for right L5 radiculopathy 1 year previously visited the pain clinic with the same symptoms that had presented again 1 month earlier. The patient could only walk for 3 min before having to stop. The benefits derived from the three rounds of caudal epidural block lasted no more than 1 week each time. MRI findings showed bilateral L5 foraminal stenosis. However, the patient's only symptom was Rt. L5 radiculopathy; therefore, balloon decompression was performed with the ZiNeu01 catheter in the right Rt. L5 foramen, preganglion, and Rt. L4–5 retrodiscal area. Due to the high probability of adhesion near the L5 traversing nerve as a result of the

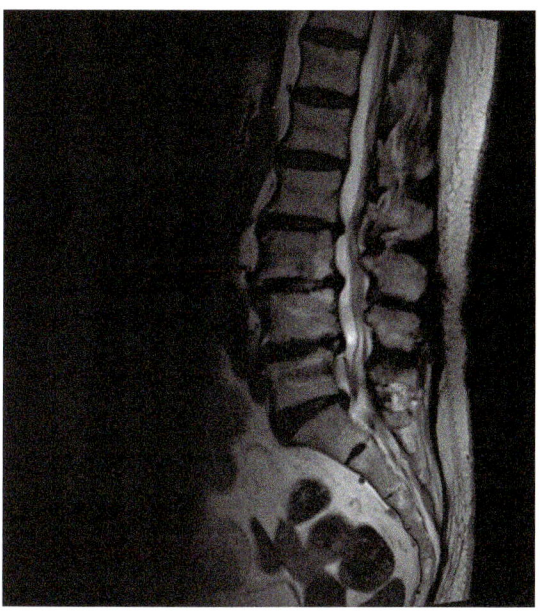

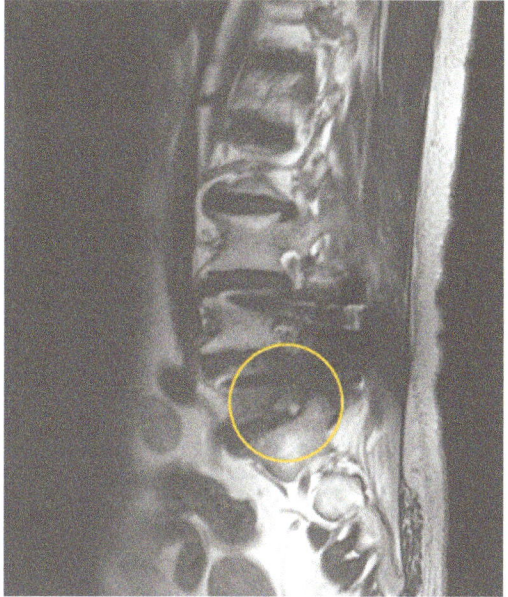

Fig. 9.5 MRI findings. L4–5 PLIF with bilateral L5 foraminal stenosis

PLIF surgery, it was determined that the procedure should also include the Rt. L4–5 retrodiscal area and that the success of the procedure depended on the Rt. L5 foramen (Fig. 9.5).

The procedure in the Rt. L5 foramen was successful. Although balloon decompression in the Rt. L4–5 retrodiscal area could not be confirmed, an L4–5 disc extrusion precluded the advancement of the catheter to that area. So, balloon decompression in the Rt. L4–5 retrodiscal area could not be performed. However, balloon decompression in the Rt. L5 preganglion area was possible (Fig. 9.6).

Following the procedure, the patient felt no pain during the following 1 month, and a pain reduction of ≥50% was sustained for up to 4 months. Despite not performing the procedure in the Rt. L4–5 retrodiscal area, the patient did not experience pain during the 1 month following the procedure. It can be assumed from these outcomes that the patient's Rt. L5 radiculopathy was caused by the Rt. L5 foraminal stenosis; thus, it was determined that if additional procedures were needed, transforaminal balloon decompression using the ZiNeuF catheter would suffice.

In such cases, whether the caudal approach with the ZiNeu catheter or the transforaminal/interlaminar approach with the ZiNeuF catheter is to be selected depends on the preferences of the operator. The author tends to perform the procedure with the ZiNeu01 catheter in patients with a history of spinal fusion surgery because such patients are expected to have extensive adhesion, and the procedure enables the treatment of a broader area or several areas. Moreover, because the success of foraminal procedure is important, the ZiNeuF catheter is also inserted if entry into the intervertebral foramen is impossible with the ZiNeu01 catheter. Thus, the general rule in this patient is to perform the procedure using the ZiNeu01 catheter in the L4–5 retrodiscal, preganglion, and Rt. L5 foramen; however, if entry into the Rt. L5 foramen is difficult, Rt. L5 transforaminal balloon decompression is to be performed with the ZiNeuF catheter simultaneously.

Because there is a high risk of dural puncture when performing the procedure in patients with a history of spinal fusion surgery, the procedure should be conducted carefully on only the area(s) associated with pain.

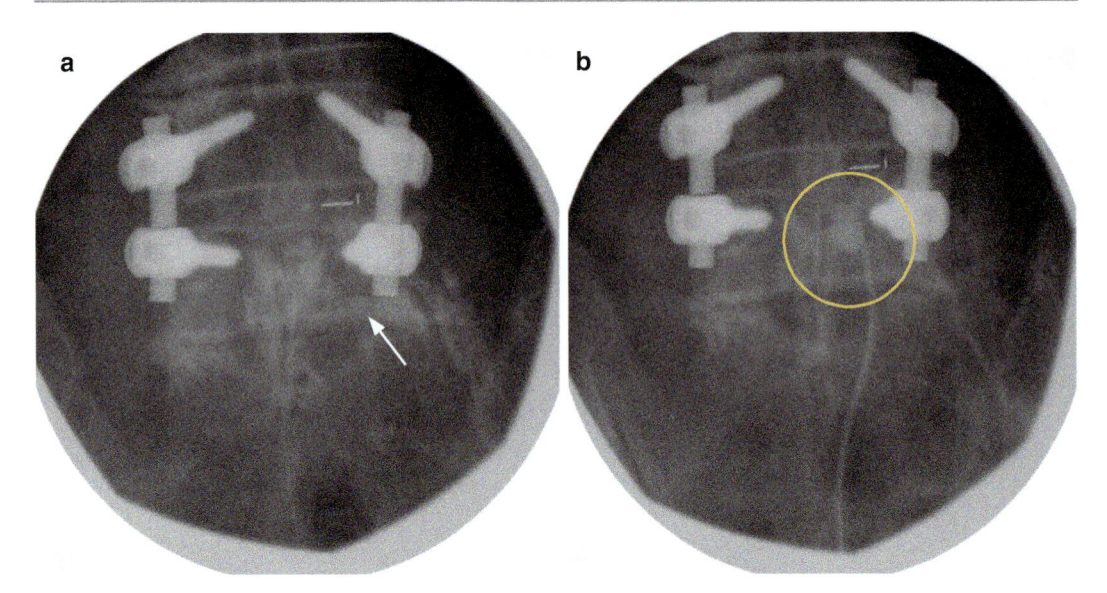

Fig. 9.6 (**a**) Image of the ZiNeu01 catheter inserted into the Rt. L5 foramen. Arrow: Catheter placed inside the intervertebral foramen. (**b**) Performance of balloon decompression in the Rt. L5 preganglion area. Yellow circle: Inflated balloon

9.2 Cases Involving Procedures in the Intervertebral Foramen

If the lesion is localized near the intervertebral foramen and symptoms are due solely to that lesion, then the catheter should be inserted only into the affected intervertebral foramen.

Case 1 A 59-year-old woman visited the pain clinic with complaints of being unable to walk for more than 15 min due to stiffness and pain in the Rt. hip and leg (Rt. L5 dermatome) that began 8 months prior (Fig. 9.7). MRI findings showed only Rt. L5 foraminal stenosis (Fig. 9.8).

The patient had previously undergone two rounds of epidural block at another hospital, and the improvement in symptoms after the procedure lasted for about 3 days each time. Subsequently performed neuroplasty did not significantly improve her symptoms. Rt. L5 transforaminal epidural block was performed at our hospital, but the improvement in her symptoms lasted for only 1 week. Accordingly, Rt. L5 transforaminal balloon decompression using the ZiNeuF catheter was performed (Fig. 9.9).

At the 1-month follow-up, the patient reported that her pain has subsided significantly and that she was able to walk and exercise for more than 40 min. At the 3-month follow-up, she reported no ambulatory limitations but occasional pain equivalent to an NRS of 3–4. The patient has been asymptomatic and has continued since then.

As the case of this patient demonstrates, if there is no suspicion of a lesion in the spinal canal but foraminal stenosis or a lesion is present, then it is advisable to perform balloon decompression by inserting the ZiNeuF catheter through the safe triangle. When inserting the guide needle, it should be inserted as close to the superior pedicle as possible so that the catheter can be inserted adjacent to the nerves' trajectory through this area.

If this patient also has a lesion in the Rt. L4–5 retrodiscal area, the ZiNeu catheter should be used to perform the procedure for all Rt. L4–5 retrodiscal, L5 preganglion, and L5 foramen areas. However, because this patient only had foraminal stenosis, the ZiNeuF catheter was sufficient.

Occasionally, a patient may exhibit L5 radiculopathy despite the lack of any severe lesions in the spinal canal or intervertebral foramen. In such cases, although L5 foraminal stenosis is

9.2 Cases Involving Procedures in the Intervertebral Foramen

Fig. 9.7 Patient's pain sites. The patient complained of pain along the Rt. L5 dermatome

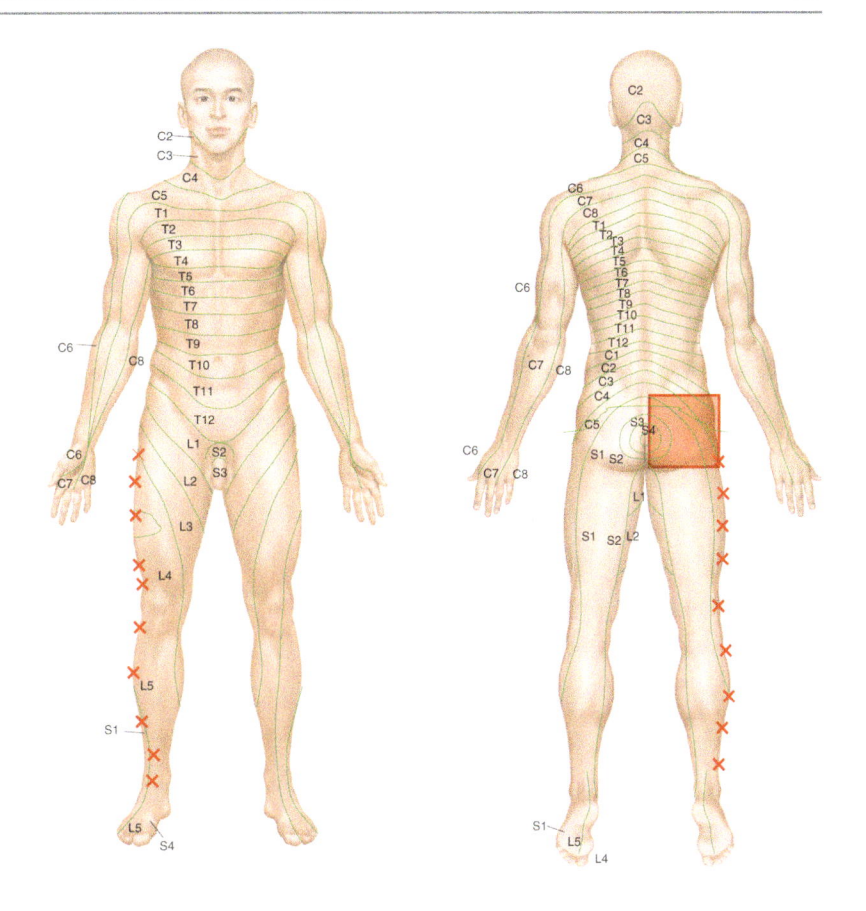

absent, the symptoms may have been caused by adhesion in the area. Therefore, L5 transforaminal block should be performed first. If the effect is temporary, then L5 transforaminal balloon decompression could be considered. However, if there is no severe lesion and L5 transforaminal block is ineffective, then balloon decompression may not show effect any improvement either. In such cases, differential diagnoses for other diseases are needed.

When treating lesions in the intervertebral foramen, it is paramount to gain entry through the superior aspect of the intervertebral foramen at the site through which the nerves pass. The following case proves this point.

Case 2 MRI findings of a 47-year-old man showed isthmic spondylolisthesis and Rt. L5 foraminal stenosis. The patient complained of Rt. hip and leg pain (L5 dermatome) that worsened while walking, rendering walking for more than 20 min difficult. Despite two rounds of Rt. L5 transforaminal block, the improvement in the patient's symptoms was sustained for only 1 week (Fig. 9.10).

The patient subsequently underwent Rt. L5 transforaminal balloon decompression with the ZiNeuF catheter. The insertion of the catheter along the nerve root was successful, and the balloon could be inflated sufficiently. The patient's symptoms improved for 6 months, but eventually recurred; the patient thus underwent the same procedure once more. This time, however, the ZiNeuF catheter could not be inserted accurately into the superior aspect of the intervertebral foramen, and the balloon was inflated in an area slightly below the intervertebral foramen. The postoperative contrast-dye findings showed that

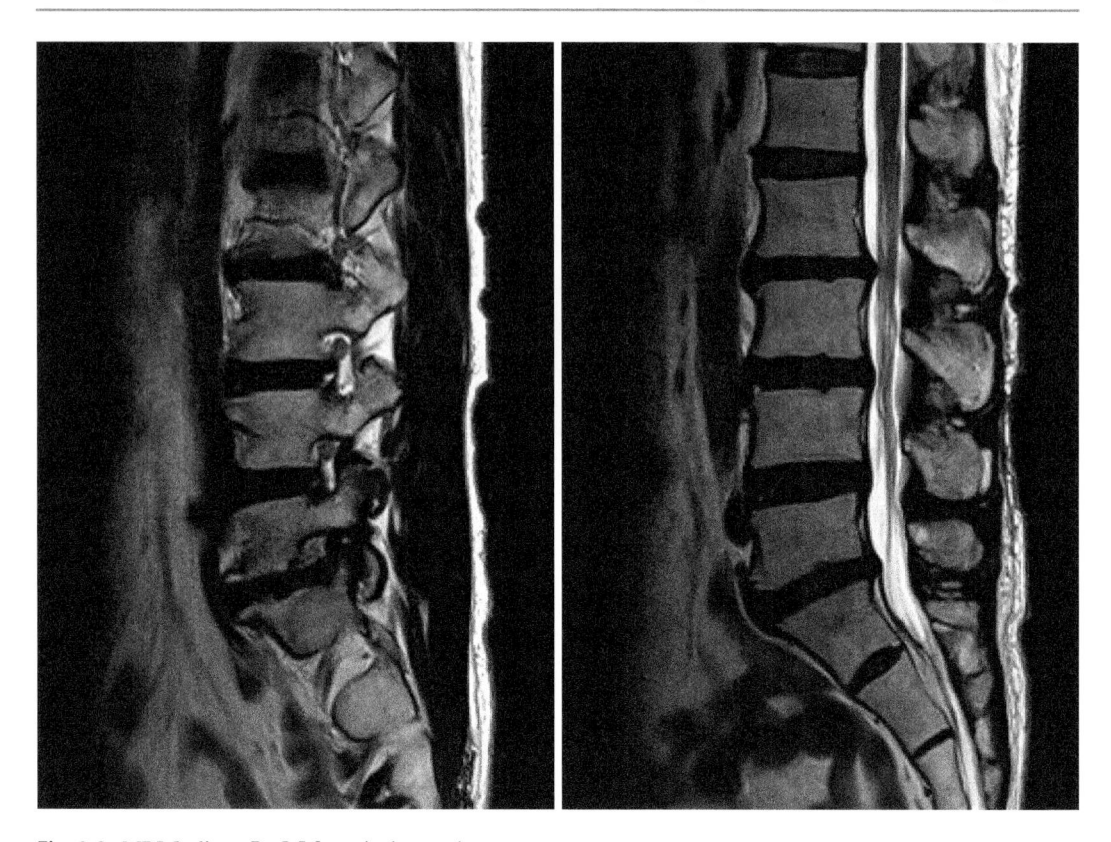

Fig. 9.8 MRI findings. Rt. L5 foraminal stenosis

the Rt. L5 filling defect remained. Because the symptoms did not improve significantly after the procedure, the patient underwent another procedure 1 month later. The catheter was inserted in the same manner as in the first procedure, and the patient had continued to do well through his last follow-up at 1 year following the procedure (Figs. 9.11 and 9.12).

This case demonstrated that when performing transforaminal balloon decompression through the safe triangle, it is essential to accurately insert the guide needle to allow the catheter to approach along the nerve root just below the pedicle.

As demonstrated by this case, if only the lesion in the intervertebral foramen area is problematic, the catheter must be inserted close to the trajectory of the nerves through the safe triangle. It should be kept in mind that simply inserting the catheter into the intervertebral foramen does not guarantee success; this consideration also applies to approaching the intervertebral foramen with other ZiNeu series catheters.

9.3 Cases Involving Procedures in the Retrodiscal Area

Case 1 A 68-year-old woman complained of Lt. L5 radiculopathy and claudication after 30 min of walking. She had undergone several rounds of Lt. L5 transforaminal epidural block, but the effect lasted only an approximate 2 weeks each time. MRI findings showed Lt. L4–5 central stenosis with Lt. L5 root compression, while epidurogram findings showed extensive filling defects on the left side (Figs. 9.13 and 9.14). Based on the determination that the symptoms were attributable to L5 nerve compression in the Lt. L4–5 retrodiscal area, balloon decompression was performed in the Lt. L4–5 retrodiscal area. The patient showed improvement in symptoms and had no problems in the 3 years following the procedure (Fig. 9.14).

In this case, Lt. L5 radiculopathy was caused not by foraminal lesion but rather by the lesion in the Lt. L4–5 retrodiscal area; therefore, this area

9.3 Cases Involving Procedures in the Retrodiscal Area

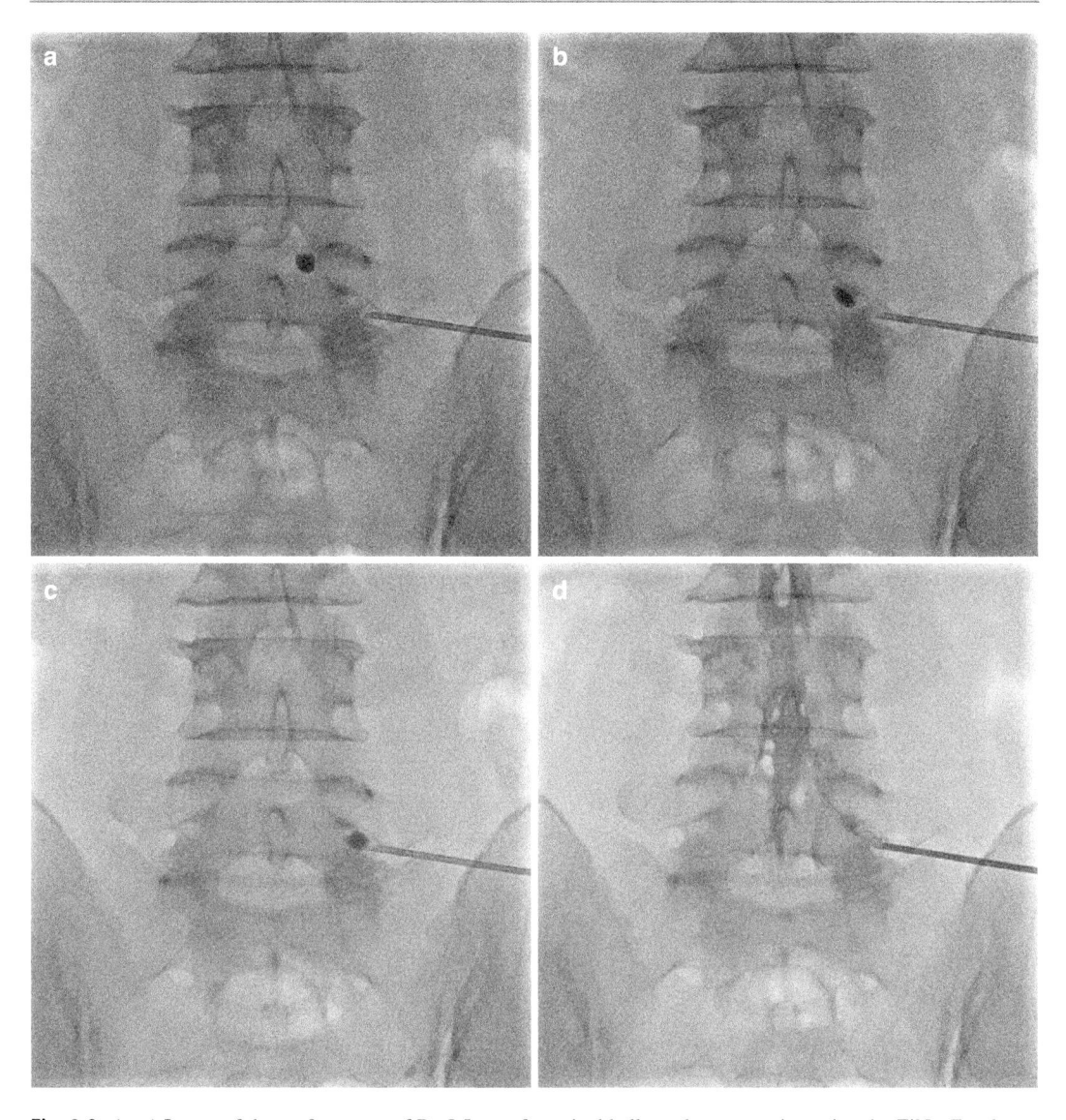

Fig. 9.9 (**a–c**) Image of the performance of Rt. L5 transforaminal balloon decompression using the ZiNeuF catheter. (**d**) Postoperative contrast-dye findings

required balloon decompression. If the procedure was meant to treat additional areas, then, time permitting, it would be advisable to also address the Lt. L5 foramen and preganglion areas as adhesion may also be present in those areas. Actually, the preganglion area was passed while approaching the retrodiscal area in this case; balloon decompression was, thus, performed only on that area, and entry into the foramen was not made.

Because there was no low back pain and posterior epidural filling defect was not observed, the procedure was not performed in the posterior epidural space. Lt. L4–5 retrodiscal balloon decompression by inserting the ZiNeuF catheter through Kambin's triangle in the Lt. L4–5 intervertebral foramen may have benefitted this patient just as much. As shown, once the target areas are determined, it is important to select the catheter that best facilitates approach to those areas.

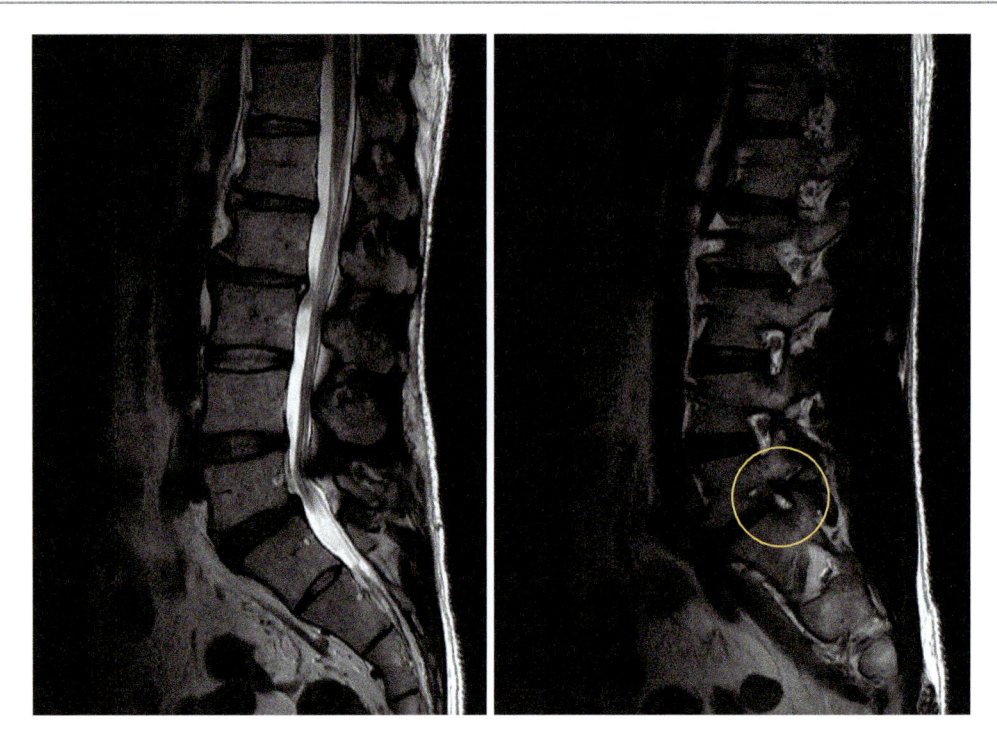

Fig. 9.10 MRI findings. Isthmic spondylolisthesis of L5 on S1 with the Rt. L5 foraminal stenosis. Yellow circle: Rt. L5 foraminal stenosis

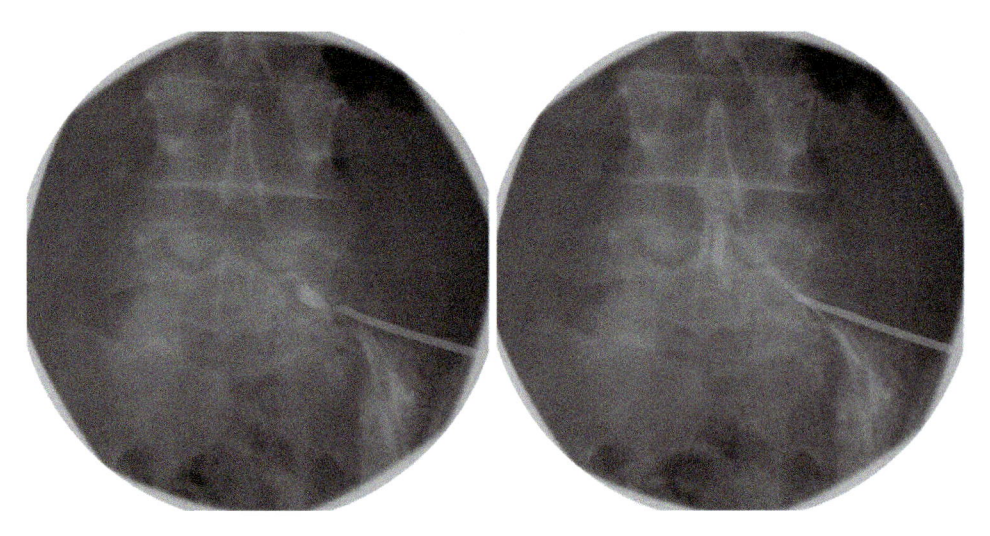

Fig. 9.11 Rt. L5 transforaminal balloon decompression through the safe triangle. The catheter enters through the superior aspect of the intervertebral foramen just below the pedicle

In summary, if the patient has L4 or L5 radiculopathy with a lesion in the upper retrodiscal area but no foraminal abnormalities, radiculopathy can be considered to be caused by lesion in the retrodiscal area and not the intervertebral foramen; accordingly, the procedure should specifically target the retrodiscal area. For such procedures, both the ZiNeu and ZiNeuF catheters could be used, and the final selection should be made by the operator after considering various other facts.

9.3 Cases Involving Procedures in the Retrodiscal Area

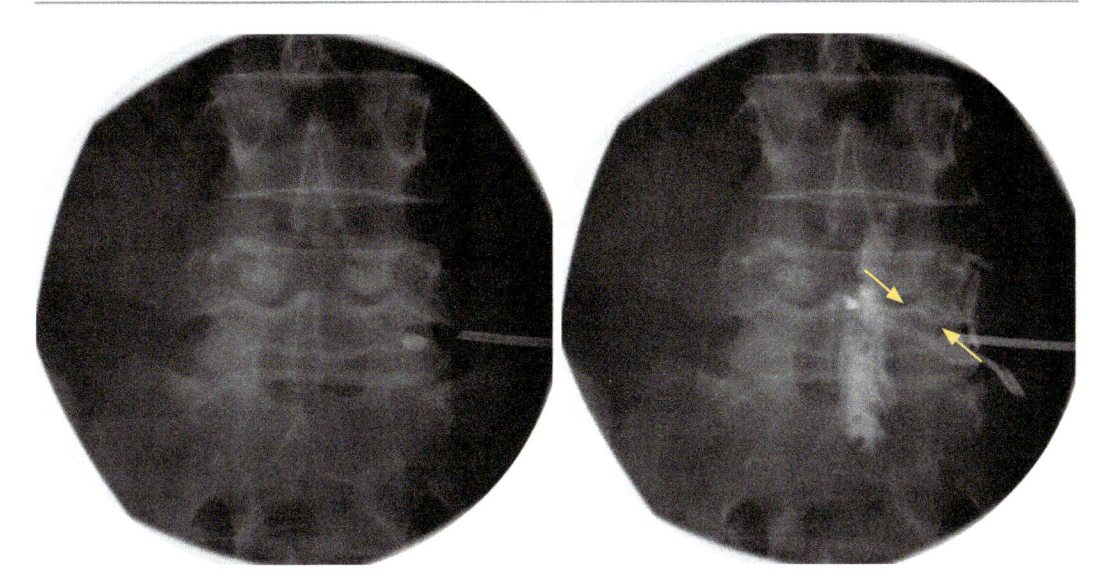

Fig. 9.12 Image of the second procedure performed 6 months after the first. Unlike the previous procedure, the ZiNeuF catheter was inaccurately guided into the superior aspect of the intervertebral foramen: instead of entering the superior aspect of the intervertebral foramen just below the pedicle, the catheter entered the inferior aspect of the intervertebral foramen. Arrow: Filling defect area. Compare this image to Fig. 9.11

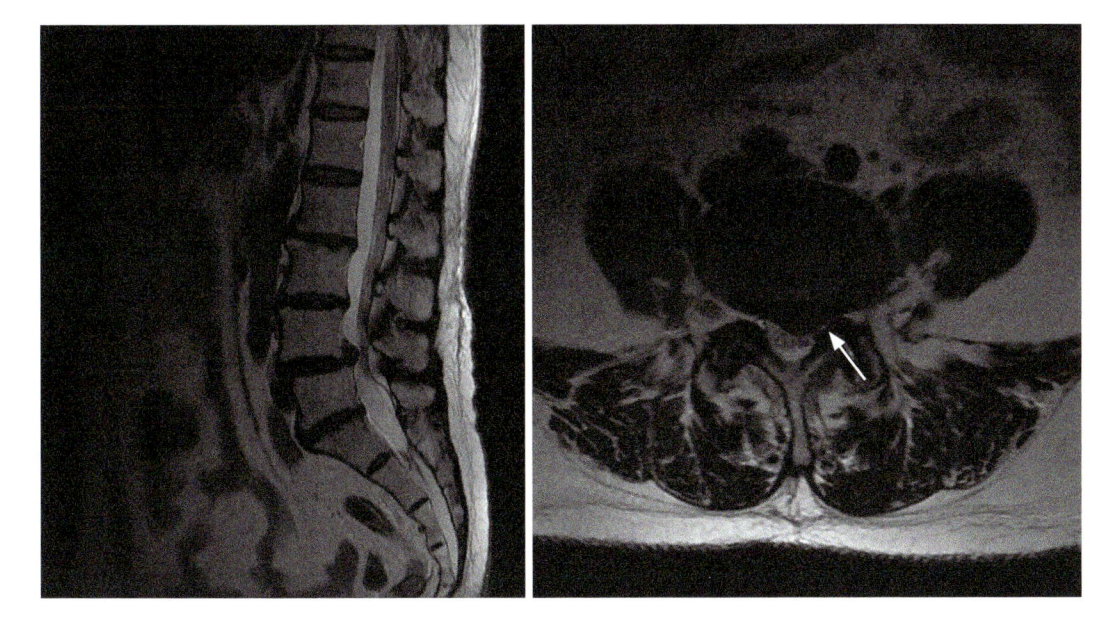

Fig. 9.13 MRI findings. Lt. L4–5 central stenosis with Lt. L5 root compression. Arrow: Compressed Lt. L5 root

Case 2 A patient who had been asymptomatic after undergoing a discectomy 13 years previously visited the pain clinic at our hospital for Rt. hip, posterior leg, and plantar pain (S1 dermatome) that had begun 4 years earlier. The patient reported that the pain grew severe after long periods of sitting or standing. MRI findings revealed that the Rt. S1 root was being compressed by the L5–S1 central protrusion. Based on the determination that the transforaminal approach would be

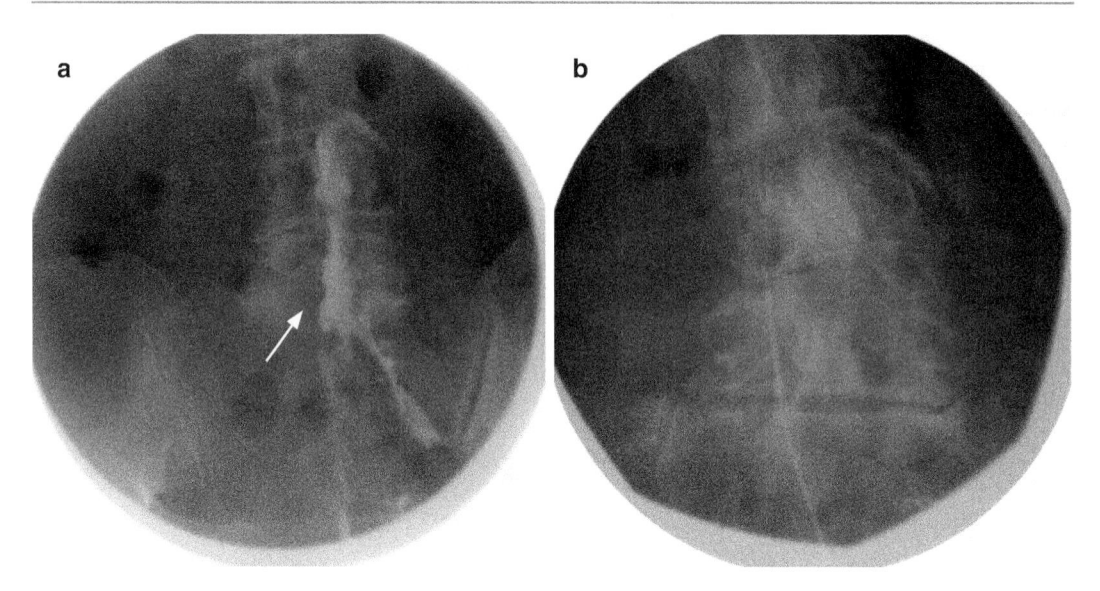

192   9 Methods for Determining the Site of Procedure According to Case

Fig. 9.14 (**a**) Extensive adhesion on the Lt. side. Arrow: Filling defect area. (**b**) Performance of balloon decompression after catheter insertion into the Lt. L4–5 retrodiscal area

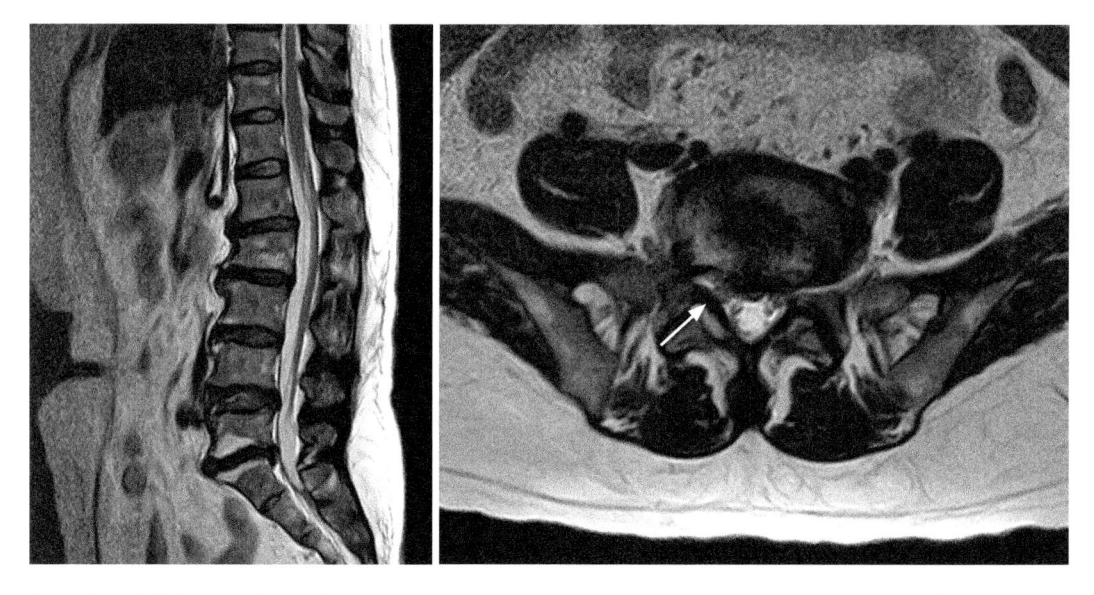

Fig. 9.15 MRI findings. Rt. L5–S1 protrusion with Rt. S1 root compression. Arrow: compressed Rt. S1 root

difficult due to the high iliac crest, the procedural plan prescribed the insertion of the ZiNeu01 catheter into the caudal epidural space to facilitate the approach to the Rt. L5–S1 retrodiscal area of the anterior epidural space and inflate the balloon for S1 root decompression (Figs. 9.15 and 9.16).

After the procedure, the patient showed 40% and 70% improvement in leg pain at the 1- and 3-month follow-ups, respectively. This improvement was sustained for approximately 1 year. If the patient did not have a high iliac crest, retrodiscal balloon decompression by the Rt. L5–S1

9.3 Cases Involving Procedures in the Retrodiscal Area

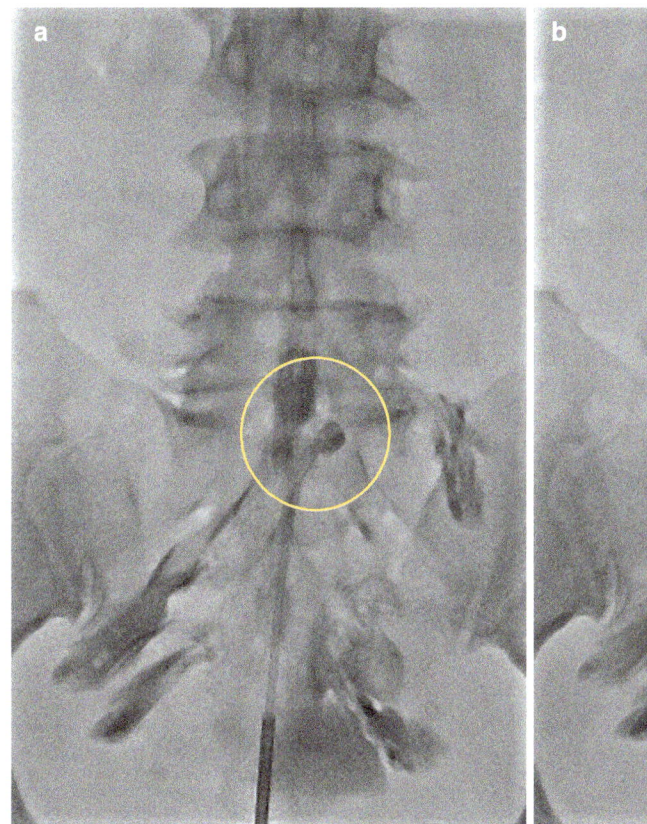

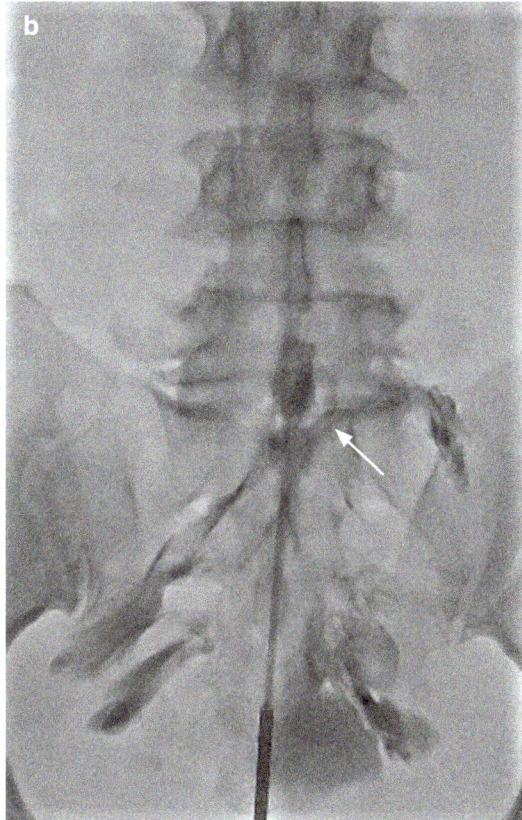

Fig. 9.16 (**a**) The inflation of the balloon near the site of nerve compression following the insertion of the ZiNeu01 catheter into the Rt. L5–S1 retrodiscal area. Yellow circle: Inflated balloon. (**b**) After deflating the balloon, the contrast dye was injected to confirm that the drug was accurately injected into the lesion. Arrow: Contrast-dye findings around the lesion

transforaminal approach using the ZiNeuF catheter would have been performed.

Case 3 The patient had undergone L4–S1 PLIF with screw fixation at another hospital 1 year previously and was treated for spondylitis 5 months earlier. The patient visited our pain clinic complaining of low back pain and Lt. leg numbness (S1 > L5 dermatome) that worsened subsequent to those treatments. While the patient exhibited no difficulty in walking, oral analgesic administration and epidural block performed at another hospital reportedly had no effect on alleviating the patient's symptoms (Fig. 9.17).

The patient's symptoms may have been caused by adhesion that developed after the PLIF surgery; however, based on a greater suspicion of L3–4 stenosis (adjacent segmental degeneration: ASD), L3–4 retrodiscal balloon decompression with the ZiNeuF catheter was performed with the transforaminal approach (Fig. 9.18).

The procedure was performed successfully around the lesion area, and the patient reported an approximate 60% improvement in the experienced symptoms following the procedure. While the operative plan allowed for the repeated performance of the procedure if the symptoms recurred, it has proved unnecessary thus far—the patient has maintained the improvements across the 7 months following the procedure.

For this patient, the procedure was performed based on the determination that the onset of symptoms was attributable to ASD-induced stenosis. If the results of this procedure yielded limited improvement, then additional Lt. L5

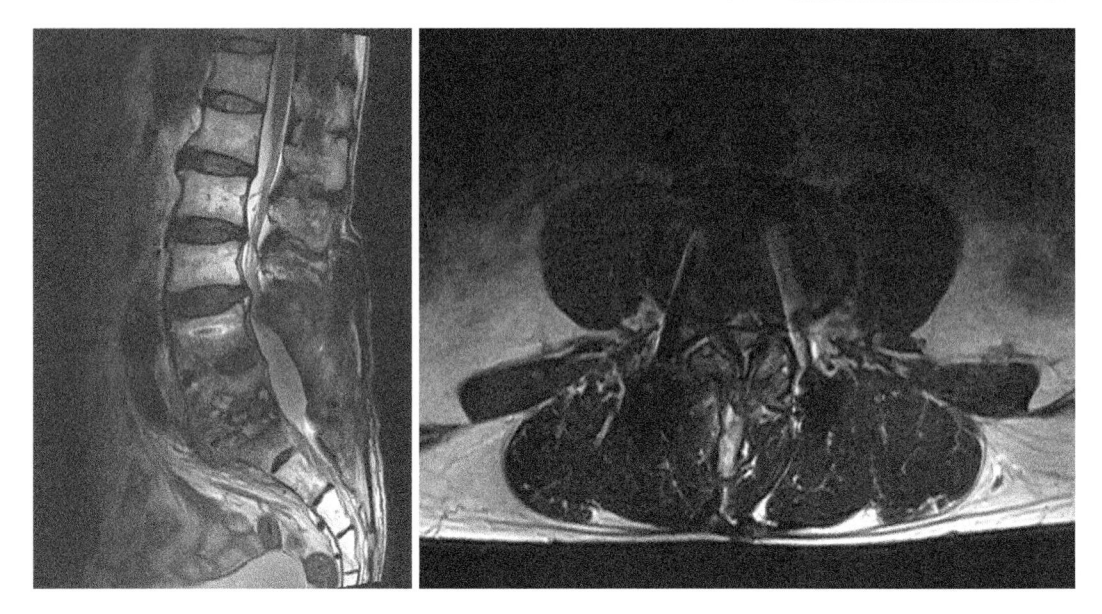

Fig. 9.17 MRI findings. S/P Decompression and PLIF at the L4–5–S1 levels, L3–4 central stenosis d/t bulging disc, and LF thickening

foraminal and Lt. side central balloon decompression with the ZiNeu01 catheter was planned. However, because the first procedure showed significant improvement, additional procedure has not been needed. It is believed that this patient developed symptoms of low back pain and Lt. leg numbness due to ASD rather than adhesion in the spinal fusion area.

In cases in which the lesion causing the symptoms is unclear, the simplest procedure should be attempted first to clarify the diagnosis.

Case 4 A 47-year-old man visited our pain clinic complaining of needing rest after just 5 min of walking due to tingling and pulling in his left leg (S1 dermatome). MRI findings showed Lt. L5–S1 extrusion with Lt. S1 root compression (Fig. 9.19). The patient reported only slight improvement during the 2–3 days following the first S1 root block. Consequently, Lt. L5–S1 retrodiscal balloon decompression was performed. Because this patient's Lt. S1 radiculopathy was caused by S1 root compression in the Lt. L5–S1 retrodiscal area, the procedure was performed only in this area.

Retrodiscal balloon decompression could be performed with any balloon catheter; the success or failure of the procedure may depend on the competency of the operator as well as the patient's condition. In this patient, balloon decompression in the anterior epidural space was attempted with the ZiNeu01 catheter. However, as shown in the figure, entry was blocked by extrusion in the anterior epidural space, making it impossible to reach the site of nerve compression in the retrodiscal area (Fig. 9.20). Accordingly, the procedure was successfully completed with the ZiNeuF catheter for the transforaminal approach (Fig. 9.21).

As evinced by the sustained improvement of his symptoms, the patient continued to do well for 7 months following the procedure. However, his symptoms recurred, requiring the procedure to be performed once more. The patient has sustained his improvements across the 4 months since the procedure was completed. If retrodiscal balloon decompression had not yielded any improvement, discectomy was to be performed. Discectomy was not performed right away because removing the disc could accelerate future

9.3 Cases Involving Procedures in the Retrodiscal Area

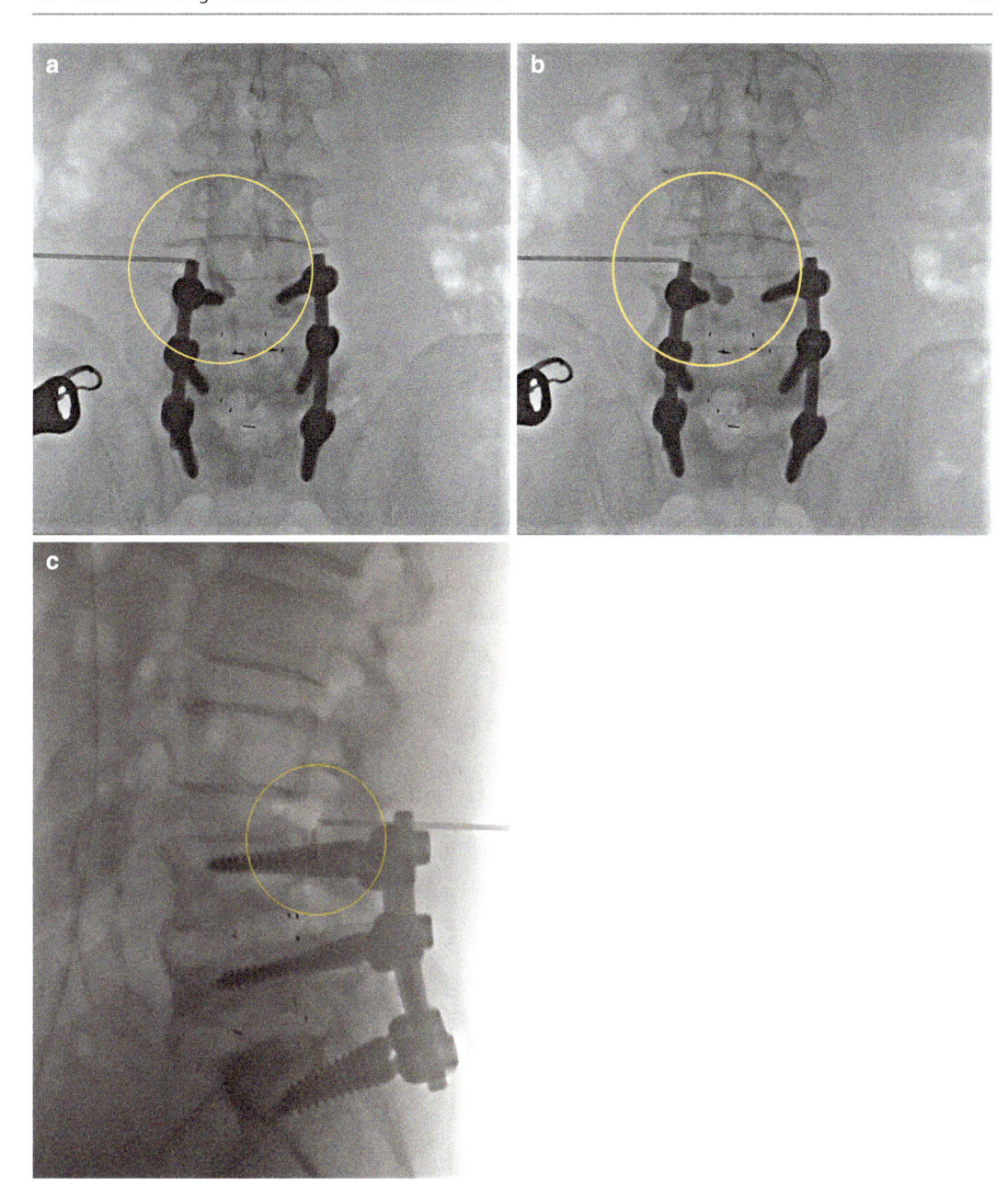

Fig. 9.18 (**a**, **b**) Inflation of the balloon after the insertion of the ZiNeuF catheter into the Lt. L3–4 retrodiscal area through the Kambin's triangle in the Lt. L3–4 intervertebral foramen. (**c**) Image of the inflated balloon in the anterior epidural space of the L3–4 retrodiscal area. Yellow circle: Inflated balloon

degenerative changes. Accordingly, the decision was made to not remove the disc; balloon decompression was attempted to improve his symptoms and allow for spontaneous resorption.

Even in cases involving severe disc disorder, surprising improvement may be achieved with epidural block or balloon decompression. Therefore, before considering endoscopic discectomy, this type of balloon decompression should be attempted. If the effect of the procedure does not last for more than 1 month, endoscopic discectomy should be considered.

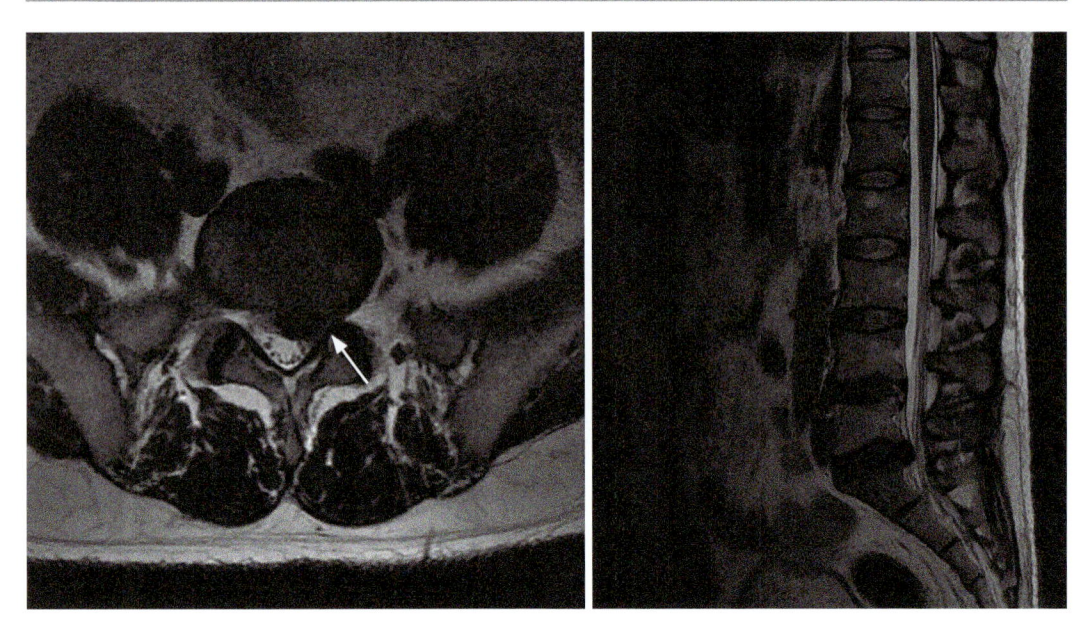

Fig. 9.19 MRI findings. Lt. L5–S1 extrusion with Lt. S1 root compression. Arrow: compressed S1 root

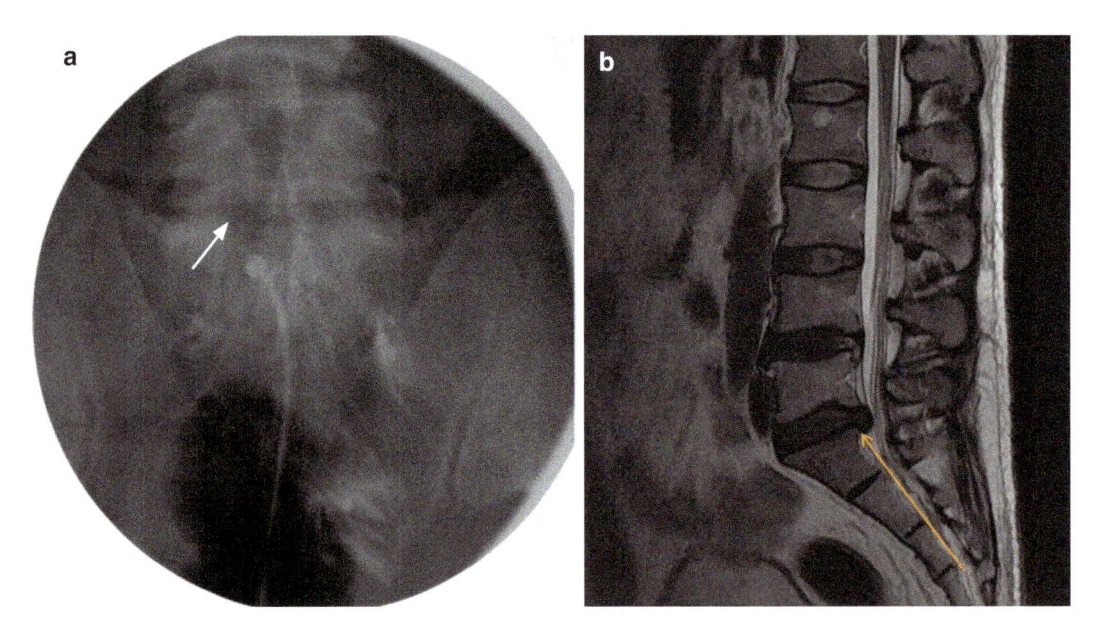

Fig. 9.20 (a) While approaching the Lt. L5 retrodiscal area with the ZiNeu01 catheter was attempted, it was unsuccessful. The operator failed to reach the target area. White arrow: Target area. (b) The catheter could not advance further due to snagging on the Lt. L5–S1 extrusion, indicated by the yellow arrow

However, if the improvement effect lasts for 3–6 months or longer, then it may be advisable to repeat the same procedure and waiting for spontaneous resorption.

In this case, wrong instruments for the procedure were chosen from the outset. The attempt was made first with the ZiNeu01 catheter; while ZiNeu01 catheter was selected because it offers

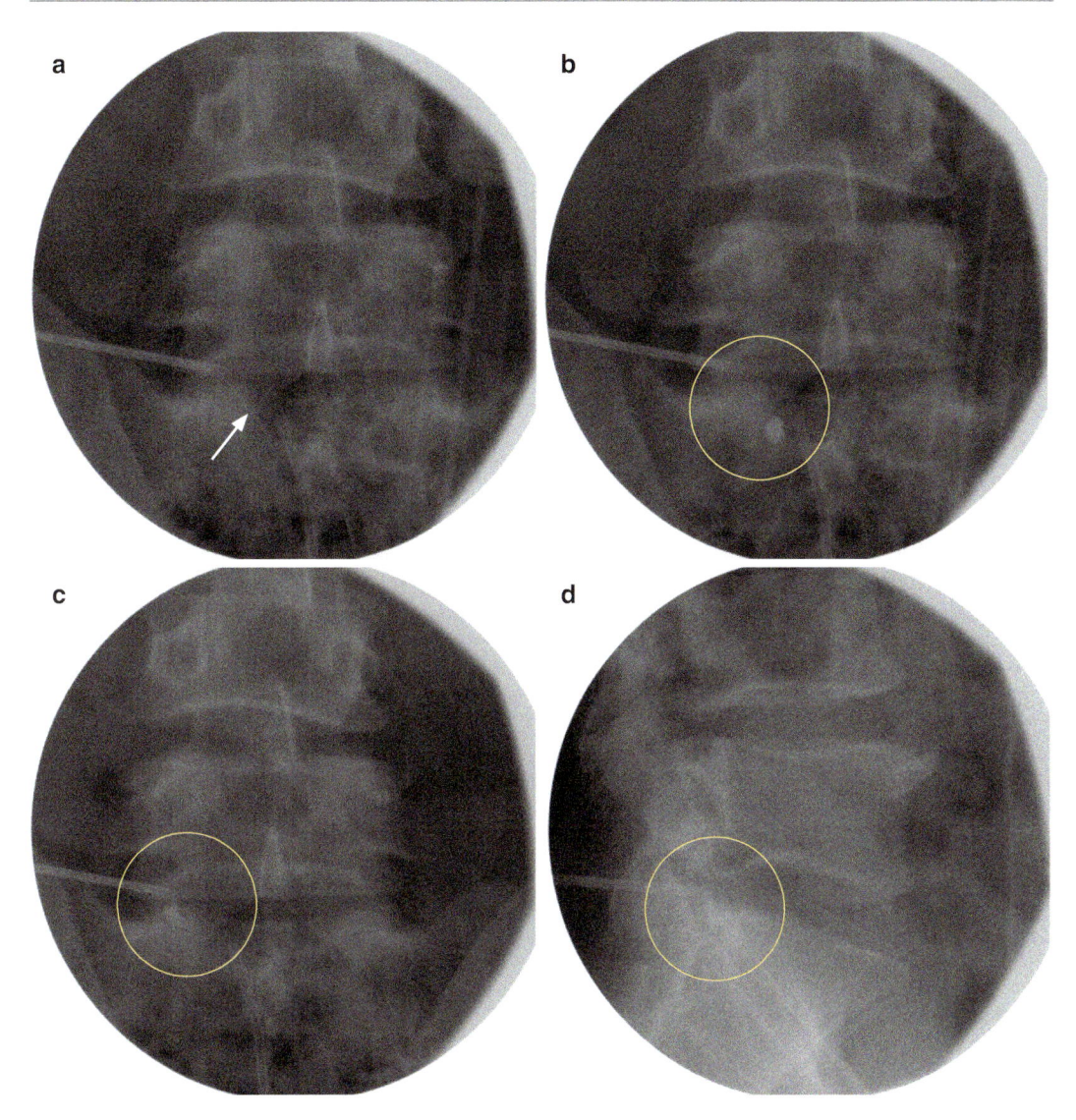

9.3 Cases Involving Procedures in the Retrodiscal Area

Fig. 9.21 (**a**) Insertion of the ZiNeuF catheter through the Lt. L5 intervertebral foramen with the ZiNeu01 catheter left in place. (**b**, **c**) Performance of decompression and adhesiolysis on the affected area by inflating the balloon from the medial aspect followed by its gradual withdrawal. (**d**) Lateral view of the balloon being inflated in the anterior epidural space. Arrow: Inserted ZiNeuF catheter. Yellow circle: Inflated balloon

better maneuverability and can be applied to a broad area, this choice ignored the MRI findings that indicated that an approach through the anterior epidural space would not allow the retrodiscal area to be reached due to a Lt. L5–S1 disc extrusion. The transforaminal approach with the ZiNeuF catheter should have been considered from the beginning. This case underscores the importance of reviewing MRI findings prior to the procedure and selecting the catheter that can best approach the affected area.

Case 5 A 53-year-old woman visited our clinic complaining of Lt. leg pain and tingling (L5 dermatome) that began 6 months prior. MRI findings showed Lt. L5 root compression caused by a retrodiscal cyst at the L4–5 level (Fig. 9.22).

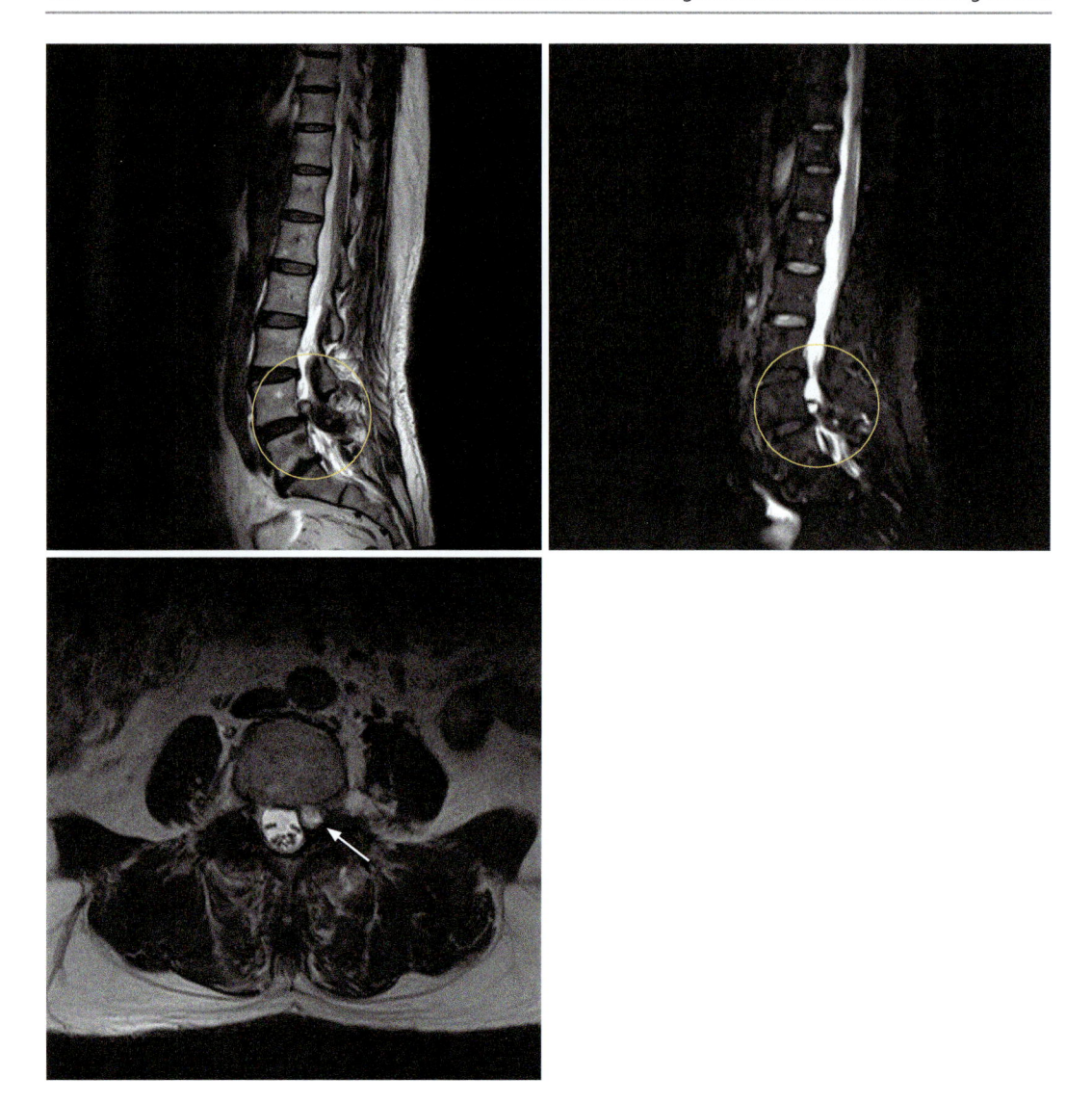

Fig. 9.22 MRI findings. Lt. L4–5 retrodiscal cyst with Lt. L5 root compression. Yellow circle: Cyst. Arrow: Cyst with Lt. L5 root compression

Because Lt. L5 transforaminal block was completely ineffective in this patient, retrodiscal balloon decompression by the transforaminal approach was attempted (Fig. 9.23).

The symptoms resolved after the procedure, and the patient has not experienced any recurrence during the 18 months following the procedure. Because the symptoms had completely dissipated after the procedure, the patient did not consent to a follow-up MRI. Therefore, whether the cyst also disappeared could not be confirmed.

The case of this patient indicates that retrodiscal balloon decompression with the ZiNeuF catheter could be useful even when cysts are present; these may rupture or decrease in size as a result of balloon inflation. Additionally, balloon inflation may cause the compressed nerve to move slightly, resulting in decompression. In such cases, balloon decompression certainly warrants an attempt.

Case 6 A 60-year-old man visited the pain clinic due to symptoms of tingling and cramp-

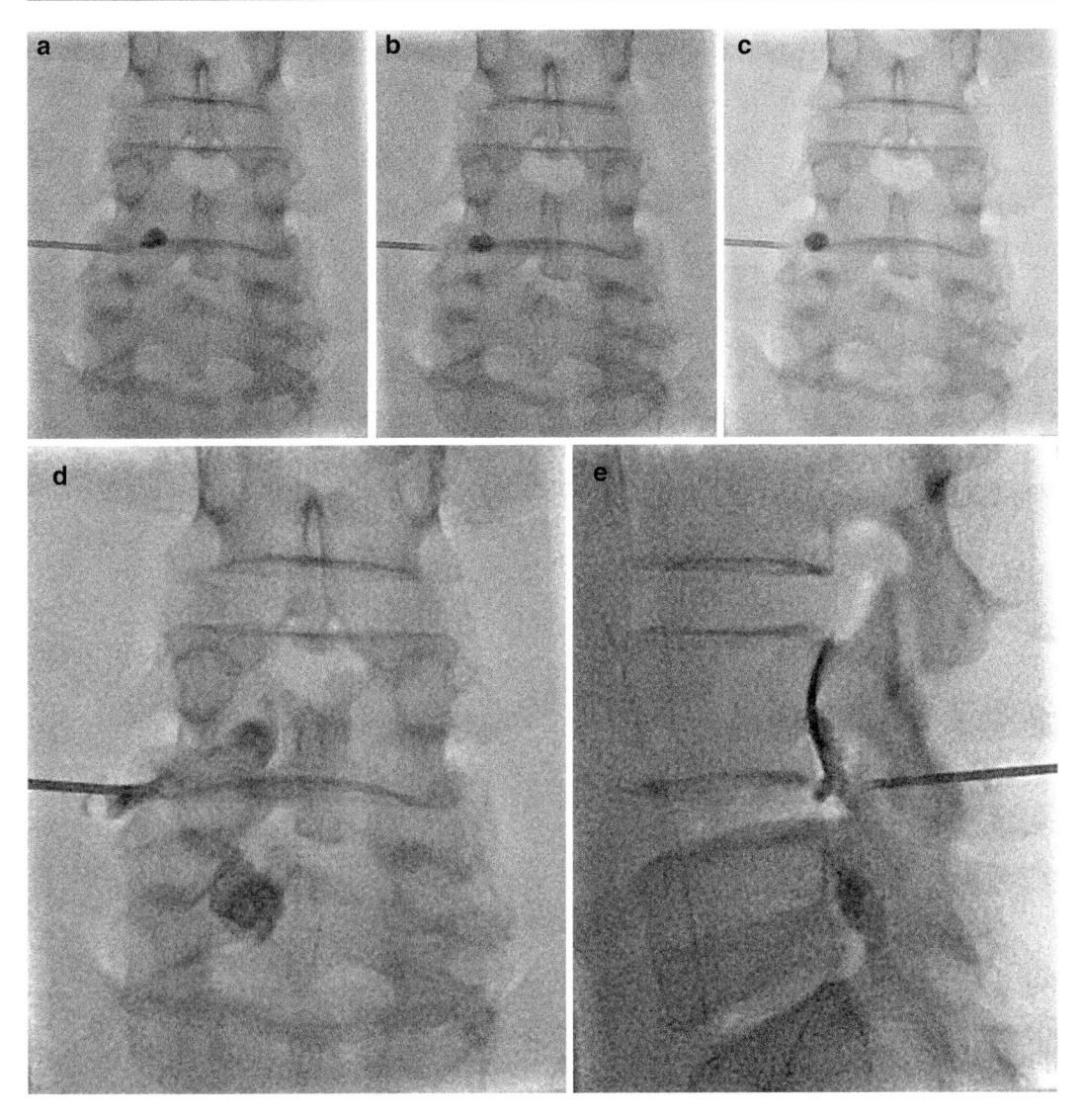

9.3 Cases Involving Procedures in the Retrodiscal Area

Fig. 9.23 (**a–c**) Balloon decompression performed in the area with the cyst in the order of **a → c**, from the medial to lateral aspects of the Lt. L4–5 retrodiscal area. (**d**) AP view of the contrast dye spreading into the affected area after the procedure. (**e**) Lateral view of the contrast dye spreading into the anterior epidural space of the affected area after the procedure

ing in the posterior bilateral legs (S1 dermatome), which had worsened across the prior year. He reported the most difficulty while standing and some difficulty while walking, but no symptoms while sitting or lying down (Fig. 9.24). The patient had previously undergone three rounds of epidural block, but the approximate 50% improvement was sustained only for 1 month each time.

MRI findings show only L4–5 central stenosis (Fig. 9.25).

Based on the determination that the symptoms were caused by L4–5 central stenosis, balloon decompression using the ZiNeu01 catheter was performed in the L4–5 retrodiscal area (Fig. 9.26).

At 1 month following the procedure, the patient reported that over 80% of the tingling had resolved and that he had experienced no diffi-

Fig. 9.24 Patient's sites of pain. Complaints of pain localized to S1 dermatome

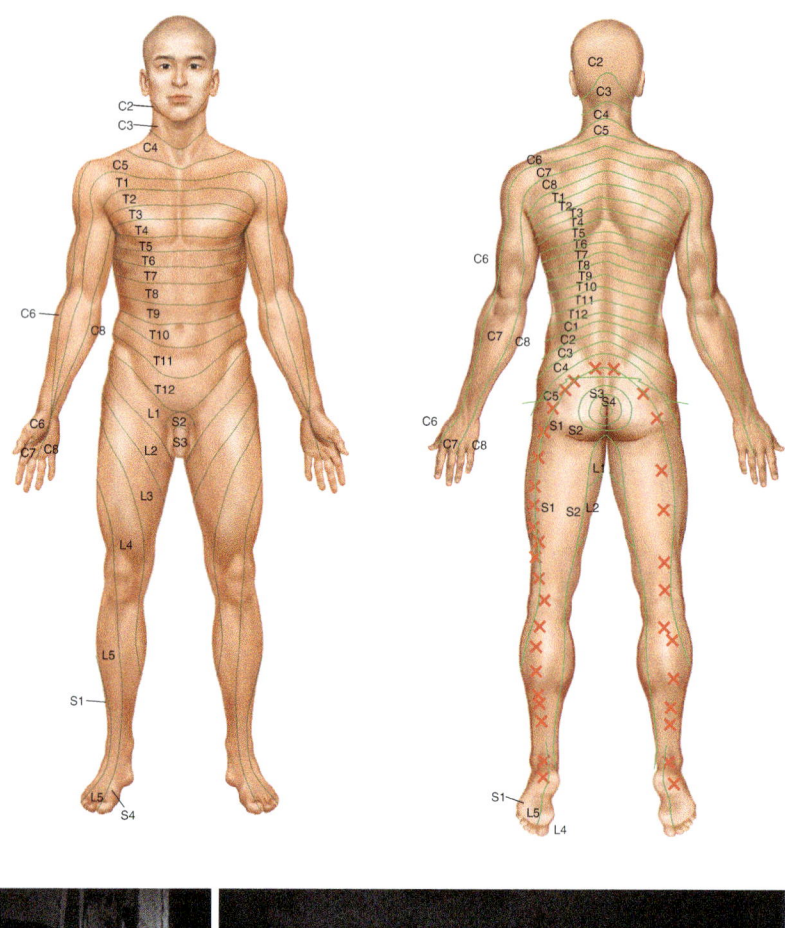

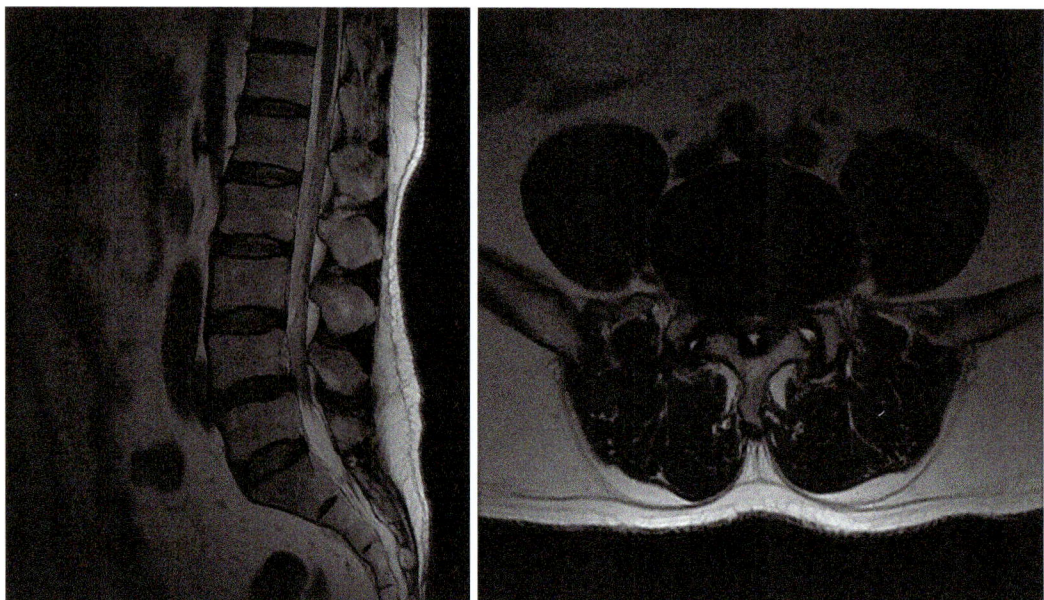

Fig. 9.25 MRI findings. L4–5 central stenosis

9.3 Cases Involving Procedures in the Retrodiscal Area

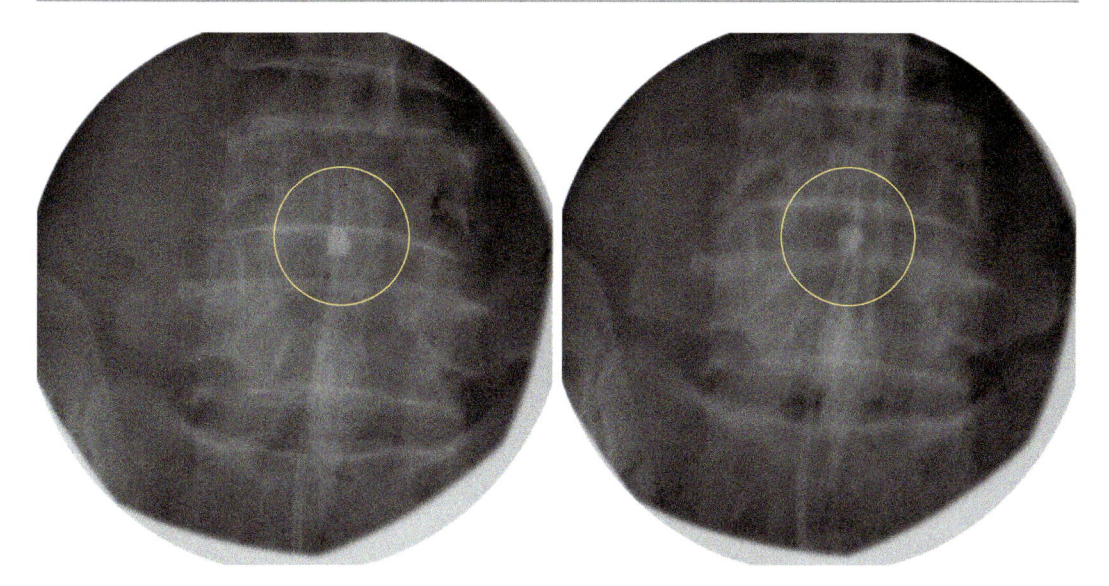

Fig. 9.26 Inflation of the balloon in the L4–5 central stenosis area. If possible, the procedure should target a laterally wide area. The procedure was performed only in the anterior epidural space

culty in walking. At 3 months after the procedure, the symptoms had reduced by 70%; by 5 months following the procedure, an improvement of over 90% was achieved and maintained with an NRS of 2 points. The patient revisited the pain clinic after 2 years, stating that while the effects of the previous balloon decompression procedure had sustained for 1 year, the symptoms gradually reappeared thereafter. As a result, he wanted to undergo the same procedure again. Because the patient did not have any problems walking or exercising at the time, the decision was made to monitor him for a few more months before committing to the procedure.

In this patient, bilateral S1 radiculopathy caused by central stenosis was the primary symptom. In such cases, performing balloon decompression in the retrodiscal area with stenosis could improve S1 radiculopathy. While some operators would insert the catheter into the S1 foramen if S1 radiculopathy is present and consider the procedure to be a success if the injected contrast dye shows a contrast-enhanced S1 nerve, S1 foraminal stenosis or adhesion is almost never present. Thus, the cause of symptoms in the S1 dermatome must be found in the central area (usually L5–S1 or L4–L5). There is no need to waste time by inserting the catheter into the S1 foramen.

Generally, procedures are often completed by inserting the catheter only into the anterior epidural space according to the belief that the posterior epidural space is not important. However, based on the experience of the author, a significant number of cases involving low back pain are caused by adhesion in the posterior epidural space. If there is no low back pain, as in this patient, there is no need for balloon decompression to include the posterior epidural space. However, if low back pain is present, then it would be advisable to perform balloon decompression in the posterior epidural space for adhesiolysis.

Case 7 A 65-year-old man had undergone manual therapy, four rounds of epidural block, and FIMS procedure for low back pain and bilateral leg pain (S1 dermatome) that had begun 3 years earlier. However, the improvement effects were minimal, and he had experienced difficulty when walking for more than 3 min. Based on MRI findings that indicated L4–5 spondylolisthesis and L3–4 and L4–5 central stenosis as well as the patient's complaints of low back pain, balloon decompression was performed in both the anterior and posterior epidural spaces of the L4–5 central area (Figs. 9.27, 9.28 and 9.29).

The patient's symptoms improved immediately after the procedure, and the patient reported no difficulty in walking. Moreover, his low back pain had also decreased significantly. At 2 years following the procedure, some tingling reappeared, but not to any extent that caused discomfort in his daily life.

Fig. 9.27 Sites to which the patient's complaints of low back and bilateral S1 dermatome pain can be attributed

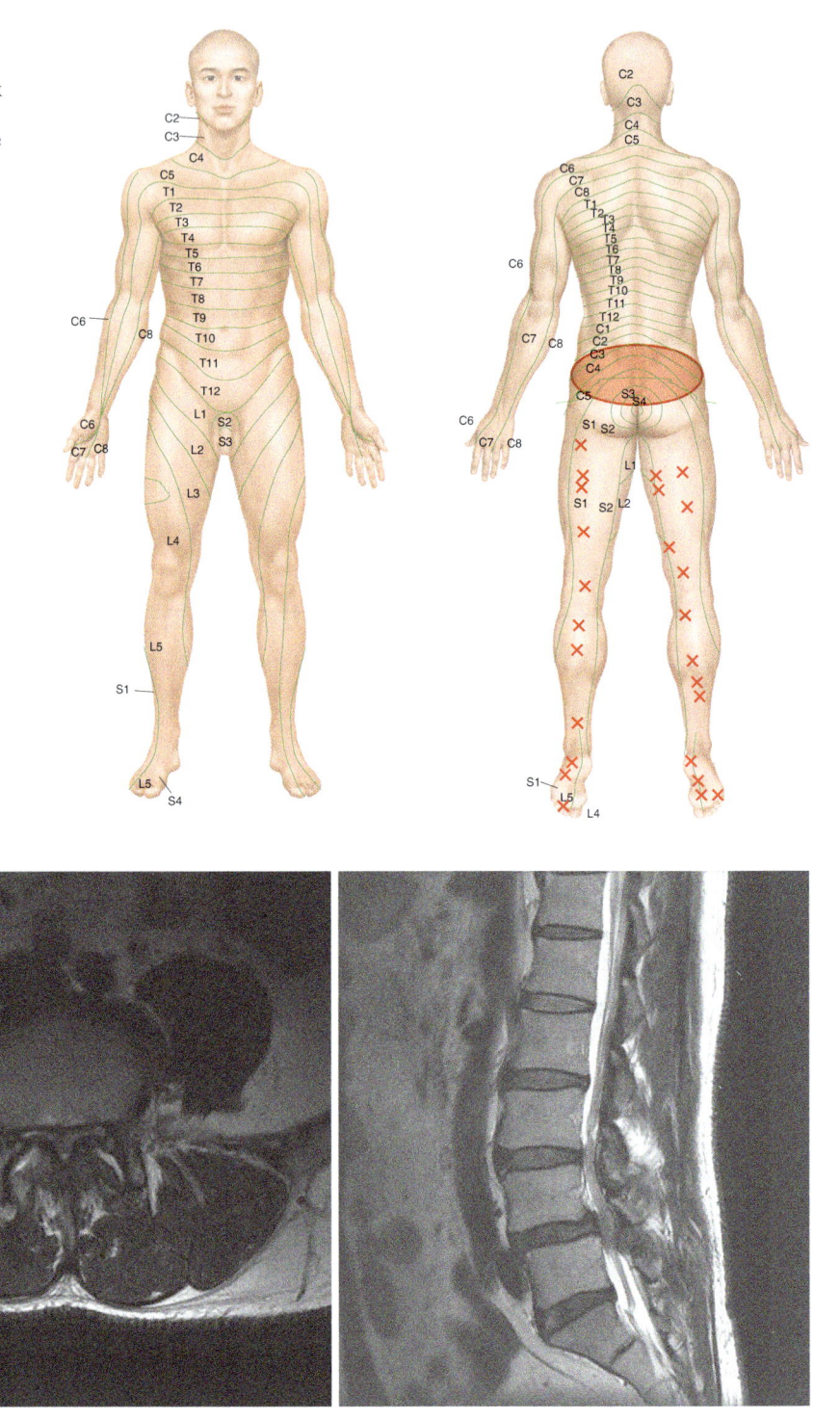

Fig. 9.28 MRI findings. L4–5 spondylolisthesis, L3–4, and L4–5 central stenosis findings

9.4 Cases Involving Procedures in Filling Defect Areas

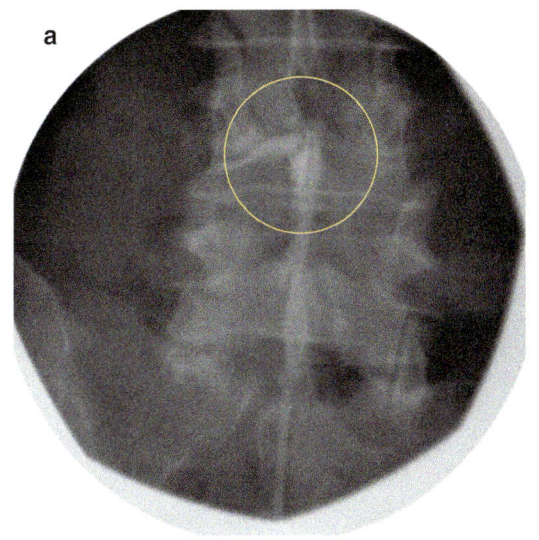

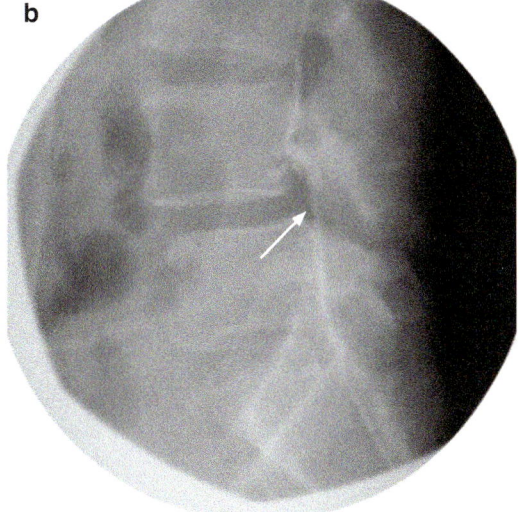

Fig. 9.29 (**a**) Performance of balloon decompression in an area slightly above the L4–5 central area. (**b**) The spread of the contrast dye into the anterior epidural space after the procedure. Although no image is available, the procedure was also performed in the posterior epidural space. Yellow circle: Inflated balloon. Arrow: Contrast-dye findings in the anterior epidural space

Accordingly, the patient is being monitored. Because adhesion in the posterior epidural space may cause low back pain, it is advisable to perform the procedure in both the anterior and posterior epidural spaces if low back pain is present. This patient also showed improvement in bilateral S1 radiculopathy despite the procedure not being performed in the left or right S1 foramen.

9.4 Cases Involving Procedures in Filling Defect Areas

Case 1 A 50-year-old woman who underwent lumbar microdecompression at another hospital 15 years earlier visited the pain clinic with various symptoms, including bilateral leg tingling (S1 dermatome) and intermittent weakness that had begun 1 year earlier, low back and hip pain when rising from a lying position, and worsening pain during hyperextension. Despite a dull sensation in the low back and hips, she did not experience any difficulty in walking. Except for mild diffuse bulging disc at L4–5–S1, MRI findings yielded no specific findings (Fig. 9.30).

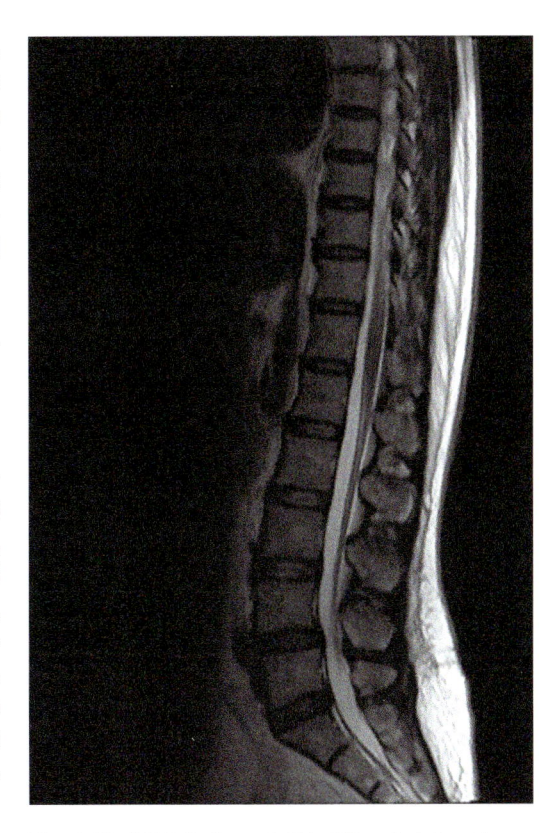

Fig. 9.30 MRI findings. Mild diffuse bulging disc at L4–5–S1

Analgesics were prescribed to slightly reduce the patient's pain but did not yield any significant improvement. Accordingly, lumbar interlaminar epidural steroid injection was performed, but this also failed to produce any significant improvement. A subsequently performed caudal epidurogram showed a distinct filling defect in the anterior epidural space (Fig. 9.31).

As the patient showed no improvement in symptoms even after 1 month, balloon decompression was performed in the anterior epidural space. Balloon decompression was performed by dividing the L4–5 retrodiscal area that had previously undergone microdecompression into three sections (Fig. 9.32). While improvement in symptoms was observed for up to 6 months after the procedure, the same procedure was performed again due to recurrence. The effect has been maintained, as evinced by a VAS of 2 points, for 9 months since the second procedure.

Epidurograms are important contributors to the diagnosis of patients for whom epidural block does not yield improvement. However, the appearance of a filling defect on an epidurogram does not always indicate a lesion. Because the contrast dye spreads in a caudal-cephalad direction, if adhesion unrelated to pain presents below the lesion, the entire upper area is not contrasted; this complicates the localization of the pain-related lesion. Moreover, it is difficult to assume that the extent of the filling defect is consistent with the severity of adhesion or disease. Therefore, determination of the pain-inducing lesion must be informed by the careful consideration of the patient's symptoms, MRI findings, and epidurogram findings.

The epidurogram showed a filling defect in the anterior epidural space, and subsequent procedure was performed only in that area, which was determined to be associated with the patient's symptoms. Because the patient did not have L5 radiculopathy, entry into the intervertebral foramen was not made. Moreover, as the contrast dye spread well into the posterior epidural space, the procedure was performed only in the anterior epidural space.

If the effect of epidural block does not last very long, as in this case, an epidurogram should be performed to confirm the presence of the filling defect and whether that area is associated with pain; if such is expected, then balloon decompression should be performed in that area.

Case 2 A 21-year-old man visited our pain clinic because he had been experiencing tingling and numbness from the Lt. hip to the plantar area

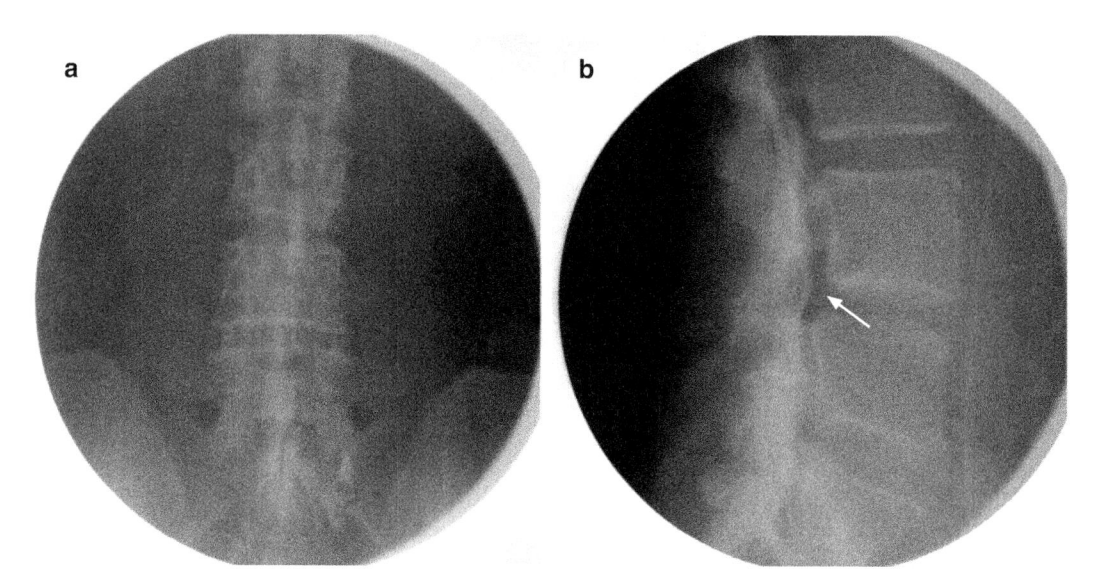

Fig. 9.31 Epidurogram findings. (**a**) Findings in the AP view are normal. (**b**) In the lateral view, a filling defect in the anterior epidural space is observed. Arrow: Filling defect area in the anterior epidural space

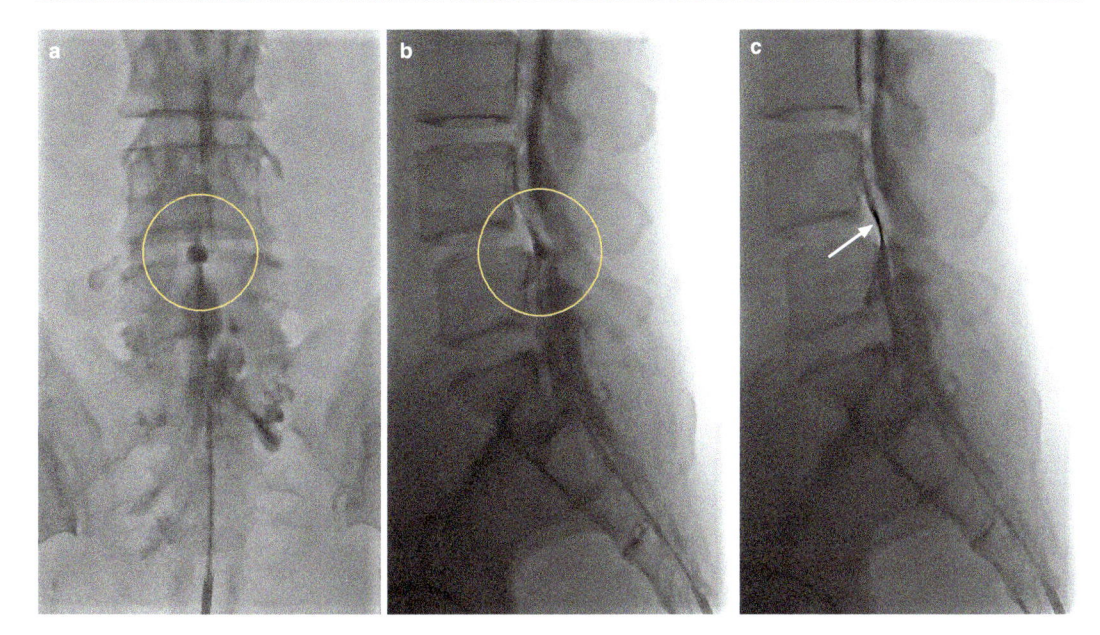

Fig. 9.32 (**a**, **b**) Balloon inflation in the L4–5 retrodiscal area. (**c**) The filling defect was resolved after the procedure. Yellow circle: Inflated balloon. Arrow: Contrast-dye findings in the anterior epidural space

after just 10 min of walking for 6 months. He had previously undergone MRI and electromyography at another hospital. However, the test results did not show any abnormal findings, and subsequently performed piriformis injection, transforaminal epidural block, and caudal epidural block also effected no improvements. The epidurogram performed at our pain clinic showed an extensive filling defect on the Lt. side. Accordingly, balloon decompression was performed in the Lt. L5 foramen and Lt. L5–S1 retrodiscal area (Figs. 9.33 and 9.34).

The patient showed immediate improvement in symptoms after the procedure and reported that he experienced no major discomfort at the 7-month follow-up.

9.5 Cases Involving Procedures in Both the Anterior and Posterior Epidural Spaces

Case 1 A 70-year-old woman reported that she had undergone more than 10 rounds of epidural block for low back pain that had persisted for 20 years. Initially, the improvements yielded by epidural block lasted about 1 month; recently, however, the injection provided no improvement at all. Her low back pain worsened in the 2 months prior to her presentation at our pain clinic. The patient reported a pulling sensation in the low back that became excessively severe after walking for just 5 min, forcing her to rest and inducing a cold sweat; the level of pain when walking was equivalent to an NRS of 8 points. She also experienced pain when standing up from a sitting position and had difficulty lifting objects from the front but no problem lifting objects to the side. Several tender points were found in the bilateral paraspinal muscles (Fig. 9.35).

Besides mild L3–4 and L4–5 central stenosis, MRI findings did not show any other pathological findings that could cause low back pain (Fig. 9.36).

An epidurogram was performed because the patient's pain was suspected to be attributable to adhesion in the epidural space. The results showed several filling defects in the anterior and posterior epidural spaces. Based on these findings, central adhesiolysis with balloon decompression was performed (Fig. 9.37).

At the 1- and 3-month outpatient visits, the patient reported that the low back pain dissipated immediately after the procedure and that the difficulties in walking had resolved. During the tele-

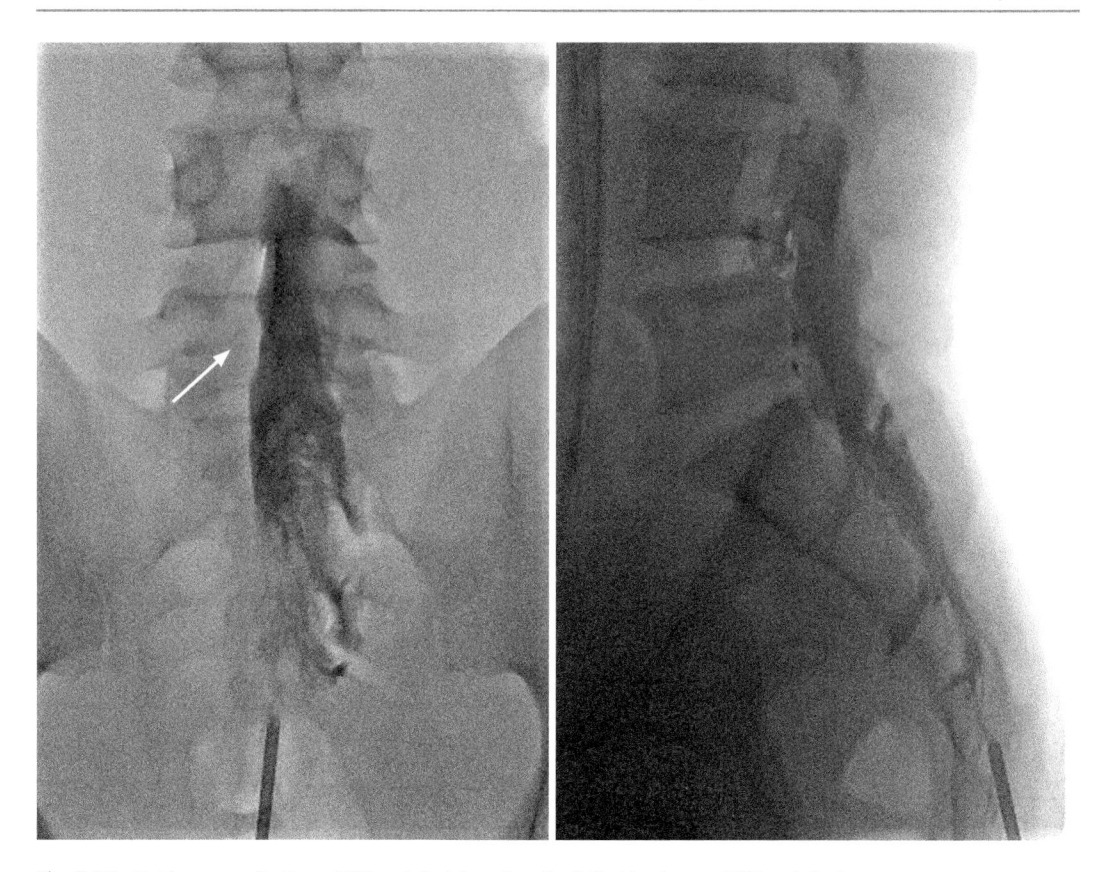

Fig. 9.33 Epidurogram findings. Filling defect found on the left side. Arrow: Filling defect area

phone follow-up performed at 1 year following the procedure, the patient reported that he was doing well and did not experience any severe low back pain.

This case indicates that if there is no pain when sitting or lying down but low back pain occurs when walking, especially a sensation of pulling, epidural adhesion should be suspected. It is recommended that the procedure should be performed on all filling defect areas in both the anterior and posterior epidural spaces.

Case 2 A 70-year-old woman visited our clinic due to low back pain that had begun 4 years earlier but had worsened in the month prior to her presentation at our clinic. The patient reported that she did not have any leg pain but that her low back pain prevented her from walking for more than 100 m. She also felt pain when standing, but she could lie down or sit without any discomfort (Fig. 9.38). She had undergone epidural block and neuroplasty at other hospitals, but the effect lasted for the following 2–3 days and 1 month, respectively.

The severe pain when walking, lack of pain when sitting as well as of specific findings from various physical examinations, and MRI findings of L4–5 central stenosis implicated central stenosis and adhesion as the cause of the patient's low back pain. Accordingly, it was expected that performing balloon decompression in the L4–5 central area alone would yield improvement (Fig. 9.39).

Epidurogram findings showed partial filling defects in the anterior and posterior epidural spaces at the L4–5 level. The procedure involved balloon decompression in both the anterior and posterior epidural spaces of the entire area with L4–5 central stenosis followed by drug administration. When performing balloon decompression, an effort was made to treat as much of the L4–5 retrodiscal area as possible (Fig. 9.40).

9.5 Cases Involving Procedures in Both the Anterior and Posterior Epidural Spaces 207

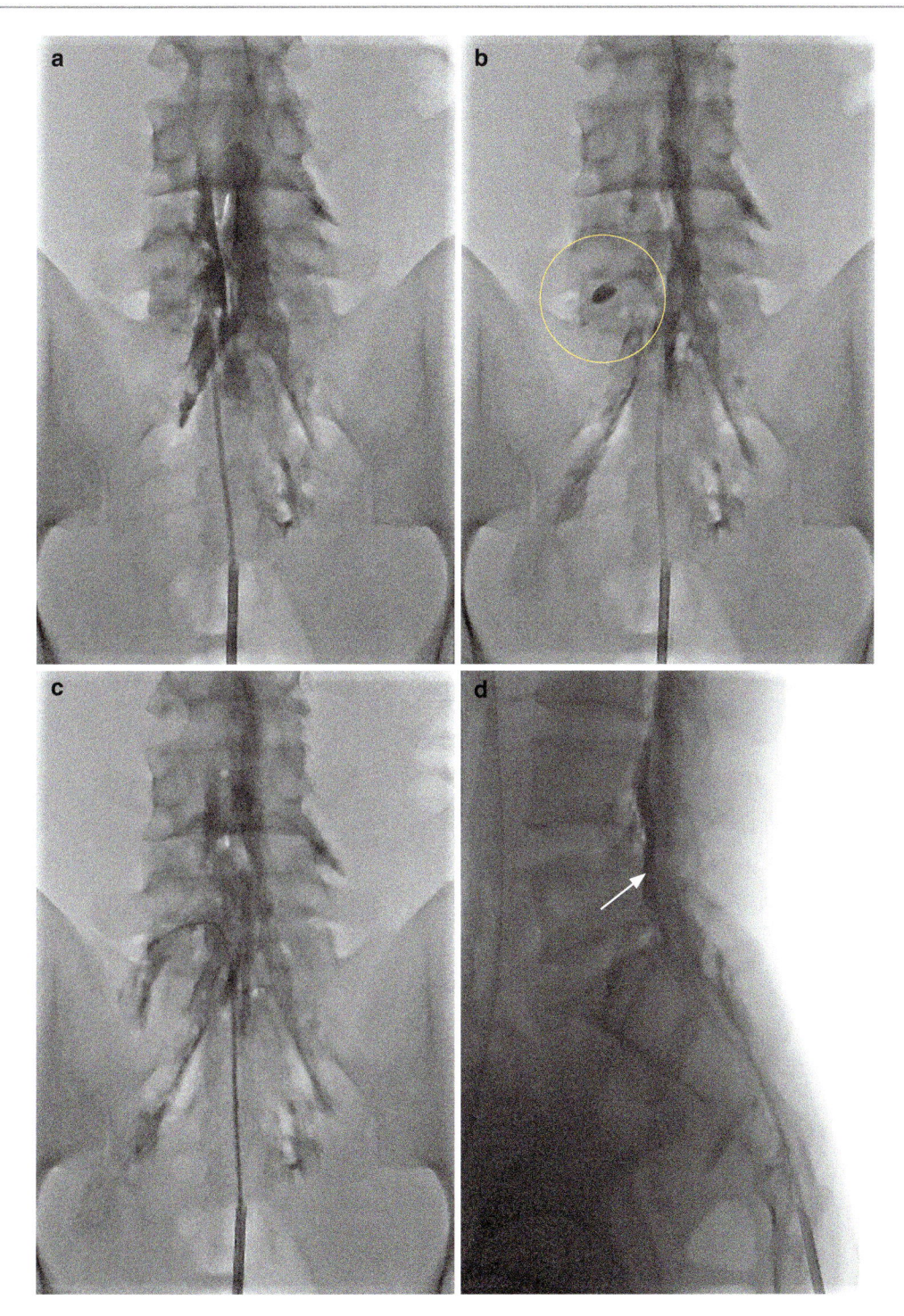

Fig. 9.34 (**a**) The filling defect on the left side resolved after balloon decompression was performed in the left anterior epidural space with the ZiNeuS catheter. (**b**) Image of balloon decompression being performed in the Lt. L5 intervertebral foramen. Yellow circle: Balloon inflated in the Lt. L5 intervertebral foramen. (**c**) The filling defect in the Lt. L5 intervertebral foramen resolved after the procedure. (**d**) The filling defect in the anterior epidural space resolved after the procedure. Arrow: Contrast-dye findings in the anterior epidural space

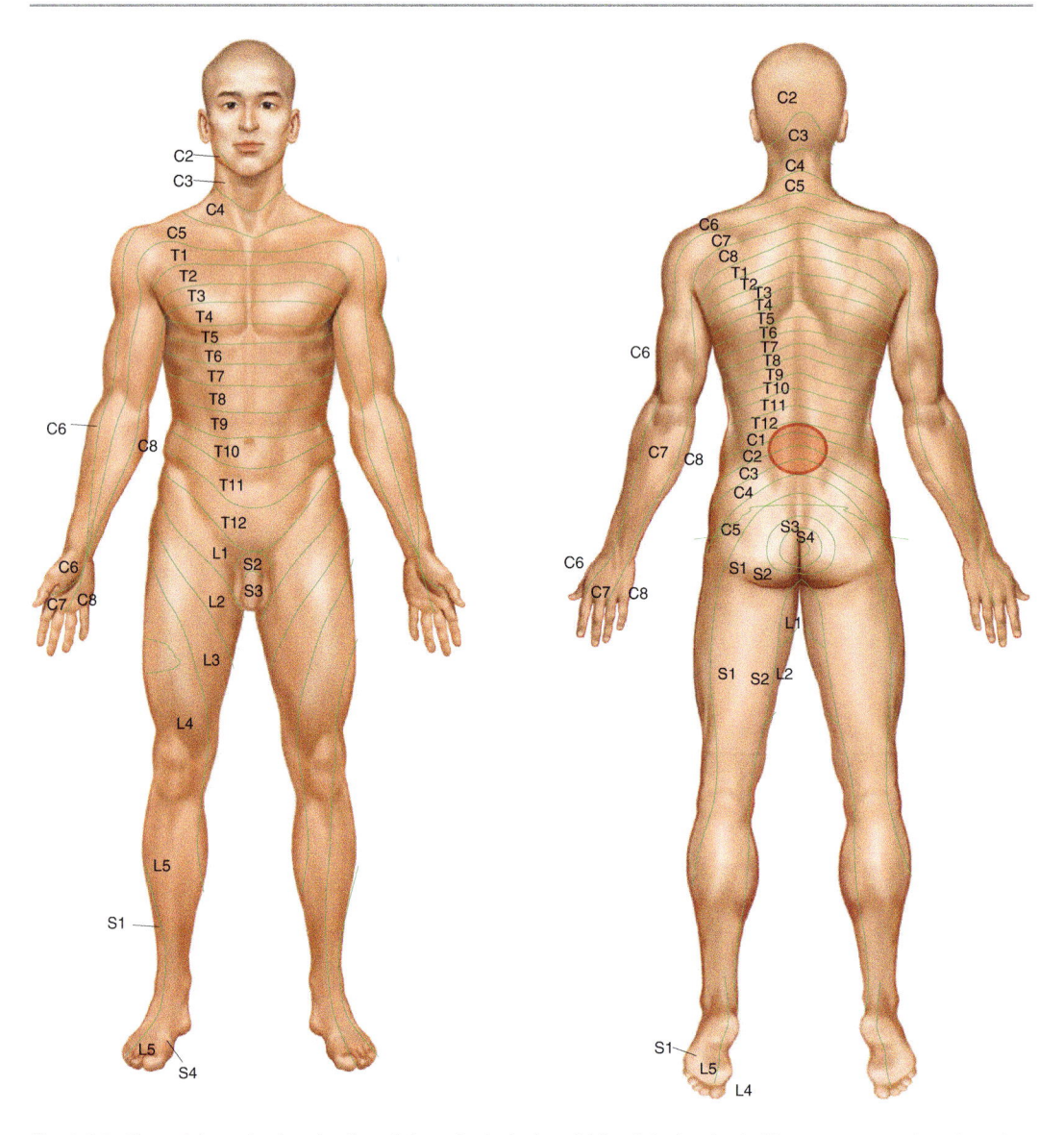

208　　　　　　　　　　　　　　　9　Methods for Determining the Site of Procedure According to Case

Fig. 9.35 Sites of the patient's pain. Complaints of pain in the middle of the low back. There were several tender points in the paraspinal muscles

After 1 month, the patient's pain improved by approximately 40%, and she was able to walk approximately 400 m without having to stop with the assistance of a cane. After 2 months, her symptoms improved even more, as evinced by an NRS of 3 points, to the point where she could walk 800 m without a cane. The patient was recommended to engage in walking for 1 h per day.

At her follow-up visit at 6 months following the procedure, it was determined that the patient had maintained an NRS of 3 points despite feeling occasional pain. She reported that she was able to perform activities of daily living without a cane.

This case demonstrates that low back pain is often caused by stenosis and adhesion, both of which should be suspected when low back pain occurs when walking. It is important in such cases to perform balloon decompression in both the anterior and posterior epidural spaces. As in this patient, continuing to engage in walking after the procedure led to even greater improvements

9.5 Cases Involving Procedures in Both the Anterior and Posterior Epidural Spaces

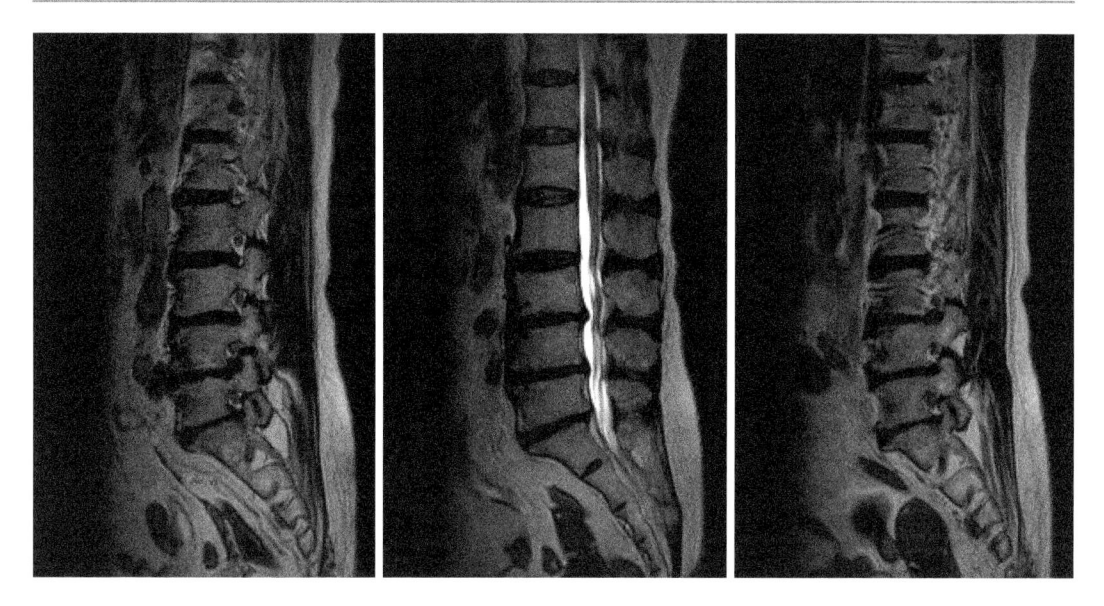

Fig. 9.36 MRI findings. L3–4: mild central stenosis and Rt. lateral recess stenosis; L4–5, L5–S1: left neural foraminal stenosis

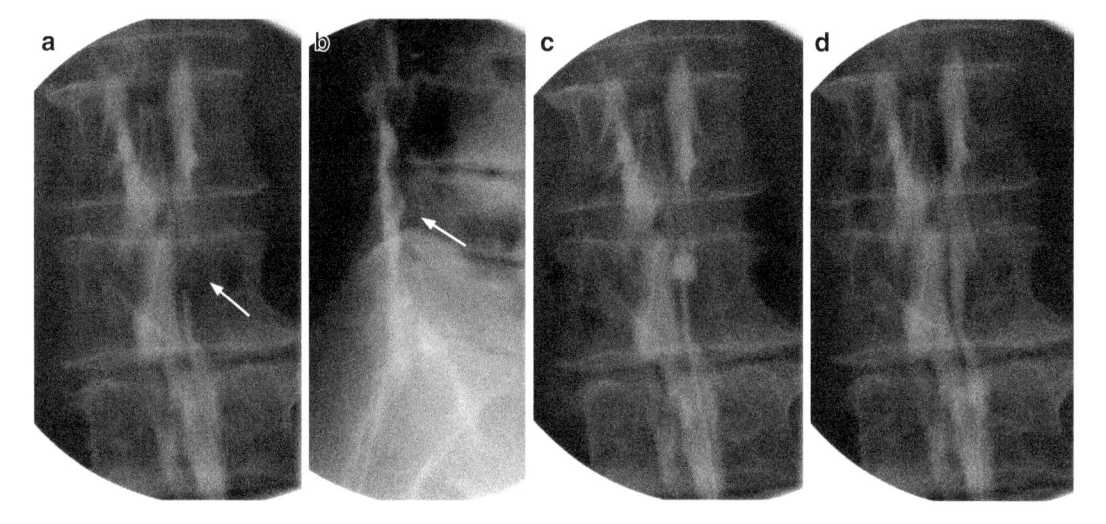

Fig. 9.37 (**a**, **b**) Several filling defects in the anterior and posterior epidural spaces. Arrow: Filling defect area. (**c**) Balloon decompression performed in the L3–5 anterior and posterior epidural spaces. (**d**) Improvement in filling defects after the procedure

over time. Therefore, patients should be instructed to increase their amount of exercise when they experience functional improvements following the procedure.

Case 3 A 72-year-old woman who had undergone L4–5 fusion surgery 14 years prior to her visit to our clinic complained of difficulty in walking due to low back pain that had begun 3 years earlier. She reported experiencing throbbing pain and heaviness when standing; these symptoms worsened when walking. Although she underwent two rounds of caudal epidural block at another hospital, the procedures did not yield any improvements. There were no suspicious findings indicative of a particular cause of her low back pain, such as spondylarthritis or muscular disorder. Meanwhile, the epidurogram

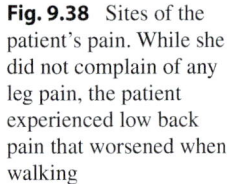

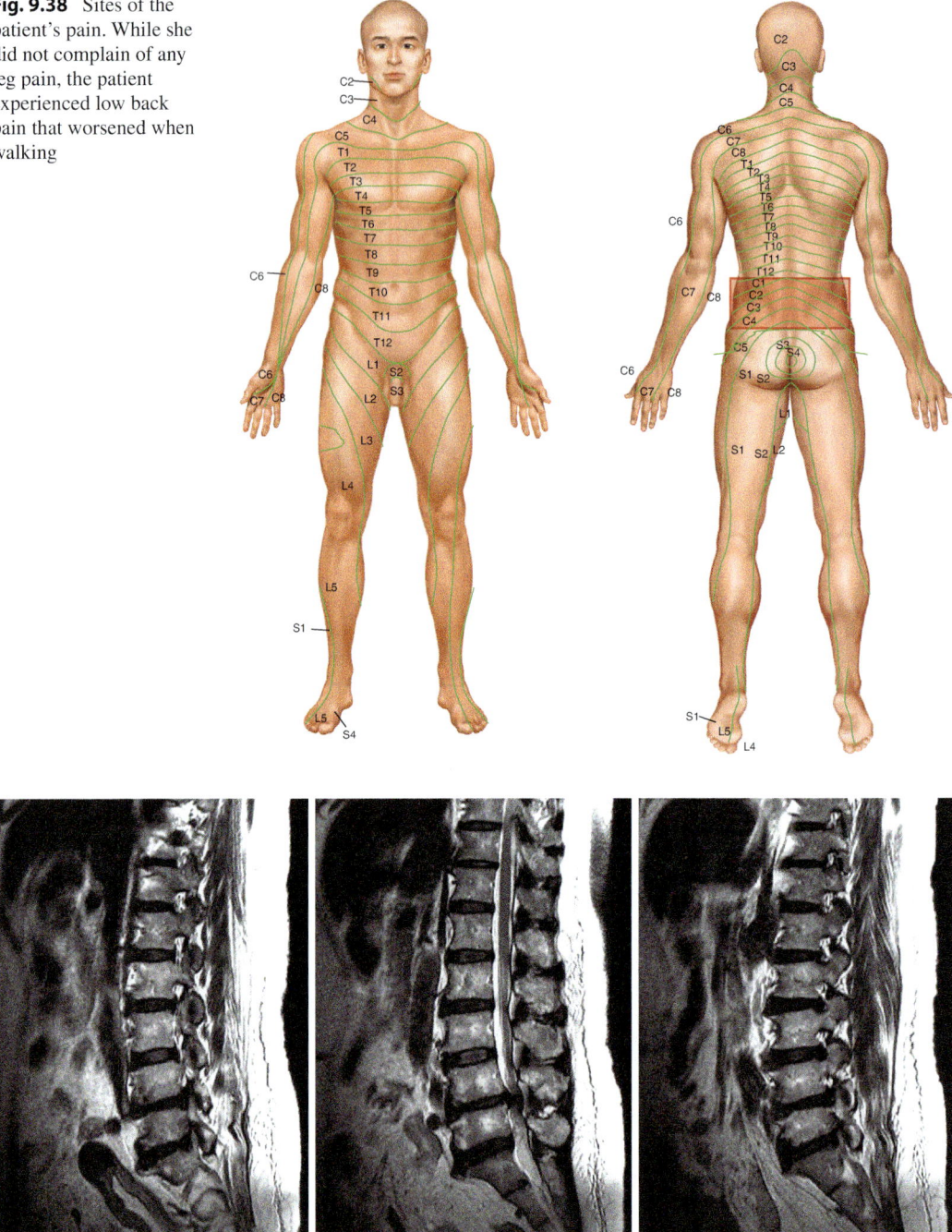

210 9 Methods for Determining the Site of Procedure According to Case

Fig. 9.38 Sites of the patient's pain. While she did not complain of any leg pain, the patient experienced low back pain that worsened when walking

Fig. 9.39 MRI findings. L4–5 central stenosis with bilateral L5 foraminal stenosis

results showed an extensive filling defect in the fusion area. Based on her complaint that the pain worsened when walking, low back pain caused by epidural adhesion was suspected, and balloon decompression was performed accordingly.

The procedure was performed by removing a satisfactory amount of adhesion in the anterior epidural space by repeatedly inflating and deflating the balloon. As a result, spread of the contrast dye was achieved. However, it was impossible to

9.5 Cases Involving Procedures in Both the Anterior and Posterior Epidural Spaces

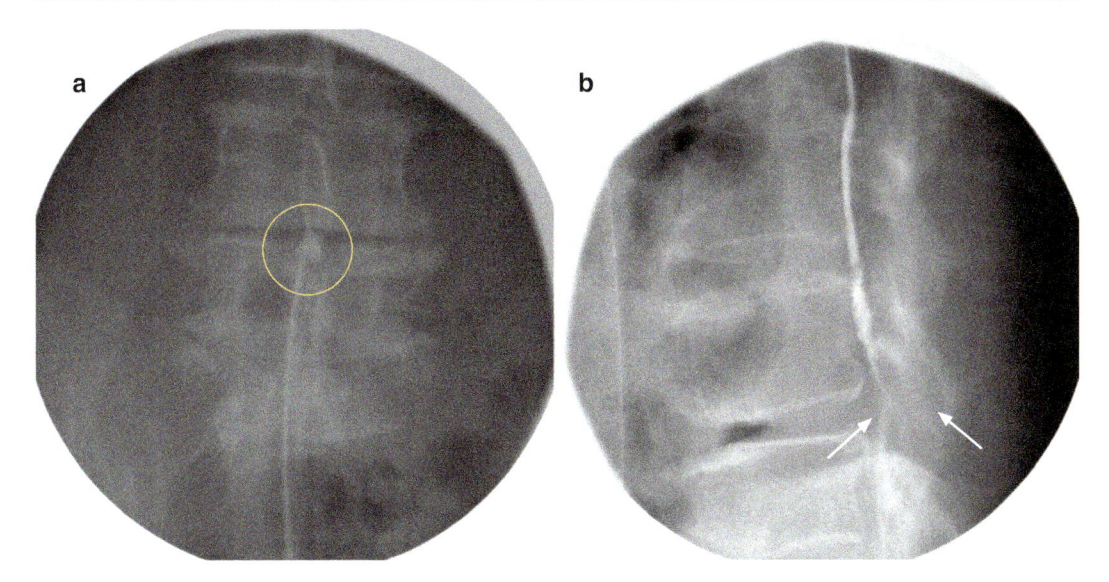

Fig. 9.40 (**a**) Balloon decompression in both the anterior and posterior epidural spaces in the area with L4–5 central stenosis. (**b**) Spreading of the contrast dye into the anterior and posterior epidural spaces after the procedure. Circle: Inflated balloon. Arrow: The anterior and posterior epidural spaces where the contrast dye spread

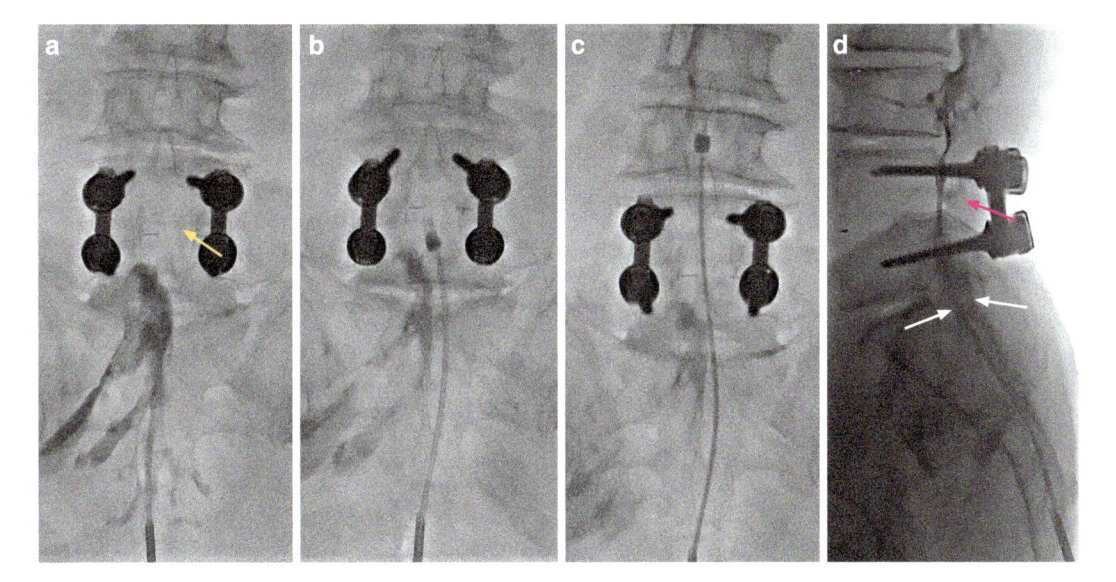

Fig. 9.41 (**a**) Filling defect in the fusion area as observed on the epidurogram. Yellow arrow: Filling defect. (**b**, **c**) Adhesiolysis was carefully attempted by approaching the cephalad from the anterior epidural space while repeatedly inflating and deflating the balloon. (**d**) Contrast dye spread after the procedure. White arrow: Contrast dye spread into the anterior and posterior epidural spaces. Red arrow: Filling defect in the posterior epidural space above the fusion area

insert the catheter into the posterior epidural space above the fusion area due to severe adhesion at the previous site of surgery; the procedure was thus completed in that state. Of note, the contrast dye did not spread upward beyond the posterior epidural space (Fig. 9.41).

At the 1-month follow-up, the patient reported that the throbbing, heavy pain had subsided significantly but that she still experienced a similar degree of difficulty in walking. The patient was recommended to walk consistently, as much as the pain has decreased. By 4 months after the procedure, the patient reported that walking had become much more comfortable.

In this case, the procedure performed in the anterior epidural space was determined to be satisfactory, but adhesion in the posterior epidural space was not sufficiently removed. Therefore, the limited level of improvement may have been an avoidable outcome.

When the case involves spinal fusion, it is rare for adhesiolysis to be performed successfully up to the posterior epidural space due to the excessive breadth of the surgical site and severe adhesion in the posterior epidural space. Therefore, it is necessary to explain to the patient prior to the procedure that a satisfactory level of improvement may not be achievable.

The onset of epidural adhesion after spinal fusion surgery can also cause low back pain. With a balloon catheter, adhesion can be removed more safely from a wider area, even in cases of severe adhesion. Although performing the procedure in both the anterior and posterior epidural spaces would be ideal, the procedure should be performed without excessive aggression. Moreover, engaging in walking after the procedure is essential.

9.6 Procedure for Patients with Bertolotti's Syndrome (Lumbosacral Transitional Vertebrae)

Bertolotti's syndrome refers to pain in the lumbosacral transitional vertebrae, i.e., pain associated with lumbarization or sacralization. It was reported for the first by Bertolotti in 1917.

The lumbosacral transitional vertebrae could be classified by the Castellvi classification, and low back and leg pain has been reportedly associated with the fusion of the L5 transverse process and sacral bone, or type II–IV, with anomalous articulation (Fig. 9.42).

Figure 9.43 presents images of the anomalous articulation or fusion of the unilateral L5 transverse process and sacral bone.

Such anomalous articulation or fusion of an excessively large transverse process and sacral bone on one or both sides could cause pain induced by degenerative changes that resemble the pain following spinal fusion surgery. Similar to adjacent segmental degeneration that frequently occurs after spinal fusion, degenerative changes, including stenosis of the upper levels,

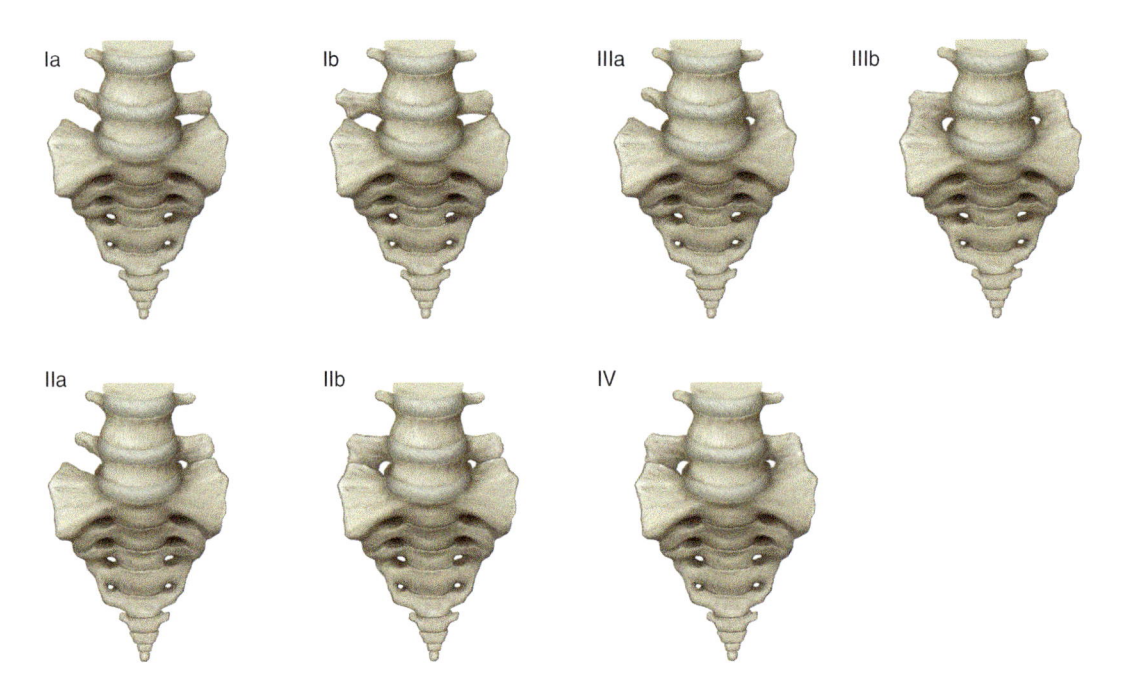

Fig. 9.42 The Castellvi classification of the lumbosacral transitional vertebrae

9.6 Procedure for Patients with Bertolotti's Syndrome (Lumbosacral Transitional Vertebrae)

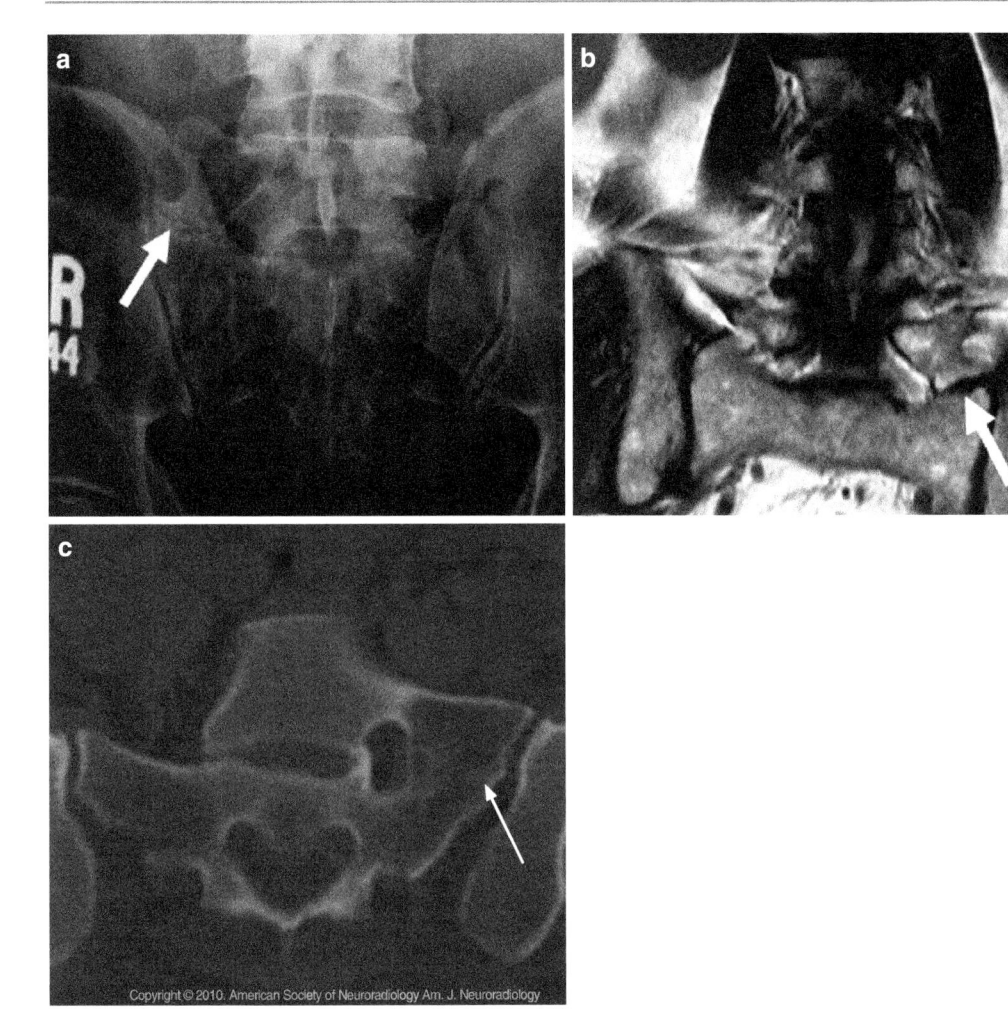

Fig. 9.43 (**a**) Type IIa. AP findings. Anomalous articulation of the Rt. L5 transverse process and sacrum. (**b**) IIa. T2 weighted coronal MR image. Anomalous articulation of the Lt. L5 transverse process and sacrum. (**c**) IIIa. Axial CT image. Fusion of the Lt. L5 transverse process and sacrum

could be facilitated. Disc disorder and facet joint syndrome associated with such changes could also occur, and, in some cases, extraforaminal stenosis due to an excessively large transverse process can also develop. Other clinically significant factors include possible differences in anatomical nerve distribution and physiological nerve functions.

Although it is unclear whether congenital L5–S1 level fusion is the cause, the anatomical L5 nerve could execute the physiological function of the S1 nerve and the anatomical L4 nerve could execute the physiological function of the L5 nerve. Normally, while the L5–S1 level is the area of the low back with the highest mobility, a fusion or anomalous articulation in this area results in the L4–5 level becoming the area with the highest mobility. Consequently, the L4 nerve may function similar to the L5 nerve—this should be considered when checking for lesions during a surgery or procedure. The following case is related to one personally experienced by the author.

Case A 58-year-old man visited our pain clinic complaining of Lt. low back and leg pain (L5 radiculopathy) that had begun 5 years prior. Although he had undergone five rounds of Lt. L5

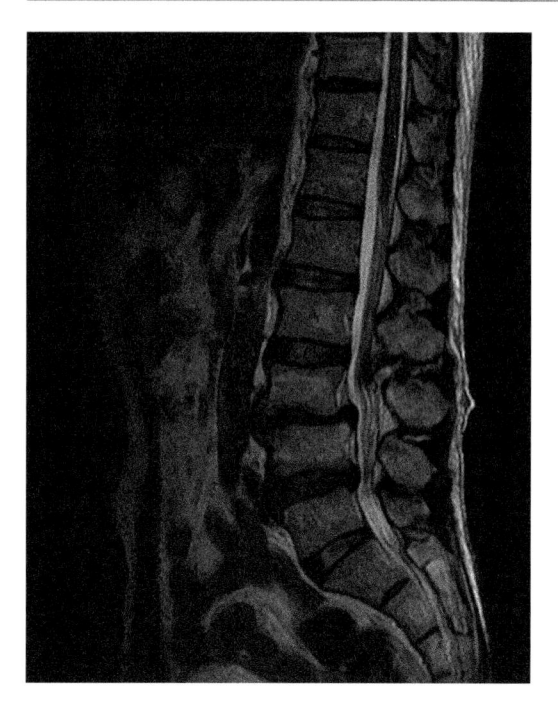

Fig. 9.44 MRI finding. L4–5 spondylolisthesis, disc space narrowing, and extrusion

transforaminal block at another hospital, the resulting improvements lasted for only 1 or 2 days each time. MRI findings indicated L4–5 spondylolisthesis, disc space narrowing, and disc extrusion but no Lt. L5 foraminal stenosis. Simple X-ray images showed anomalous articulation of the Lt. and Rt. L5 transverse process and sacral bone, but it was not a major concern. Accordingly, adhesiolysis and balloon decompression were performed with the ZiNeu catheter (Figs. 9.44 and 9.45).

During balloon decompression with the ZiNeu catheter, when the catheter was inserted into the Lt. L5–S1 intervertebral foramen and the balloon was inflated, the patient complained of S1 dermatome stimulation. When the catheter was inserted into the Lt. L4–5 intervertebral foramen and stimulation was applied, the patient complained of Lt. L5 dermatome stimulation and stated that the sensation was consistent with the site of that pain that he usually felt. The procedure was completed by performing balloon decompression that specifically targeted the L4–5 intervertebral foramen (Fig. 9.46). The patient's pain completely disappeared after the procedure, and the patient has maintained the improvement since the completion of the procedure 3 years previously.

At another hospital, Lt. L5 transforaminal block was performed based on the patient's symptoms; however, because adhesion was actually found around the nerves emerging from the Lt. L4–5 intervertebral foramen, the procedure was ineffective. When performing the procedure, it is useful to conduct a provocation test around the affected area to confirm the site of the lesion, especially in cases involving patients with Bertolotti's syndrome because the anatomical nerve of such patients may be different from the actual physiological nerves.

9.7 Procedure for Patients Who Are Not Expected to Benefit from Balloon Decompression

A 74-year-old woman visited the pain clinic due to low back, hip, and bilateral leg tingling (S1 dermatome) and pain that had begun 3 years prior. The patient reported that she felt tingling even when lying down and that she could not walk for longer than 5 min due to severe tingling and pain. She was receiving treatment for diabetes, hypertension, and Parkinson's disease and had received Cyberknife treatment for a brain tumor 2 years prior.

Although she had undergone epidural block and neuroplasty at other hospitals, the procedures effected no improvement, not even for a day. MRI findings showed L3–4, L4–5 central stenosis with bilateral L5 foraminal stenosis (Fig. 9.47). Based on the determination that significant improvement may not have been achievable from balloon decompression with the ZiNeu catheter, simple L4–5 level balloon decompression with the ZiNeuF03 catheter was performed. Local anesthesia was then applied, and 4 cc of 5% hypertonic saline was administered. Because the case involved bilateral S1 radiculopathy, insertion of the catheter into the intervertebral foramen was unnecessary and balloon decompression was performed only in the central area.

9.7 Procedure for Patients Who Are Not Expected to Benefit from Balloon Decompression 215

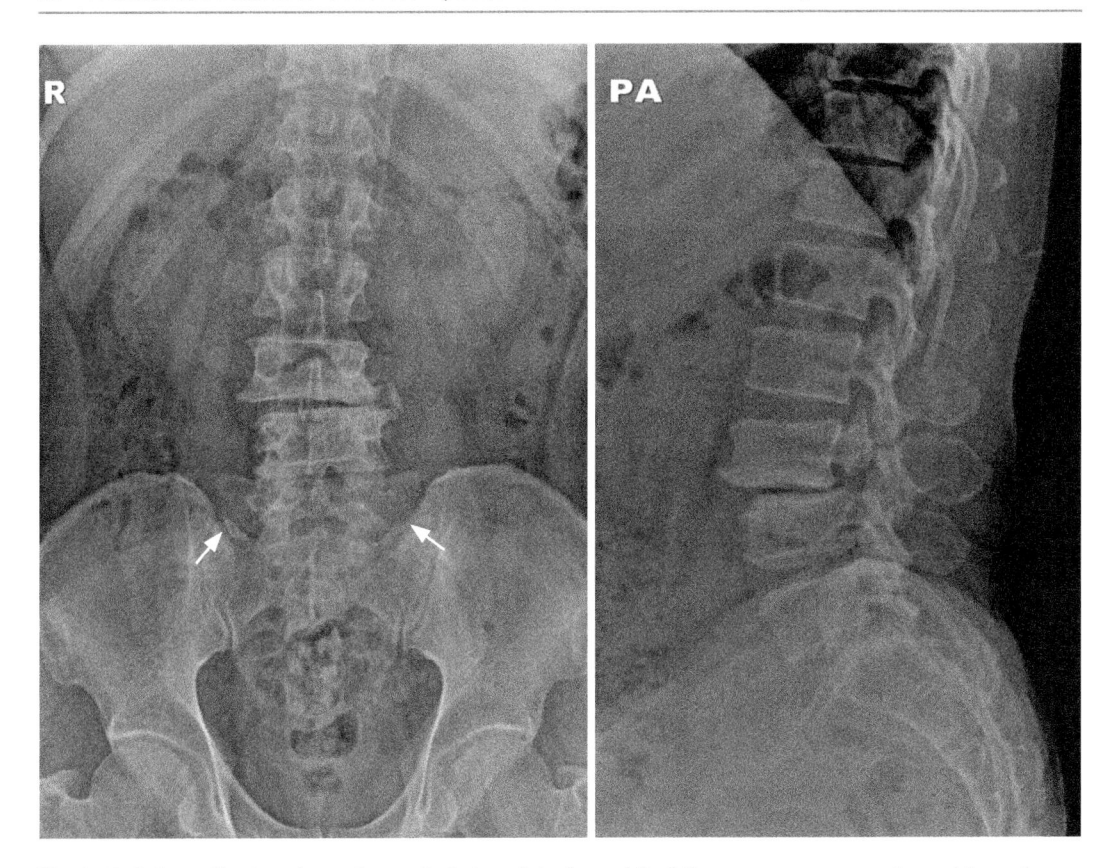

Fig. 9.45 L5 sacralization. Anomalous articulation of the Lt. and Rt. L5 transverse process and sacral bone. Arrow: Anomalous articulation

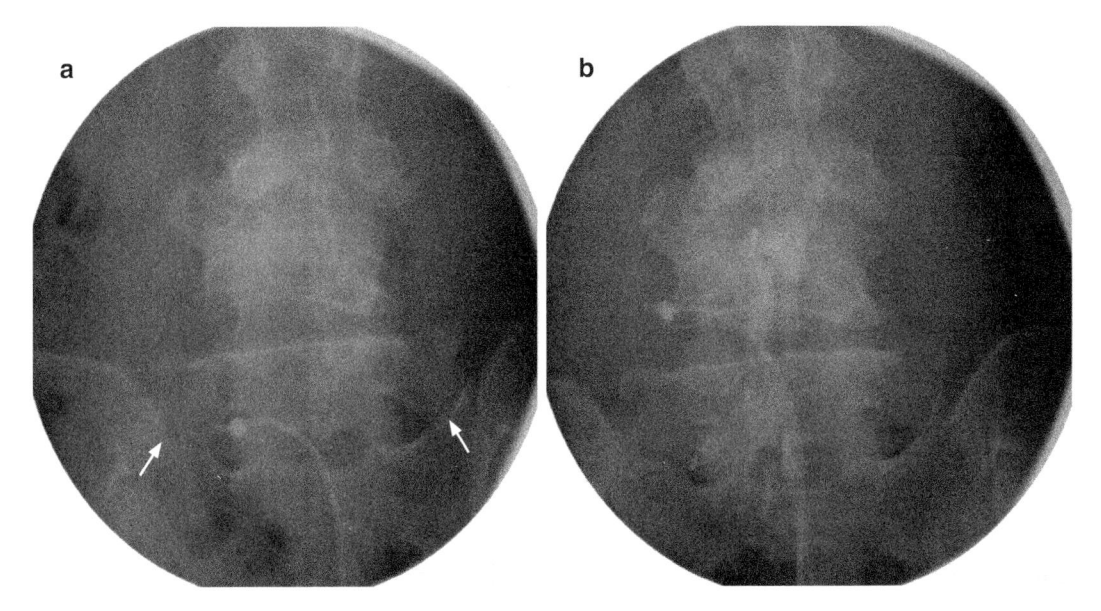

Fig. 9.46 Provocation test during balloon decompression. (**a**) The patient complained of Lt. S1 dermatome stimulation when the balloon was inflated in the Lt. L5 intervertebral foramen. (**b**) The patient complained of Lt. L5 dermatome stimulation when the balloon was inflated in the Lt. L4 intervertebral foramen. Anatomical L4 nerve demonstrated the adoption of the physiological function of the L5 nerve. Arrow: Anomalous articulation

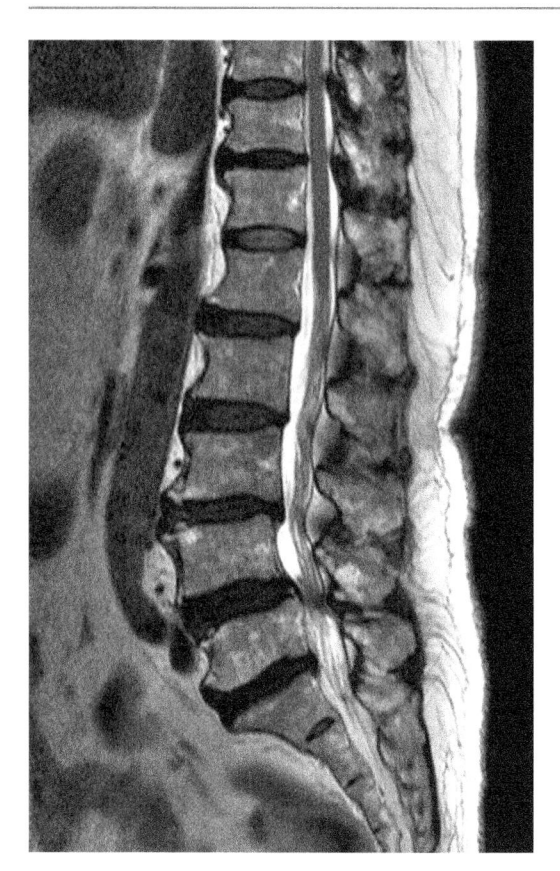

Fig. 9.47 MRI finding. L3–4, L4–5 central stenosis with bilateral L5 foraminal stenosis

A dose of 4 cc of 5% hypertonic saline was administered twice more at 2-h intervals and twice again at 2-h intervals on the following day. The catheter was then removed. Because the patient had reported that her diabetes was not well regulated, steroid was not administered (Fig. 9.48).

Approximately 2 months after the procedure, the patient reported an improvement of approximately 30%. Accordingly, the procedure was performed once more. The patient was monitored for the following 3 months.

Multiple factors could have caused the limited improvement effect after the procedure. For example, tingling that occurs while lying down could be considered a form of neuropathic pain, while diabetes, as explained in the Introduction section, can lower the probability of a successful spinal procedure. Parkinson's disease is a neurologic condition that diminishes the improvement effect after the procedure. In particular, if previously received neuroplasty achieves no improvement, it is likely that balloon decompression would also yield low improvement. As explained earlier, if epidural block or neuroplasty is effective, but the level of improvement is not significant or the effect is sustained for only a short time, there is a high likelihood of balloon decompression achieving excellent, sustained improvement. However, if such procedures were completely ineffective, then there is a high likelihood that balloon decompression will be ineffective as well.

For cases similar to this patient, the patient and guardian should be warned that the treatment will involve mostly exercise and drug therapy, rather than the procedure. However, if the patient is unable to exercise due to severe pain, the operator should consider performing the procedure with the ZiNeuF03 catheter, which is useful for the administration of hypertonic saline; as a less expensive alternative, this option could reduce at least some of the severe pain. If the employment of the ZiNeuF03 catheter effects satisfactory improvement, then conducting the operation with a ZiNeu series catheter, which could achieve an even greater improvement, should be considered in case of recurrence.

In conclusion, achieving pain reduction with the repeated administration of hypertonic saline may be a more cost-effective option for intractable patients than expecting an improvement in symptoms with physical adhesiolysis or stenosis alleviation.

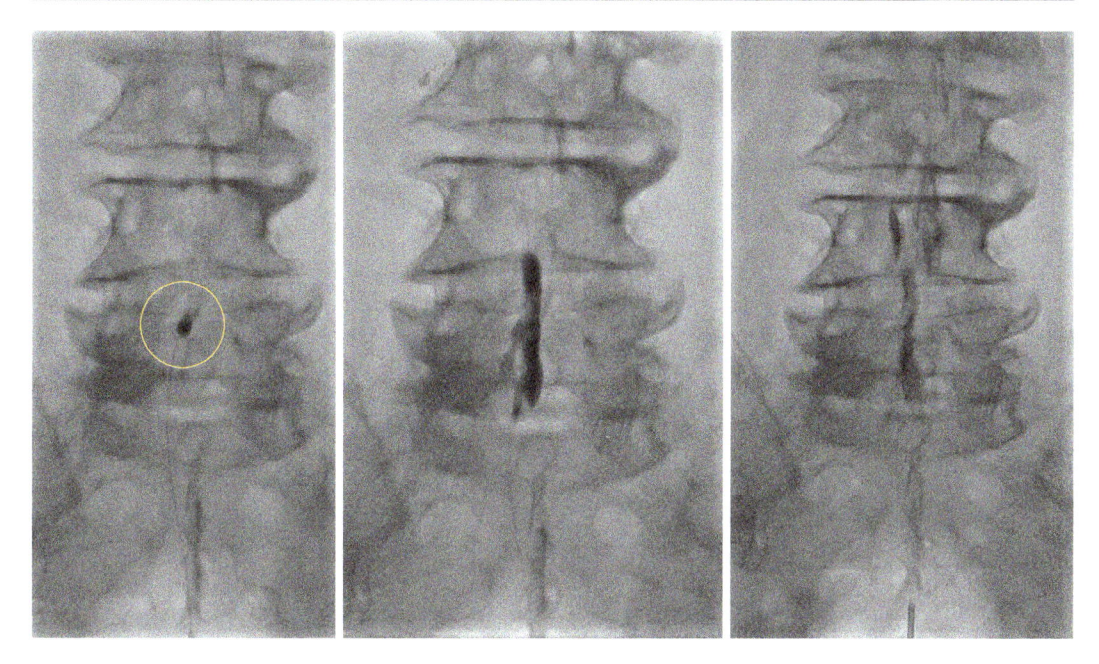

9.7 Procedure for Patients Who Are Not Expected to Benefit from Balloon Decompression

Fig. 9.48 Balloon decompression in the L4–5 central area with the ZiNeuF03 catheter followed by the administration of 5% hypertonic saline. Circle: Inflated balloon

Summarizing the Aforementioned Cases
1. With respect to the areas targeted for intervention, the patient's symptoms, physical examination, and MRI and epidurogram findings should be reviewed comprehensively to inform the selection of only the areas that require treatment.
2. For example, if Rt. L5 radiculopathy is present with lesions in the Rt. L4–5 retrodiscal area, then balloon decompression with the ZiNeu catheter should be performed in the Rt. L4–5 retrodiscal area, Rt. L5 preganglion, and Rt. L5 foramen to treat all affected sites. When performing the foraminal procedure in such cases, the catheter must be inserted into the superior aspect of the intervertebral foramen along the trajectory of the nerves through this area.
3. For example, if Rt. L5 radiculopathy is present but there are lesions in the Rt. L4–5 retrodiscal area, balloon decompression should be performed with the ZiNeuF catheter only in the superior aspect of the Rt. L5 foramen along the trajectory of the nerves through this area.
4. For retrodiscal lesions, both the caudal approach with the ZiNeu series catheter and transforaminal approach with the ZiNeuF catheter should be implemented.
5. If L5 radiculopathy is present but MRI findings show no particular retrodiscal or foraminal lesions, and transforaminal epidural block yields only temporary improvement, there is a high likelihood of foraminal adhesion. In such cases, foraminal balloon decompression should be performed. On the other hand, if transforaminal epidural block is completely ineffective, other causes need to be identified.
6. If the improvement with epidural block lasts only for a short time, an epidurogram should be obtained to check for filling defects and to confirm whether the target area is associated with the patient's symptoms. If evidence for this is acquired, balloon decompression

should be performed only on the area(s) with the filling defect.
7. S1 dermatome symptoms are mostly caused by lesions in the retrodiscal area of the spinal canal; thus, there is no need to insert the catheter into the S1 foramen (S1 radiculopathy is mostly caused by central stenosis or adhesion).
8. If there are no L4 and L5 dermatome symptoms, insertion of the catheter into the intervertebral foramen is unnecessary.
9. The onset or worsening of low back pain when walking is often caused by spinal stenosis or adhesion; thus, they must always be considered in the context of differential diagnoses. If spinal adhesion is suspected, it is advisable to perform the procedure in both the anterior and posterior epidural spaces.
10. Leaving the drug-injection epidural catheter in place after balloon decompression and performing neuroplasty with hypertonic saline for 1–2 days can help to maximize the therapeutic effect.
11. For patients in whom multiple factors could compromise the likelihood of achieving significant improvement with balloon decompression, the ZiNeuF03 catheter should be used in consideration of cost-effectiveness. Repeated balloon inflation while the catheter is retained can also help to maximize the therapeutic effect.

Post-Procedural Care and Prognosis

10.1 Post-Procedural Care

The use of any medication, such as an antithrombotic agent, that was temporarily discontinued for the procedure should be resumed from the day following the procedure.

Aspects of post-procedural care that warrant the most attention are infection and pain. Should the ZiNeu series catheter have been used or the drug-injection epidural catheter was left in place for 2–3 days, antibiotics should be administered intravenously before and after the procedure and oral antibiotics and analgesics should be delivered together for 3 days after the procedure to prevent infection and control pain. The patient and guardian should be instructed to contact the hospital immediately if symptoms such as infection occur after the procedure. Fortunately, the author has yet to encounter any case of infection after balloon decompression.

On the other hand, it is common for some patients to experience persistent pain for 3–5 days after balloon decompression. Although such pain may be due to the rigid catheter tip causing tissue damage and nerve irritation during the procedure, nerve compression caused by the balloon could be implicated to some degree in the onset of post-procedural pain. According to the author's experience, such pain does not last very long and typically dissipates within 10 days; in some cases, however, it may persist for up to 1 month. The possibility of such pain should be explained in advance to the patient and guardian prior to the performance of the procedure.

Minimizing the induction of pain during the procedure is critical to reducing post-procedural pain. To achieve this, the operator should consider using ≤1% Lidocaine for epidural anesthesia before the procedure and maneuvering the catheter itself as slowly and smoothly as possible during its insertion. Severe pain occurring during the procedure can be caused by the irritation of an inflamed area and indicate tissue damage. Therefore, the importance of reducing the incidence of pain during the procedure cannot be understated. Of course, it is advisable not to touch any area that is not directly associated with the patient's lesions.

Any effort to reduce pain during the procedure can help to eliminate or shorten the duration of transient pain that could occur after the procedure. Despite such efforts, if the patient complains of severe pain after discharge and the pain cannot be managed with the administration of analgesics alone, then the patient should be instructed to visit the hospital once more to undergo epidural block under local anesthesia: a sodium channel blocker, this can be very helpful as it can reduce the excitability of the nerves that become sensitive due to irritation borne during the procedure. Steroids can also be used if neurogenic inflammation is suspected, but they are not always necessary.

Some patients complain of severe post-procedural pain in the sacral hiatus region where the guide needle was inserted; such pain can reach the point of preventing the patient from sitting. In most of these cases, pain occurs from inflammation or weakening of the sacrococcygeal ligament that was damaged during guide needle insertion. Injecting a small amount of a mixture containing steroids and local anesthetics into the area with the most severe pain can quickly reduce pain.

As will be explained further in the Prognosis section, maintaining the therapeutic effect following a procedure and achieving even further improvement depend on self-care practiced by the patient. If post-procedural pain is not severe, the patient should be instructed to engage in increasing amounts of exercise, starting from the day after the procedure, in proportion to the degree of symptom improvement. In particular, patients should be reminded that increasing their amount of walking will yield further improvement over time. Sometimes, patients who find it difficult to walk on account of being overweight or those with knee pain are recommended to walk in a swimming pool as walking in water reduces the strain of weight on the low back or knees.

The author always reminds patients that if they feel pain while walking, they should discontinue the activity and take a moment to stop and rest. The author recommends this type of walking for at least 1 h every day. If patients do not engage in walking, recurrence may occur more quickly and walking will become even more difficult over time.

10.2 Prognosis

Factors that have the most significant influence on prognosis include selection of the target patient and competency of the operator. It is important to choose patients whose condition could improve significantly following balloon decompression; for patients who may benefit little from the procedure, it should only be performed after they have been explained the reason for the likely inefficacy of the procedure as well as their prognosis. It is important for less experienced operators to build familiarity with the procedure by performing the operations that require relatively uncomplicated iterations of balloon decompression. By doing so, it becomes possible, at some point, to predict the amount of improvement that can be expected from the procedure according to the patient's condition.

Satisfactory improvement could be achieved only if areas where the procedure needs to be performed are accurately identified and the procedure is performed successfully in all those areas. As explained in the Concept section, the low procedural success rate in the target area indicates less improvement of shorter duration. Targets for balloon decompression include adhesion and stenosis caused by degenerative spinal diseases, including disc herniation. Factors that determine the relative likelihood of improvement in the patient's condition after the procedure are as follows:

Factors influencing the relative likelihood of improvement following balloon decompression
1. Younger patients with single lesions have a higher likelihood of improvement than elderly patients with multilevel lesions.
2. Patients with stenosis caused by soft structures, such as a disc or ligament, have a higher likelihood of improvement than those with hard stenosis attributable to bone tissue.
3. Patients whose symptoms improve after receiving epidural block, no matter how temporary the improvement, have a higher likelihood of improvement than those who gain no improvement from epidural block at all.
4. Cases involving less severe lesions have a higher likelihood of improvement.
5. Among patients with spondylolisthesis, while symptom improvement effect tends to be excellent, the recurrence rate is higher than among those without spondylolisthesis, which may be due to spinal instability.

6. Patients without diabetes have a higher likelihood of improvement than those with diabetes.
7. Patients without systemic diseases, such as Parkinson's disease, fibromyalgia, rheumatoid arthritis, or ankylosing spondylitis, have a higher likelihood of improvement.
8. Cases involving psychological issues, such as depression and compensation, have a lower likelihood of improvement.
9. Cases involving neuropathic pain have a lower likelihood of improvement.
10. Among patients with postspinal surgery pain, those with greater areas or extents of spinal surgery have a lower likelihood of improvement.
11. Among patients with chronic spinal stenosis, those for whom MRI has revealed redundant nerve roots may have a relatively low likelihood of improvement.

Table 10.1 Douleur Neuropathique en 4 Questions (DN4) questionnaire

DN4 questionnaire		
Please read the following questions and answer each item with "Yes" or "No":		
Question 1. Does your pain present one or more of the following characteristics?		
1—Pain feels like burning	Yes	No
2—Sensation of painful cold	Yes	No
3—Pain feels like an electric shock	Yes	No
Question 2. In the same area, is your pain associated with one or more symptoms?		
4—Tingling	Yes	No
5—Pins and needles	Yes	No
6—Numbness	Yes	No
7—Itching	Yes	No
Question 3: Is there pain located in the area indicated by the examination results?		
8—Hypoesthesia to touch	Yes	No
9—Hypoesthesia to pinprick	Yes	No
Question 4: Is the pain provoked or increased by the following?		
10—Pain after brushing	Yes	No

Scores of ≥4/10 indicate neuropathic pain

While these factors may be equally relevant to all spinal procedures and surgeries, as well as balloon decompression, their applicability may differ slightly according to the degree of procedural difficulty, price, and the expected degree of effect and its period of sustainment.

Degenerative spinal disease is often accompanied by neuropathic pain caused by mechanisms such as central sensitization as it persists as a chronic disease. Such neuropathic pain does not improve immediately once the lesion is removed; thus, the pain may persist even if the procedure or surgery was successful. In fact, the pain may be exacerbated due to irritation caused by the procedure or surgery. A significant portion of patients with pain following spinal surgery may exhibit persistent neuropathic pain that already presented before the surgery. Therefore, the presence of neuropathic pain should be thoroughly checked prior to the performance of any spinal surgery. If there are findings suspicious of pre-procedural neuropathic pain, then the patient and guardian should be informed of such findings and reminded that immediate improvement in symptoms after the procedure might be improbable.

Table 10.1 is called the DN4 questionnaire, which is used to determine the presence of neuropathic pain based on a 10-point scale, where scores of ≥4 affirm neuropathic pain. Of course, this metric does not guarantee 100% certainty, but it is worth using in clinical practice and research as it supplies a basis by which to inform suspicions of neuropathic pain.

In the following case, balloon decompression was performed in a patient who was suspected of having neuropathic pain.

Case 1

A 78-year-old man visited the pain clinic complaining of low back pain, tingling sensation below both knees (L5 and S1 dermatome), and dysesthesia that had begun 3 years earlier. The patient reported that he only felt slight tingling when lying still, but he had to stop after walking just 5 m due to leg tingling, cold sensation, the feeling of stepping on sand, and burning. While the pain diminished the most when sitting or lying down, even standing decreased the pain.

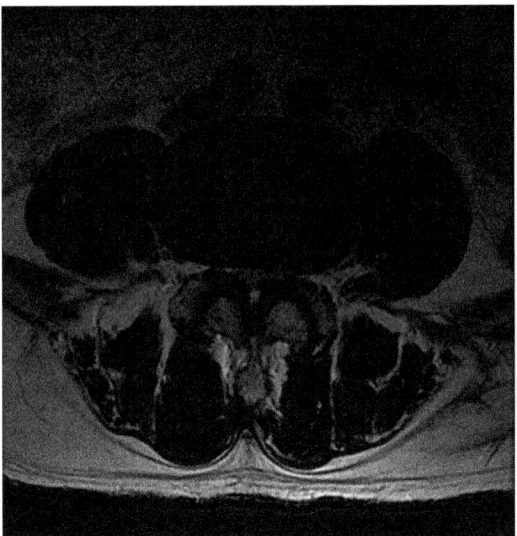

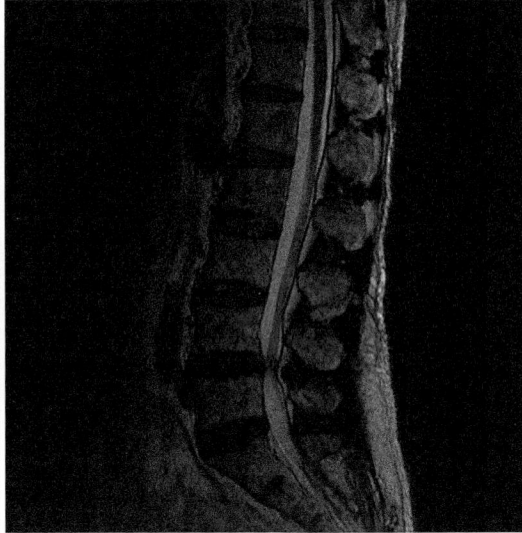

Fig. 10.1 MRI findings. L4–5 central stenosis

MRI findings showed only moderate central stenosis in the L4–5 level (Fig. 10.1).

Although he had undergone several rounds of epidural block and neuroplasty at other hospitals, any improvement gained therefrom was temporary. He was taking oral medications—Neurontin (300 mg tid), Enafon (10 mg bid), and Tridol (50 mg tid)—however, the improvements in his symptoms were weak.

Based on the presence of symptoms indicative of neuropathic pain, the patient was told that balloon decompression might not mitigate his symptoms. The patient still wanted to receive the procedure. Balloon decompression was performed in both the Lt. and Rt. L5 foramen, preganglion, and retrodiscal area, and the contrast dye was found to spread satisfactorily. Subsequently, 3 cc doses of a steroid/local anesthetic mixture were injected into each target area (Fig. 10.2).

At the 1-month follow-up, the patient reported the lack of any improvement. Accordingly, he was prescribed pharmacotherapy and physical therapy for neuropathic pain with no additional procedures.

The following may account for the lack of efficacy of balloon decompression in this patient.

1. The patient's symptoms were suspicious of neuropathic pain. Most patients with spinal stenosis tend to be asymptomatic when lying still, but this patient complained of a tingling sensation even when lying still. Moreover, cold sensation in the legs, plantar dysesthesia, and burning sensation could all be suspected as symptoms of neuropathic pain.

2. The patient reported almost no improvement in symptoms despite taking Neurontin (300 mg tid), Enafon (10 mg bid), and Tridol (50 mg tid) prescribed by another hospital. Patients with neuropathic pain-related symptoms often show relatively less improvement with analgesics.

3. The patient reported that he did not benefit from several rounds of epidural block and neuroplasty at other hospitals. If the patients have many factors associated with neuropathic pain, such procedures may not yield any improvement. Balloon decompression is very effective in patients who have shown at least some improvement, even if temporary, after receiving epidural block or neuroplasty. Although it is not always the case, a lack of any improvement from epidural block or neuroplasty indicates that balloon decompression will likely not affect any improvement either. This patient's symptoms may not have improved even if he had undergone surgery.

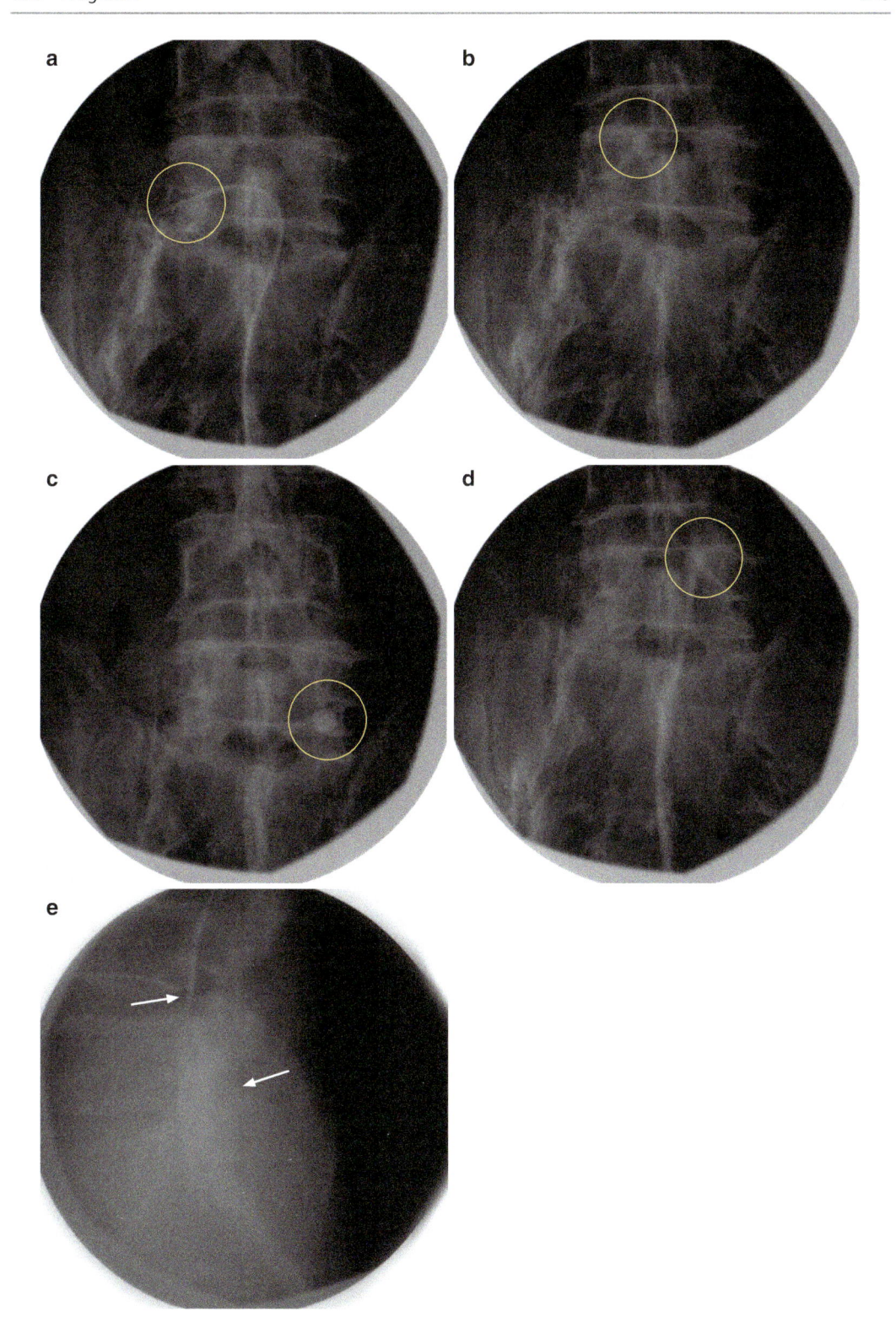

Fig. 10.2 (**a**) Performance of the procedure in the Lt. L5 foramen. (**b**) Performance of the procedure in the Lt. L5 preganglion area. (**c**) Performance of the procedure in the Rt. L5 foramen. (**d**) Performance of the procedure in the Rt. L5 preganglion area. (**e**) Spread of the contrast dye after procedure in the retrodiscal area. Circle: Inflated balloon. Arrow: Anterior and posterior epidural spaces

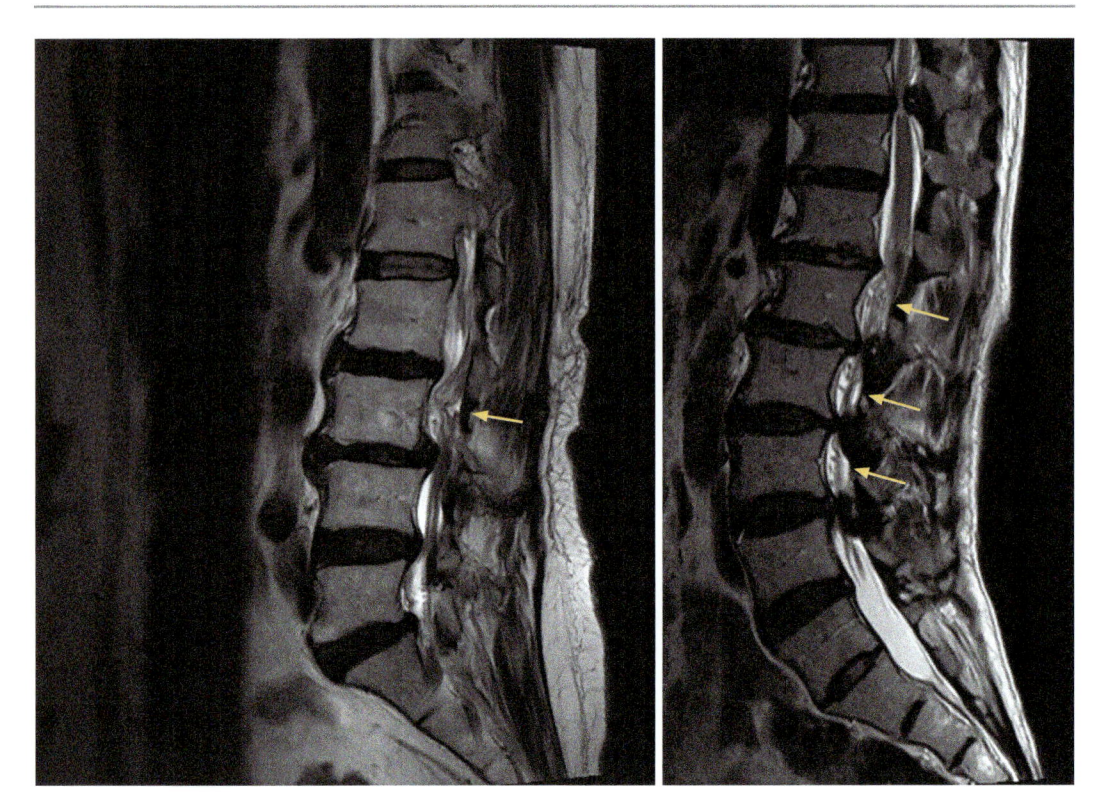

Fig. 10.3 Thin, long, convoluted redundant nerve roots found in a patient with spinal stenosis. Arrow: Redundant nerve roots

Because of these three reasons, the procedure yielded very little or no improvement effect, despite MRI findings indicative of a mild lesion. Prior to performing the procedure, such factors must be checked.

A brief explanation will be given concerning the presence of redundant nerve roots shown in MRI findings described in (11) on page 221.

As shown in Fig. 10.3, redundant nerve roots refer to long, thin, convoluted nerves that appear in the intradural space near the area with severe spinal stenosis. These are indicative of degenerative change consequent of the stretching of nerves induced by movement of the spine, such as flexion and extension, when the spinal nerves are already constricted and compressed by severe spinal stenosis.

Redundant nerve roots can be eliminated by spinal surgery, in which case, the prognosis is expected to be favorable. However, most cases are considered to involve irreversible changes that cannot be resolved with surgery.

In tissue biopsy, redundant nerve roots typically show findings indicative of nerve damage, such as demyelination of nerve tissues, endoneural fibrosis, and proliferation of Schwann cells.

Redundant nerve roots are reportedly associated with older age, symptoms that have been present for longer periods, and the presence of severe neurological symptoms; however, these associations remain contested in the literature. Regardless, redundant nerve roots indicate that prognosis following epidural block and surgery will likely be poor; this may be due to the high likelihood of redundant nerve roots being accompanied by neuropathic pain caused by neurological degenerative changes and deformation.

Similarly, balloon decompression would also effect little improvement in patients with such findings. Whether the procedure should be performed should only be determined after this is fully explained to the patient.

In cases that involve other factors (e.g., history of previous spinal surgery and comorbidities, such as neurological or musculoskeletal diseases), the cause of pain is very complex, and the pain may thus persist as not all problems causative of the pain could be resolved with balloon decompression alone. If the area in which the procedure is being performed is the primary cause of pain, then balloon decompression can produce significant improvement. As that may not be the case, sufficient explanation must be provided to the patient and guardian prior to receiving their agreement to undergo the procedure.

As explained earlier, exercising after the procedure has an important impact on the patient's prognosis.

Some physicians instruct patients with pain induced by spinal stenosis to not engage in excessive amount of walking; while this may reduce pain in the short term, the lack of exercise weakens the muscles, tendons, and ligaments as well as exacerbates adhesion. These effects will ultimately cause the disease to worsen. Walking can help to strengthen and stabilize the musculoskeletal system, improve nutrient supply and blood circulation, and resolve inflammation. Therefore, engaging in walking can provide critical utility in treating spinal diseases, including spinal stenosis.

If the patient is able to exercise owing to alleviation of his or her symptoms by drug therapy, epidural block, or physical therapy, then the patient may not need balloon decompression. On the other hand, if the patient has difficulty exercising, balloon decompression should be performed to enable to patient to engage in walking, and the patient should be instructed to increase the amount of exercise in proportion to his or her level of improvement to ensure that the improvement effect is sustained.

Therefore, the most important patient-related factors following the procedure are self-care and walking.

10.3 General Questions About the Procedure

The questions mentioned below are informed by situations often encountered in clinical practice or during instruction in the performance of balloon decompression. As the readers of this book may have similar questions and many patients may actually ask these questions, the author's responses to these sample questions have been prepared as follows:

10.3.1 If the Balloon Compresses a Nerve, Could It Cause Nerve Damage or Dysfunction?

When balloon decompression was first developed and underwent review for the New Medical Technology Certification, this uncertainty engendered the most questions and greatest concern with respect to safety and some reviewers opposed granting the technique certification on account of this very issue.

A literature review performed by the author found that articles employing conditions similar to those used in the clinical performance of balloon decompression observed that while the procedure may cause nerve damage or compromise nerve conduction, it is safe so long as the balloon pressure is raised slowly and the induced pressure is released within 2 h. Accordingly, as the author developed balloon decompression, the following recommendations to prevent nerve damage have been gathered: Inflate the balloon gradually. Do not continue to apply pressure for more than 5 s at a time and reduce the extent of balloon inflation according to the patient's pain level. Silicon balloons tend to rupture when inflated with a pressure that is strong enough to cause nerve damage. This also contributes significantly to the safety of the procedure. If the balloon does not rupture, the procedure might not have received the New Medical Technology Certification.

Along with the rupturing characteristic of silicon, as long as the aforementioned recommendations for the procedure are followed, there is no possibility of nerve damage.

10.3.2 Can the Intervertebral Foramen Actually be Expanded With a Balloon?

With the balloon, the stenosed area cannot be expanded as much as is possible with surgery. However, the primary cause of claudication is circulatory impairment, and balloon decompression is more than capable of alleviating stenosis to improve blood circulation; this capacity has been shown by published reports. The procedure could produce greater levels of improvement in cases involving soft stenosis caused by degenerative disc disorders than in those from hard stenosis. Similarly, the procedure is more effective in cases of mild stenosis than severe stenosis. If the procedure does not yield functional improvement or pain reduction, surgery should be considered.

10.3.3 How Long Can the Expansion of the Balloon be Maintained?

MRI findings indicative of severe stenosis do not imply accompanying symptoms. Even with severe stenosis, the patient may be asymptomatic, or symptoms may be mild. Therefore, it is not necessary to alleviate the stenosis as shown in MRI findings for the procedure to be effective.

The duration over which the free space created by the balloon can be maintained has not been studied yet. However, the shrinkage of space subsequent to expansion does not imply the recurrence of symptoms. There are some patients with MRI findings indicative of severe stenosis whose symptoms improved after balloon decompression and continued to improve further over several years. Continuing to engage in exercise after the procedure often ensures that symptoms do not reappear, even if stenosis or adhesion develops again. If there is only temporary improvement, repeating the procedure once more to achieve further improvement could be warranted.

Balloon decompression can improve motor function, such as walking, by increasing the distance that the patient is able to walk. By continuing to exercise, recurrences can be prevented to a certain degree. Another possibility is spontaneous resorption. It has been reported that once the pain is reduced and the patient can walk with normal posture, spontaneous resorption rate in degenerative disc disorders increases. Because balloon decompression can increase the distance that the patient can walk with good posture, it is able to sustain the therapeutic effect for a relatively long time by increasing the opportunity for spontaneous resorption and natural healing.

In the study conducted by the author, 40% of intractable patients sustained the improvements mediated by balloon decompression for over 1 year after just one procedure. In another recent study, the improvement effects on pain, motor function, and satisfaction level were maintained at the 1-year follow-up in patients for whom balloon decompression had been successful; motor function, in particular, was reported to have improved even more over time. It is believed that balloon expansion improves motor function, which in turn allows for further improvements in motor function over time. This is an important outcome that is not found in other procedures.

10.3.4 What Should the Patients be Told Concerning the Duration of Sustained Effect?

The duration of sustained effect varies significantly between patients and is thus difficult to determine in advance.

The patient is typically told that if the effect is sustained for more than 3 months after the procedure, continuing to exercise could increase the likelihood that the therapeutic benefit will be sustained for over a year. Of course, patients are also told that reintervention may be necessary in case of recurrence. However, if there is no effect or the effect lasts no more than 1 month, surgery is recommended rather than another round of the same procedure because the latter may not achieve a lasting effect even after another round.

Therefore, it is advisable to explain to the patient, in advance, that there may be no effect or the effect may be temporary if neuropathic pain or spondylolisthesis is present or the case involves multilevel stenosis and/or postspinal surgery pain syndrome.

10.3.5 Even Balloon-Less Catheters Allow for Good Contrast Dye Spread After the Procedure. How Are They Different Then from Balloon Catheters?

It may be difficult to identify the differences solely from the spread of contrast dye after the procedure. Therefore, the author uses the 3D reconstructed views of contrast dye spread for accurate quantitative comparison. The results show significant differences in the diameter and volume of spread of the contrast dye. Increases in the diameter and volume of spread of the contrast dye are indicative of increases in free space and, more accurately, greater improvements in blood circulation.

The success of the procedure should not be determined based simply on whether the contrast dye has spread; the difference in the extent of contrast dye spread in the area with adhesion or stenosis across the procedure is more important.

10.3.6 How Many Times Can This Procedure be Performed in 1 Year on the Same Patient?

Depending on the case, repeated procedures may help to improve the patient's symptoms. However, if steroids are used during the procedure, more than 3–4 times a year is not recommended.

If a steroid is not used, performing repeat operations should not be problematic, but such a determination should also consider the cost effectiveness.

If improvement is achieved after the procedure, the patient should continue to exercise. When exercise becomes difficult, the procedure should be performed again to help improve his or her walking ability.

> **Extraneous Knowledge 10**
> **Blood supply in the lumbar spinal cord**
> Blood from the aorta passes through the lumbar and segmental arteries before being supplied to the spinal cord. After bifurcating to the anterior and posterior radicular arteries in the intervertebral foramen and supplying blood to the spinal root, a single anterior spinal artery and two posterior spinal arteries connect together to supply blood to the spinal cord. However, sometimes the segmental artery is connected to the radiculo-medullary artery (Adamkiewicz artery) rather than the radicular artery to supply blood to the root, after which it connects to the anterior spinal artery.
> The Adamkiewicz artery is a major source of blood supply for the anterior spinal artery and is responsible for blood flow into the anterior two-thirds of the lumbosacral area. Therefore, caution should be exercised as damage to this artery can cause anterior spinal cord syndrome and consequently paraplegia.
> As 69–85% of the Adamkiewicz artery exits from the left side, whereas 75%, 15%, and 10% are found between T9-L2, T5–8, and L1–2, respectively, caution should again be exercised when performing the procedure at the Lt. T9-L3 level to ensure that this artery is not damaged.
> Angiographic findings indicate that the Adamkiewicz artery has a hairpin shape and that 97% of the artery passes through the safe triangle of the intervertebral foramen. Therefore, for any procedure that requires an approach through the safe triangle area of the Lt. T9-L3 level, one must consider the risk of damaging this artery. When performing a procedure in this area, particulated steroids that can induce embolisms in the Adamkiewicz artery must never be used. If a steroid must be used, then a non-particulated steroid, such as dexamethasone, should be used.

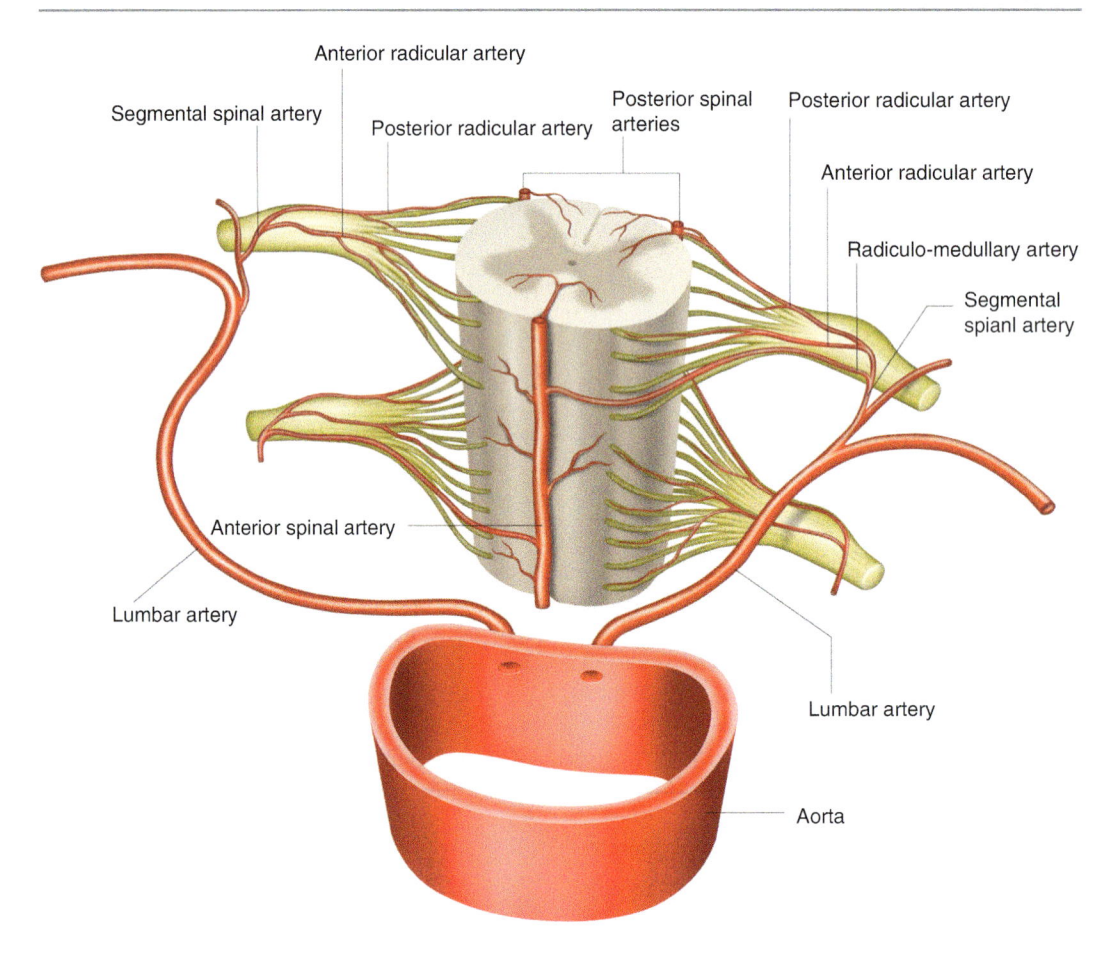

Fig. E1 Blood supply in the lumbar spinal cord. Aorta → lumbar artery → segmental artery → anterior and posterior radicular arteries → anterior and posterior spinal artery. Aorta → lumbar artery → segmental artery → radiculo-medullary artery (Adamkiewicz artery): root blood supply → anterior spinal artery

10.3 General Questions About the Procedure

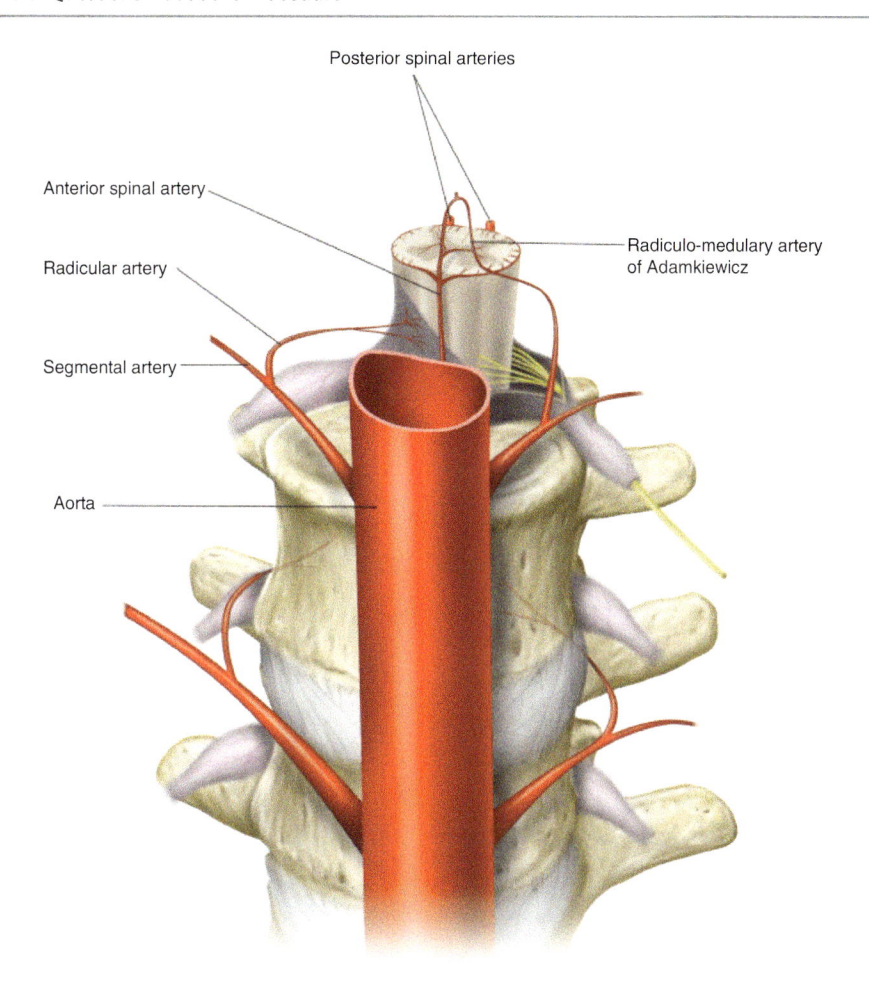

Fig. E2 Schematic of the radicular artery and radiculo-medullary artery (Adamkiewicz artery)

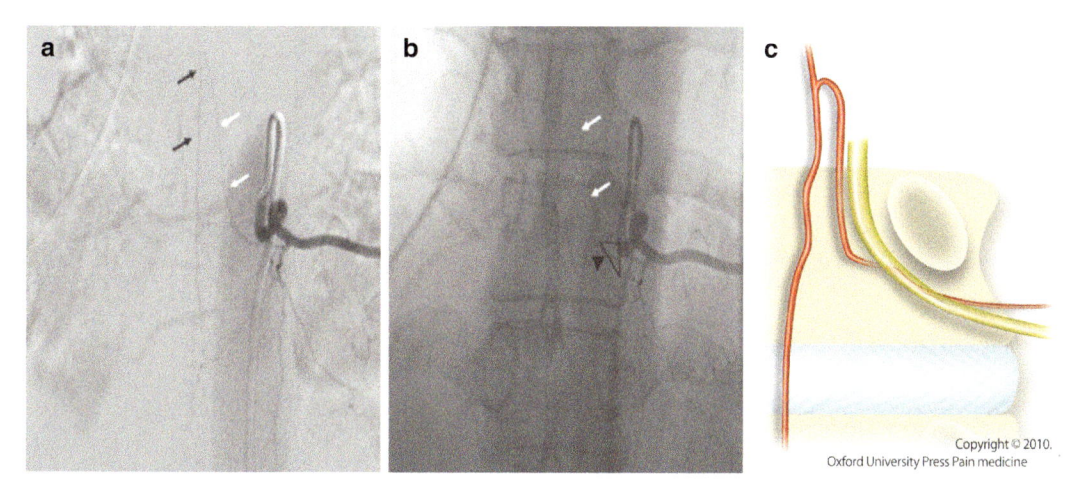

Fig. E3 97% of the Adamkiewicz artery passes through the safe triangle area. (**a**) Selected digital subtraction angiogram. (**b**) Same image without subtraction. (**c**) The Adamkiewicz artery passes through the safe triangle area. Black arrow: Anterior spinal artery. White arrow: Adamkiewicz artery. Black arrowhead: Safe triangle

Extraneous Knowledge 11

Neurogenic claudication vs. Vascular origin claudication

Neurogenic claudication, a typical symptom of spinal stenosis, must be differentiated from claudication of vascular origin. If claudication of vascular origin is mistakenly treated as a symptom of spinal stenosis, not only would symptom improvement be impossible but also it can even lead to a medical malpractice lawsuit. Therefore, caution is needed.

The following table summarizes the means by which these two diseases may be easily differentiated. If vascular origin is suspected, then the ankle brachial index (ABI) must be measured.

Symptoms	Neurogenic	Vascular
Low back pain	Common	Rare
Pain alleviation	When sitting or bending at the waist Not enough alleviation when standing or resting Slow alleviation speed (over 5 min)	No relation to posture Alleviation when standing Quick alleviation
Uphill vs. downhill	Severe when walking downhill	Severe when walking uphill
Cycling	No pain	Pain

Extraneous Knowledge 12

Ankle Brachial Index (ABI)

The ABI is an objective means of informing the diagnosis of peripheral arterial diseases, such as peripheral arterial stenosis and occlusion.

When the blood pressure in all four limbs is measured while the patient is lying down, the blood pressure in the legs is generally the same as or higher than that in the arms. However, if arterial stenosis or occlusion is present, the blood pressure in the legs is lower. The ABI is based on this principle.

To calculate the ABI, the highest systolic blood pressure (SBP) measured in the unilateral posterior tibial and dorsalis pedis arteries is divided by the highest SBP measured in the bilateral brachial arteries. The reason for using the highest SBP in the posterior tibial and dorsalis pedis arteries and not the lowest is because even if one of the posterior tibial and dorsalis pedis arteries is maintained, symptoms of peripheral arterial disease do not occur.

This test should be performed if vascular claudication is suspected. The test is noninvasive and simple and requires approximately 15–20 min to complete.

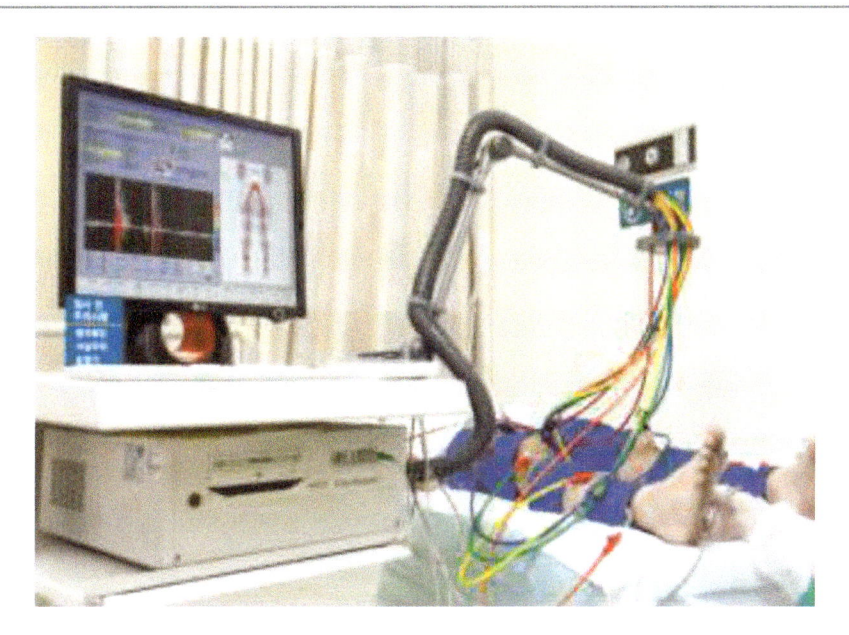

Fig. E4 Performance of the ABI test

Bibliography

1. Basaran A, Topatan S. Spinal balloon nucleoplasty: a hypothetical minimally invasive treatment for herniated nucleus pulposus. Med Hypotheses. 2008;70(6):1201–6.
2. Bouhassira D, Attal N, Alchaar H, Boureau F, Bruxelle J, Cunin G, et al. Comparison of pain syndromes associated with nervous or somatic lesions and development of a new neuropathic pain diagnostic questionnaire (DN4). Pain. 2005;114:29–36.
3. Bouhassira D. The DN4 questionnaire: a new tool for the diagnosis of neuropathic pain. Douleurs. 2005;6:297–300.
4. Olmarker K, Holm S, Rydevik B. Importance of compression onset rate for the degree of impairment of impulse propagation in experimental compression injury of the porcine cauda equina. Spine (Phila Pa 1976). 1990;15(5):416–9.
5. Olmarker K, Rydevik B, Holm S, Bagge U. Effects of experimental graded compression on blood flow in spinal nerve roots. A vital microscopic study on the porcine cauda equina. J Orthop Res. 1989;7(6):817–23.
6. Olmarker K, Rydevik B, Holm S. Edema formation in spinal nerve roots induced by experimental, graded compression. An experimental study on the pig cauda equina with special reference to differences in effects between rapid and slow onset of compression. Spine. 1989;14(6):569–73.
7. Pedowitz RA, Garfin SR, Massie JB, Hargens AR, Swenson MR, Myers RR, Rydevik BL. Effects of magnitude and duration of compression on spinal nerve root conduction. Spine. 1992;17(2):194–9.
8. Rorabeck CH. Tourniquet-induced nerve ischemia: an experimental investigation. J Trauma. 1980;20(4):280–6.

Genicular Nerve Radiofrequency Ablation

11

This chapter will introduce genicular nerve radiofrequency ablation (RFA): introduced for the first time in by the author of this book, this technique helps to improve intractable knee pain.

Dr. Yong-Up Kang from Chung Sol Pain Clinic in Busan conceived of this procedural technique and permitted the author of this book to research the technique and report the resultant findings. As an academic working in the field of pain medicine, it was a tremendous honor to have the article published in *Pain,* the most prestigious magazine in our field, in 2011. I would like to extend my gratitude once again to all who helped with this endeavor.

Research papers

Radiofrequency treatment relieves chronic knee osteoarthritis pain: A double-blind randomized controlled trial

Woo-Jong Choi [a], Seung-Jun Hwang [b], Jun-Gol Song [a], Jeong-Gil Leem [a], Yong-Up Kang [c], Pyong-Hwan Park [a], Jin-Woo Shin [a,*]

[a] *Department of Anesthesiology and Pain Medicine, Asan Medical Center, University of Ulsan College of Medicine, Seoul, Republic of Korea*
[b] *Department of Anatomy and Cell biology, Asan Medical Center, University of Ulsan College of Medicine, Seoul, Republic of Korea*
[c] *Chung sol Pain Clinics, Pusan, Republic of Korea*

After the publication of the article, this technique gained recognition as a novel treatment modality by which to resolve intractable knee pain and has become widely used by physicians worldwide. As of the end of 2018, the technique had already been cited in over 140 articles.

Many data and videos about this procedural technique have been published on YouTube and other websites (Fig. 11.1).

Recently, the cooled RFA method was incorporated into this technique, resulting in pain improvement of greater magnitude and duration. Consequently, a specific medical device for

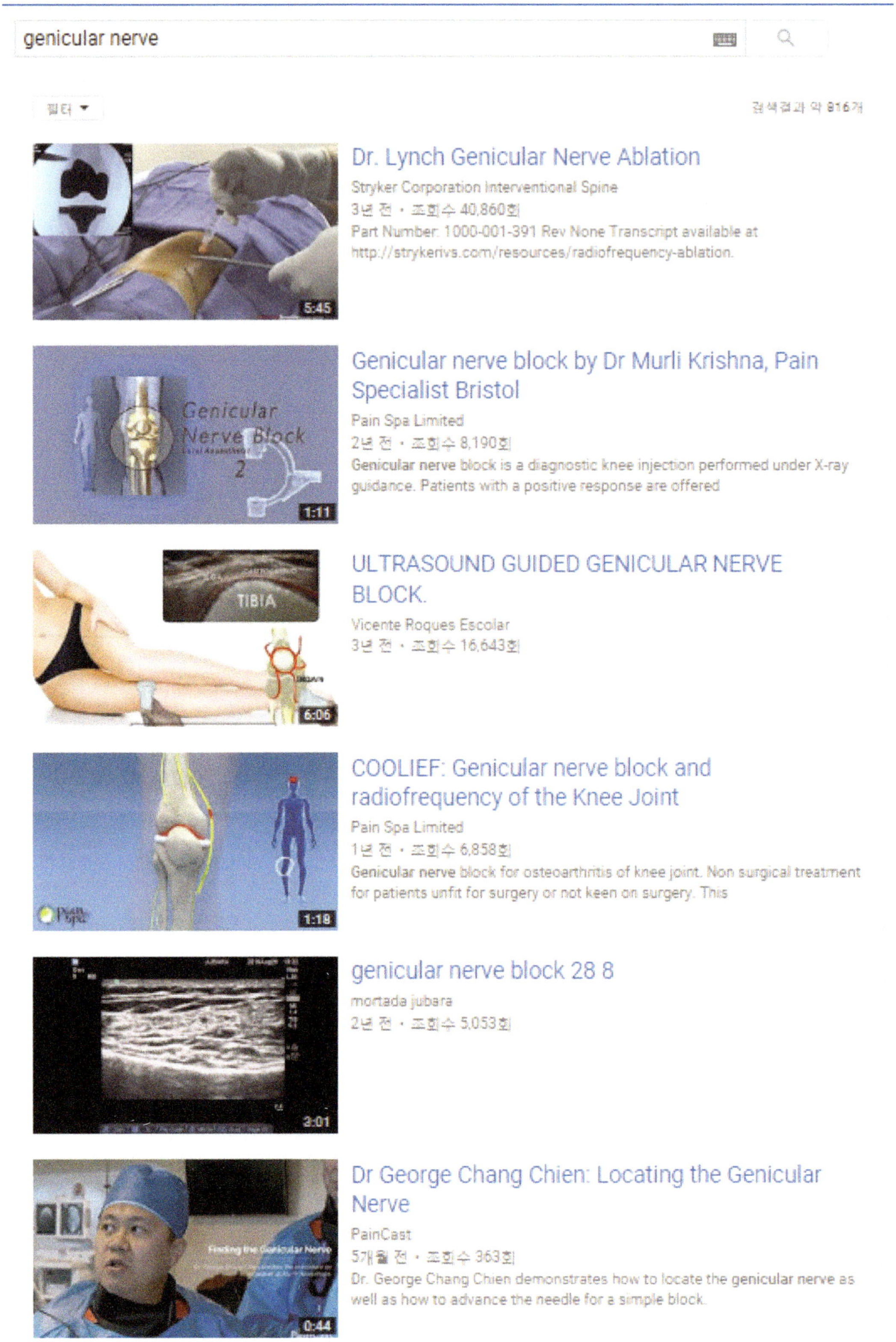

Fig. 11.1 Screenshot of the results of a YouTube search for "genicular nerve"; over 800 videos were yielded by the search

cooled RFA has been developed exclusively for this procedure.

It is expected that both cooled and conventional RFA will be recognized in the future as a basic treatment modality for intractable knee pain. The author also provided a brief introduction to this procedural technique in "Keystone of Pain Intervention," which was published by the Korean Pain Society.

11.1 Indications and Contraindications

This procedural technique is not designed to treat knee pain by removing the cause of pain; rather, it is a method by which to mitigate the amount of pain felt by the patient by blocking nerve conduction in the articular branches, pure sensory nerves that play an important role in the transmission of knee pain. Accordingly, the procedure is used only to reduce pain when the patient has shown no improvement after any other intervention, including surgery, or either cannot or elects to not undergo surgery.

11.1.1 Indications

Chronic knee pain caused by degenerative osteoarthritis.
Post-knee-surgery pain.
Other chronic knee pain that is nonresponsive to general treatments.

11.1.2 Contraindications

Pyogenic arthritis.
Patients with coagulopathy or those taking coagulants.
Patients taking immunosuppressants.
Neuropathic pain.

11.2 Anatomy

The nerves associated with knee pain include the sciatic, femoral, and obturator nerves. The sciatic nerve bifurcates into the tibial nerve (TN) and common peroneal nerve (CPN) near the popliteal fossa (Fig. 11.2).

TN further splits into articular branches that connect to the superomedial genicular nerve

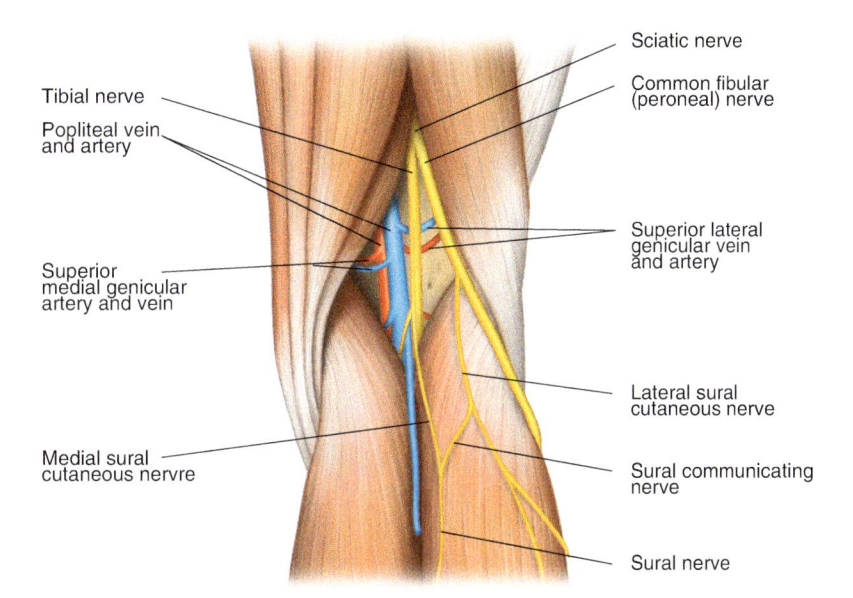

Fig. 11.2 The sciatic nerve bifurcates into the tibial nerve and the common peroneal nerve

Fig. 11.3 Major bone structures in the knee

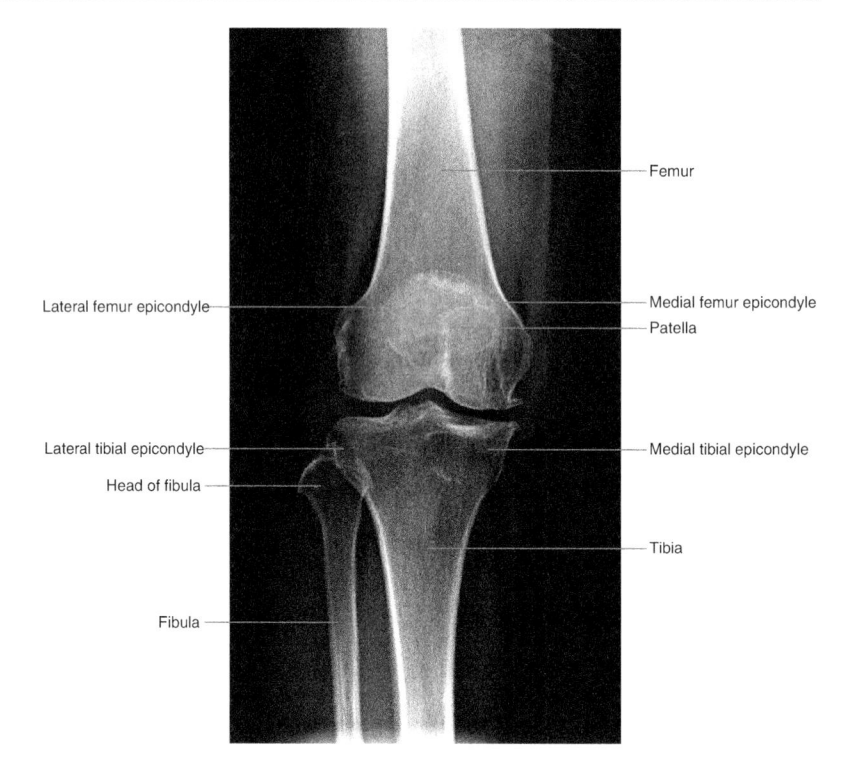

(SMGN) and middle genicular nerve. Articular branches also originate from the CPN and the saphenous nerve, which branches off from the femoral nerve: the former connect to the superolateral genicular nerve (SLGN), inferolateral genicular nerve, and tibial recurrent genicular nerve; the latter, to the inferomedial genicular nerve (IMGM). Among these articular branches, only the SMGN, IMGN, and SLGN are targeted by the genicular nerve procedure.

The following provides a summary.

1. Sciatic nerve	→ 1. Tibial nerve	→ Superomedial genicular nerve: **SMGN**
		→ Middle genicular nerve
	→ 2. Common peroneal nerve	→ Superolateral genicular nerve: **SLGN**
		→ Inferolateral genicular nerve
		→ Tibial recurrent genicular nerve
2. Femoral nerve	→ Saphenous nerve	→ Inferomedial genicular nerve: **IMGN**
3. Obturator nerve		

The SLGN, SMGN, and IMGN run uniformly across the area connecting the femoral and tibial epicondyle and shaft to the genicular vessels sharing the same name. Therefore, the locations of these vessels are helpful in ascertaining the locations of the aforementioned nerves (Figs. 11.3 and 11.4). The inferolateral genicular nerve passes through the lateral aspect of the fibular head, and, as a result, a large variation and the CPN are also situated in the adjacent area. Accordingly, the procedure does not target the inferolateral genicular nerve due to the high risk of damage.

In summary, RFA or nerve block target only the SLGN, SMGN, and IMGN, which run across the area connecting the femoral and tibial epicondyle and shaft (Fig. 11.5).

Genicular nerves comprise the major articular branches in the knee. While other types of articular branches are also present in the knee, procedures in clinical practice are not performed on the inferolateral or tibial recurrent genicular nerves. Therefore, pain can be reduced, but not completely eliminated, by performing RFA on the SLGN, SMGN, and IMGN.

11.2 Anatomy

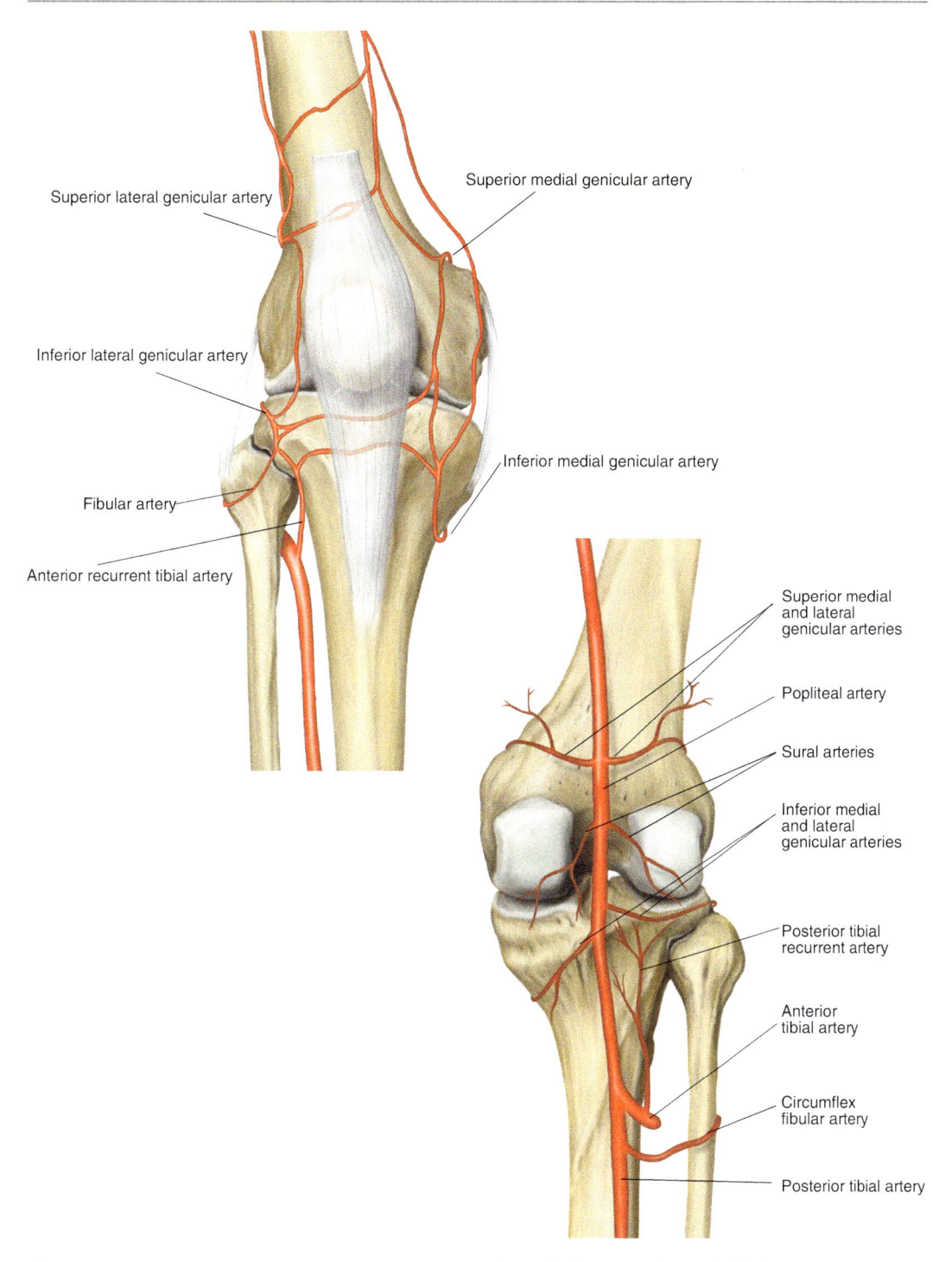

Fig. 11.4 Major blood vessels around the knee. Superior medial, superior lateral, and inferior medial genicular vessels run together with the genicular nerves; thus, the locations of these vessels are helpful in ascertaining the locations of the nerves

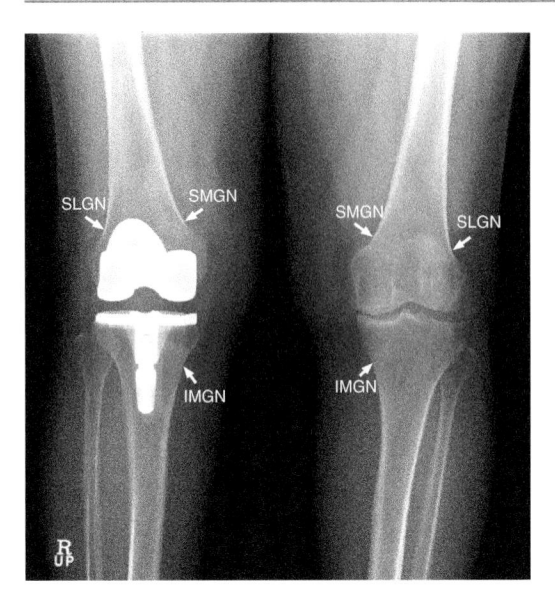

Fig. 11.5 The superolateral genicular nerve (SLGN), superomedial genicular nerve (SMGN), and inferomedial genicular nerve (IMGM) pass through the area connecting the femoral and tibial epicondyle and shaft (Arrow: Target points of SLGN, SMGN, and IMGN where the procedure will be performed)

During study of this procedural technique, the authors realized that while the characteristics of genicular vessels have been well elucidated, there were almost no data or evidence for the existence of genicular nerves. Accordingly, two fresh cadavers were dissected to confirm the presence of these nerves and their exact trajectories. As the first cadaveric dissection report on the pathways of the genicular nerves, it was ascertained that genicular nerves run very close to the genicular vessels attached to the periosteum (Fig. 11.6).

11.3 Techniques

Similar to the requirements of a typical nerve block, genicular nerve procedures may employ steroids and local anesthetics; alternatively, RFA or cooled RFA may be used during genicular nerve procedures. However, because administering the steroid/anesthetic mixture alone results in a relatively temporary effect, the use of RFA or cooled RFA is preferred. These techniques are examined in detail below.

11.3.1 C-Arm-Guided Genicular Nerve RFA

While the patient in the supine position, a tall cushion is placed beneath the knee that is being treated, and the knee is oriented to form a right angle relative to the operating table. The true AP view, with the patella situated at its center, is found in C-arm AP images. Placing a tall cushion beneath the knee causes the knee to flex naturally, facilitating the obtainment of the true AP view and preventing the opposite leg from obscuring the field of view in the lateral aspect.

Target points for the performance of a nerve block on the SLGN, SMGN, and IMGN can be found in the AP X-ray view. After applying local anesthesia, the 10-mm active tip of the 10-cm 22G curved RF cannula is inserted vertically (tunnel view) toward a target point (Fig. 11.7a). The cannula should be inserted toward the target point, with its curved part facing inward. Once it reaches the periosteum in the area where the epicondyle and shaft connect (Fig. 11.7b), the cannula should be rotated by 180°; this allows the cannula to slide while the periosteum area is scraped as the cannula is advanced to an additional depth of 1 cm (Fig. 11.7c). Having the direction of entry closer to the lateral aspect of the periosteum from the beginning of the procedure facilitates the sliding of the cannula after it is rotated. To widen the surface of contact with the nerve as much as possible during RFA, the curved part of the cannula is rotated again to face inward (Fig. 11.7d).

In this state, the true lateral view is checked to ensure that the cannula tip has been inserted to the intended depth and make any required adjustments. It is important that the tip of the cannula be in contact with the periosteum when the cannula is placed in its final position; this allows the cannula to be sufficiently adjacent to the genicular nerve without damaging other nerves. Adjusting the position of the cannula while referencing the true lateral view could cause the position of the cannula tip to change; hence, fine adjustments should be made, if necessary, while looking at the AP view (Figs. 11.8 and 11.9).

11.3 Techniques

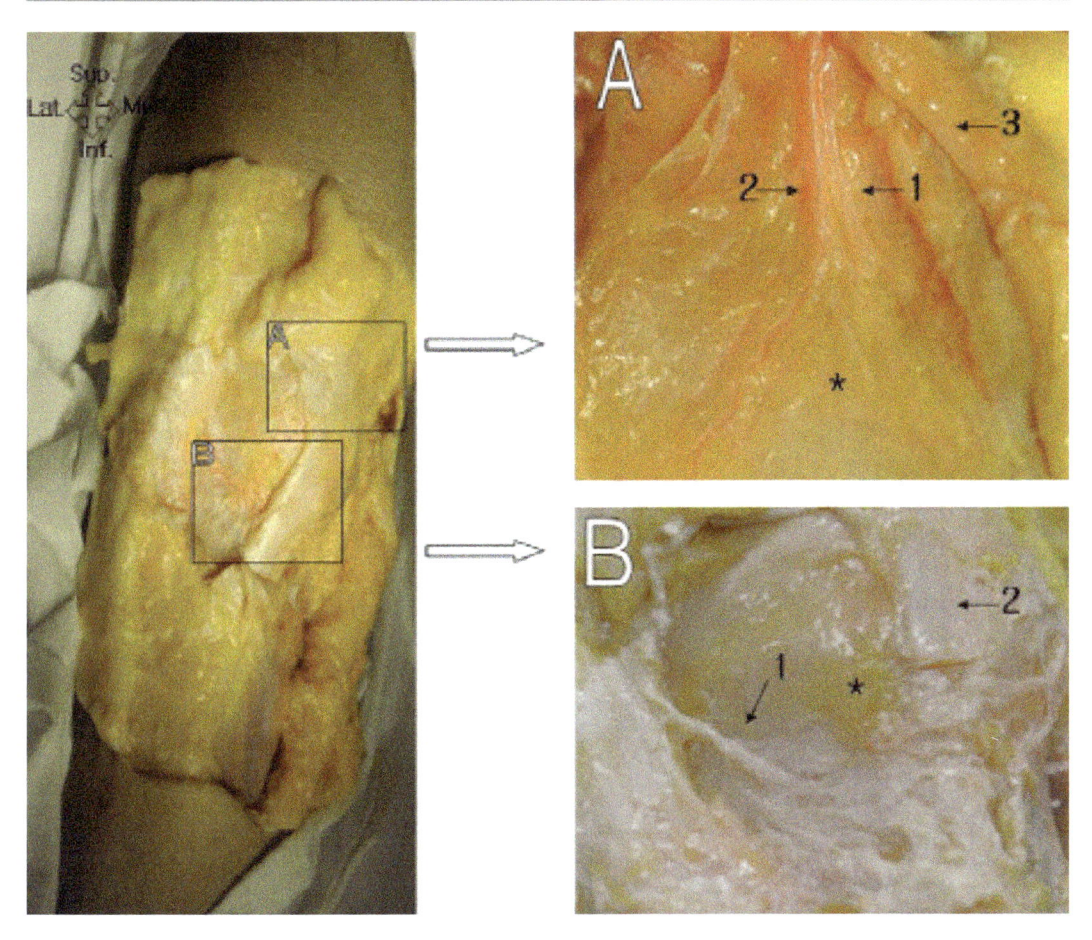

Fig. 11.6 Dissection findings of the right knee. (**a**) The superomedial genicular nerve (1) runs together with the genicular vessel (2) and superior to the femoral medial epicondyle (asterisk). The adductor magnus (3) is attached to the medial condyle and the medial aspect of the femur.

(**b**) The inferior medial genicular nerve (1) runs inferior to the tibial medial epicondyle (asterisk). The tibial collateral ligament (2) is attached to the medial condyle and the medial aspect of the tibia

The genicular nerve is found by delicately adjusting the cannula until an abnormal or heavy sensation is felt in the knee when a sensory stimulation of 0.6 V at 50 Hz is applied. To avoid damage to nearby motor nerves, the RFA is only performed after confirming that stimulation of 2.0 V at 2 Hz induces no leg or muscle movement around the knee.

The genicular nerve is small and may not, therefore, respond directly to any sensory stimulation. Among adults of less than 60 years of age, sensory stimulation is expressed as a feeling of the entire knee becoming heavy or as an abnormal feeling indicative of slight pain. However, among those of more than 60 years of age, it is often not found since abnormal sensation is not easily felt due to the application of overly weak stimulation being too weak (claiming that it is tolerable, some patients withstand it). If it is determined that the exact location has been found, even though the patient did not feel the sensory stimulation, RFA is performed after applying the 2-Hz motor stimulation. The tip of the cannula must be in contact with the periosteum. As the author has experienced many cases in which the patient showed improvement after receiving RFA despite the abnormal sensation to sensory stimulation not having been registered, it

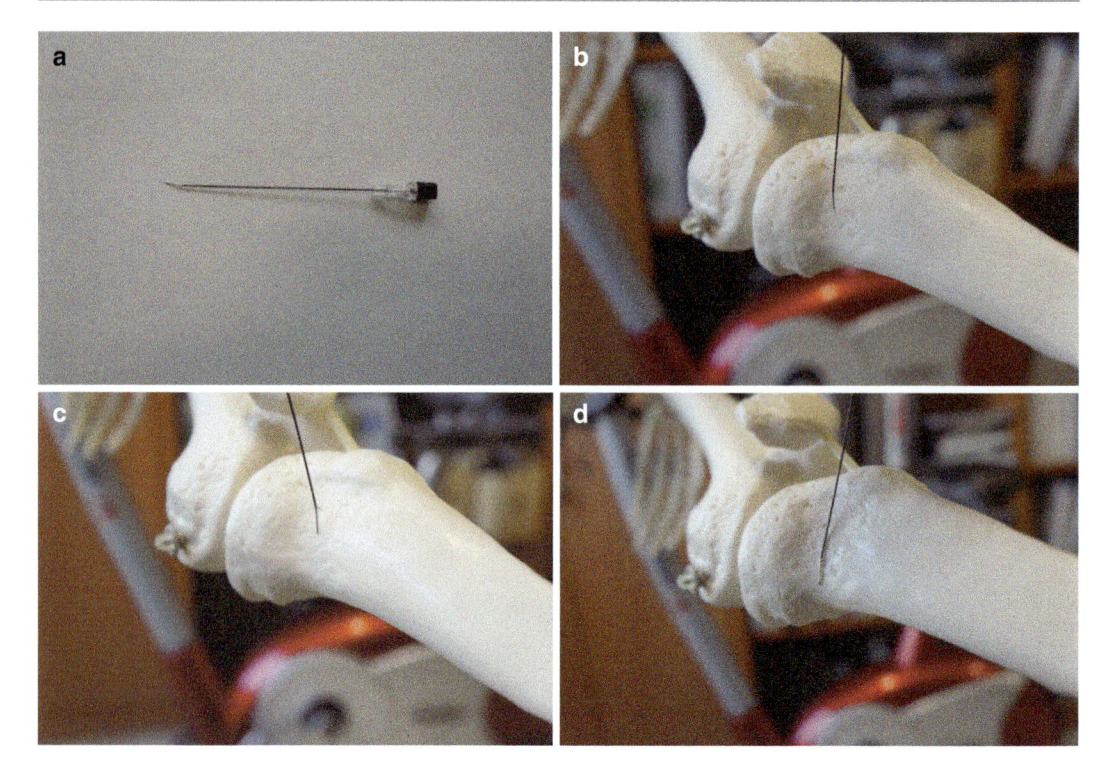

Fig. 11.7 (**a**) The cannula should be bent as shown. (**b**) The cannula is inserted toward the target point in the tunnel view, with its curved part facing inward. (**c**) Once the cannula reaches the periosteum in the area where the epicondyle and shaft connect, the cannula should be rotated by 180° to allow it to slide and scrape the periosteum area as it is advanced to an additional depth of 1 cm. (**d**) Once the cannula has been accurately placed in the target area, it is rotated again by 180°

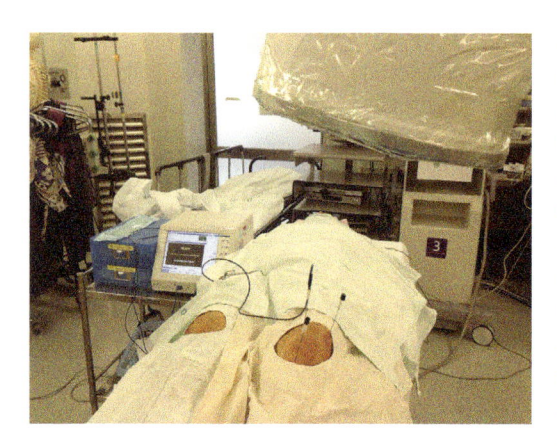

Fig. 11.8 The RF cannula is placed near the target area for the RFA of the SLGN, SMGN, and IMGN

is recommended that the operator not spend too much time trying to find sensory stimulation.

While the method of RF lesioning may vary by physician, it typically follows the same principles as those that inform the performance of RFA in other areas. Because the pain induced during RFA is severe, the author usually conducts RF lesioning after injecting approximately 2 cc of a mixture containing local anesthetic through the cannula. If the patient still complains of severe pain, RF lesioning is performed after gradually increasing the RF lesioning temperature from 50° according to the pain level or injecting additional anesthetic at a different angle toward the active tip of the cannula; because the target area is close to the skin, it is not difficult to inject the anesthetic toward the cannula tip by using the blind technique. The author typically performs the procedure for 90 s at 70° at each target point.

RF lesioning could be performed by placing cannulas at all three target points or in a one-by-one sequence. The author believes that the placement of the cannula itself could cause

11.3 Techniques

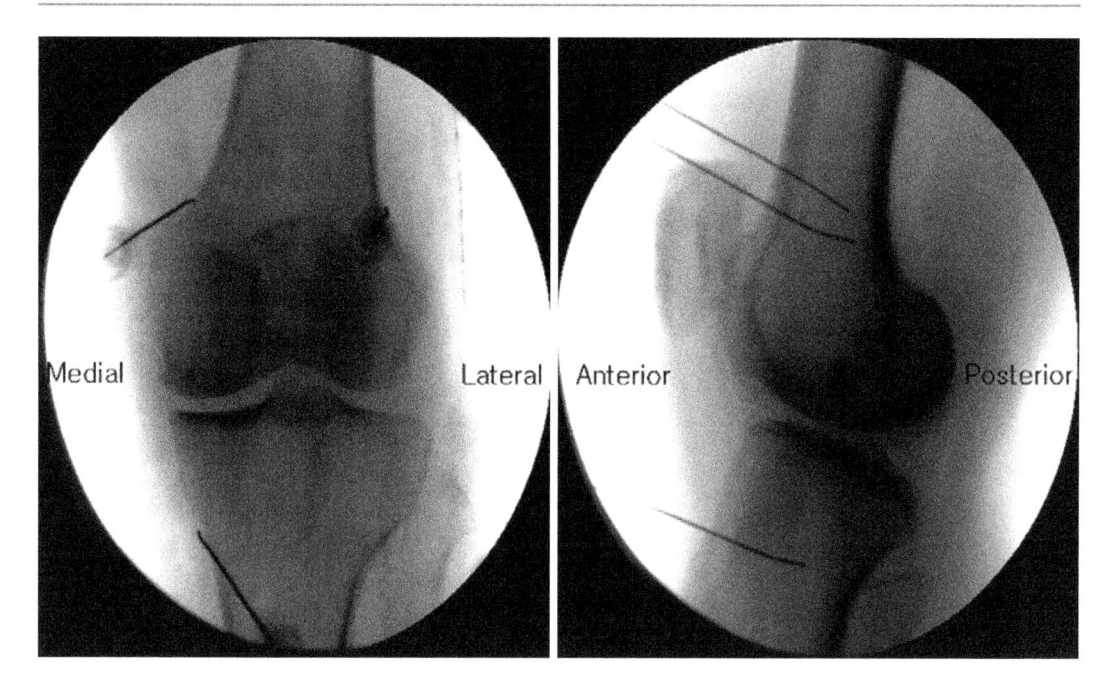

Fig. 11.9 The AP and lateral views of the cannula tip are accurately placed in the target area for the RFA of the SLGN, SMGN, and IMGN of the left knee. The curved RF cannula is accurately placed, and the active tip is in contact with the area where the epicondyle and shaft connect

pain; hence, it is recommended that the procedure be conducted in a one-by-one sequence.

For reference, in addition to the three genicular nerve points mentioned above, some have opined that ablation should also be performed in the area where the nerve emerging from the rectus intermedius muscle connects to the subpatellar plexus at a spot approximately 2 cm from the upper patellar margin (Fig. 11.10). While the academic basis for this claim remains lacking, its performance may be worth considering as it entails low risk.

11.3.2 C-Arm-Guided Genicular Nerve Cooled RFA

Cooled RFA has been recently introduced as a method by which to overcome the limitations of conventional RFA and already features widespread global use; its approval in Korea is already in progress.

Based on the word "cooled," it is easy to assume that the procedure requires cold temperatures and may thus induce nerve degeneration. However, it actually refers to the maintenance of the temperature of the tip at a constant level (usually 60°) by cooling the tip of the electrode continuously with water. This mechanism allows the procedure to supply more energy than existing methods. As a result, it creates a circular burn that is 5 times larger than that of conventional RFA (Fig. 11.11a).

With conventional RFA, the burn around the cannula tip is oval-shaped (Fig. 11.11b). Therefore, to accurately widen the lesion applied to the target nerve as much as possible, the cannula must be placed parallel to the path of the nerve. Although this is a factor determinant of the success of the procedure, actually placing the cannula parallel to the nerve is difficult. On the other hand, the larger circular lesion generated by cooled RFA precludes the need to place the cannula parallel to the nerve; hence, only the distance between the active tip and the nerve is important. In other words, sufficient ablation is possible even if the active tip is placed perpendicular to the nerve. The success rate of the procedure and the duration of the effect are increased thereby (Figs. 11.11, 11.12 and 11.13).

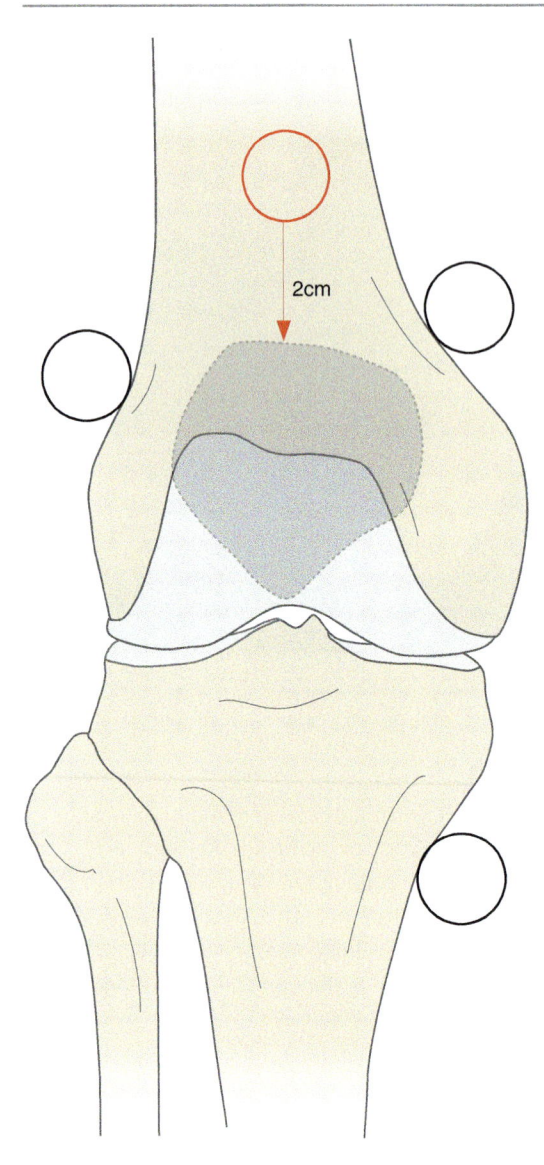

Fig. 11.10 Black circle: Area where genicular nerve RFA is performed. Red circle: Area at 2 cm superior to the upper patellar margin. Additional RFA may be performed in this area

RFA could feature enhanced utility, especially in application to genicular nerve lesioning (Fig. 11.13).

Recently, a company called HALYARD has developed and is selling a kit exclusive for genicular nerve cooled RFA. In countries outside of Korea, most procedures are being performed with this kit (Figs. 11.14 and 11.15). Korea should also be able to use this kit to perform genicular nerve cooled RFA in the near future.

The author recently performed a cooled RFA procedure on a 63-year-old male patient with persistent, intractable knee pain despite total knee replacement arthroplasty (TKRA). Cooled RF lesioning at 60° was performed for 2.5 min at each target point on the genicular nerve (Fig. 11.16).

Reporting a pain reduction of over 90% at 1, 3, and 6 months following the procedure, the patient has been satisfied with the outcome. The patient's improvement currently persists at 15 months following the procedure.

Based on the author's experience, the effect of conventional RFA tends to be much lower in patients with a history of knee surgery than in those without such history. It is believed that this may be attributable to the inability to perform RFA accurately on the genicular nerve due to the changing of the location as a result of surgery. However, this patient showed significant pain reduction and high satisfaction despite a history of TKRA. Since the size of the lesion generated by cooled RFA is large, it is believed that the procedure may have been successful even if the location of the genicular nerve had changed.

Recently, cooled RFA was performed on patients with intractable knee pain who had previously benefited little from conventional RFA; cool RFA yielded excellent improvement in all of these patients. Hence, theoretically or empirically, cooled RFA appears to be more effective than conventional RFA in genicular nerve lesioning.

Farrel et al. performed cooled RFA (60°) for 2.5 min on the genicular nerve of a patient with chronic degenerative knee arthritis. The investigators reported an improvement that was sustained for more than 6 months. The report

The genicular nerve is small and the size of the lesion generated is also small even when the active tip is placed parallel to the nerve during conventional RFA. These could cause the procedure to fail. On the other hand, cooled RFA generates a large burn; as a result, the success rate of the procedure is higher, and the effect is sustained longer even if the tip is placed perpendicular to the nerve. Therefore, it is believed that cooled

11.3 Techniques

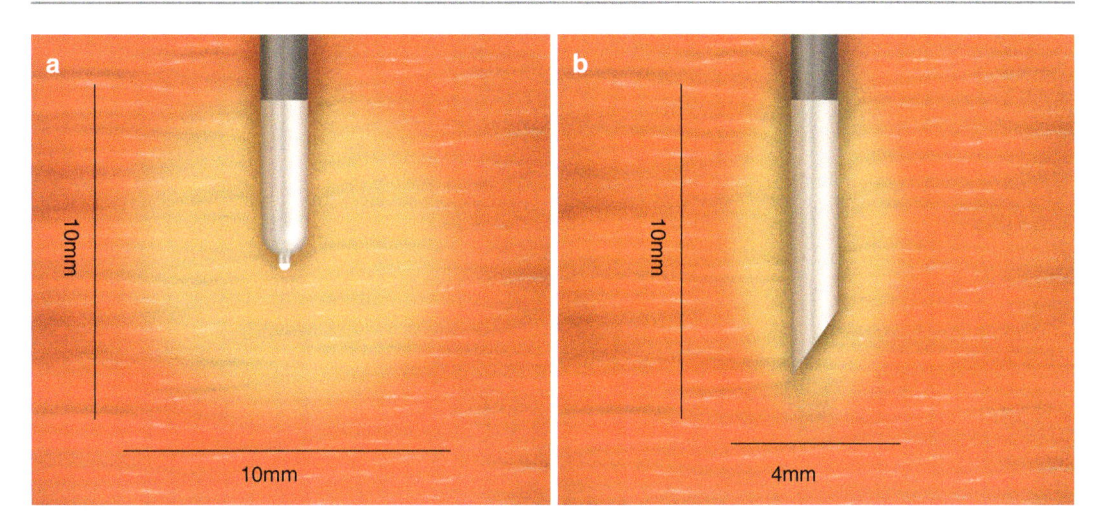

Fig. 11.11 Comparison between conventional and cooled RFA. (**a**) Cooled RFA generates a relatively large circular lesion. (**b**) Conventional RFA generates a small oval-shaped lesion near the active tip

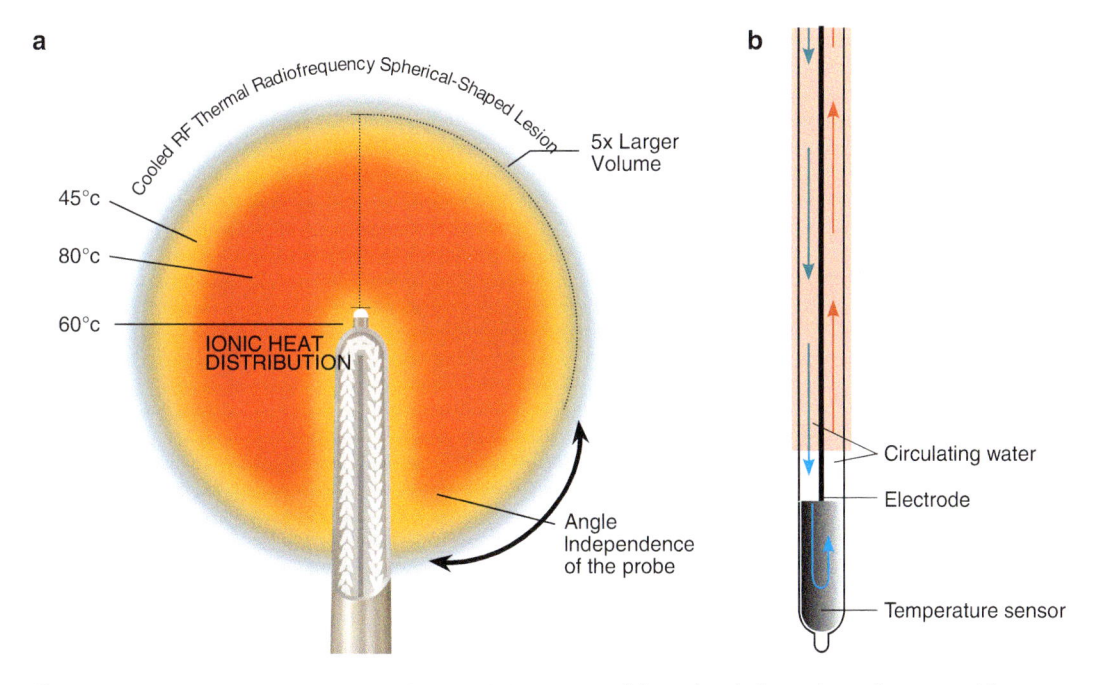

Fig. 11.12 (**a**) Temperature distribution of circular lesion generated by the cooled RF active tip. Although the temperature of the electrode tip is maintained at 60°, an 80°-ablation is generated at the lesion. (**b**) The temperature of the active tip is continuously measured by a temperature sensor, and the circulating water maintains the temperature of the electrode tip at 60°

included the post-procedural MRI findings; as shown in Fig. 11.17, the cooled RFA generated lesions approximately 12.5 mm in diameter, which were large enough to be visible on the MRI images.

Walega et al. published a case report describing the performance of cooled RFA on the thoracic medial branch of a 61-year-old female patient, who, with a BMI of 21.8 kg/m^2 and a history of C3-T1 posterior instrumented fusion surgery, was suspected of having thoracic facet

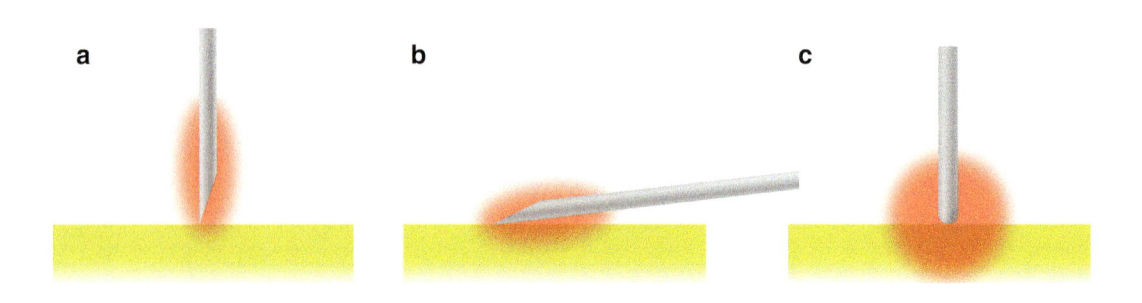

Fig. 11.13 (**a**) Conventional RFA with the cannula placed perpendicular to the nerve. Because the size of the burn is small, the effect may be small as well. (**b**) With conventional RFA, a larger lesion can be generated if the nerve and active tip are placed parallel to each other. (**c**) Cooled RFA with the cannula placed perpendicular to the nerve. Because the size of the burn is large, the success rate is high regardless of the angle of approach

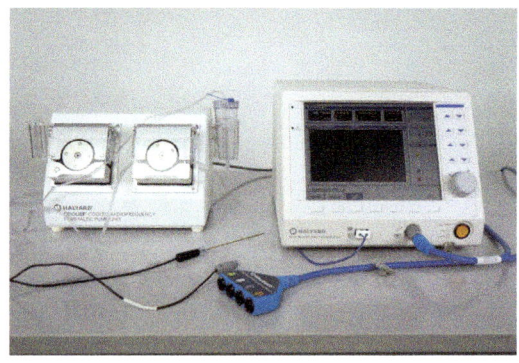

Fig. 11.14 RF generator and water cooling peristaltic pump developed by HALYARD

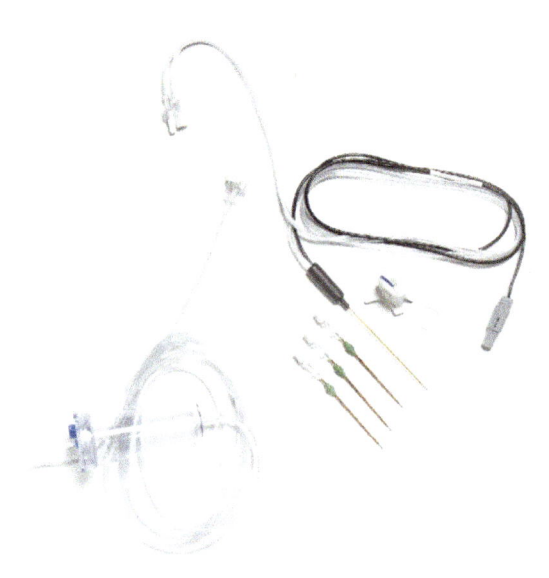

Fig. 11.15 Kit for genicular cooled RFA developed by HALYARD

syndrome. Because the patient was very thin, it was difficult to maintain the cannula where it had been placed during the procedure. Accordingly, the investigators performed cooled RFA while holding the cannula with one hand. However, the patient complained of severe pain during the procedure, and subsequent examination revealed that she had suffered a third-degree burn on her skin (Fig. 11.18).

If the distance between the lesion and the skin is shallow, as in this patient, cooled RFA should be performed with caution. The lesion induced by the cooled RFA is typically 12.5 mm in size. If

11.3 Techniques

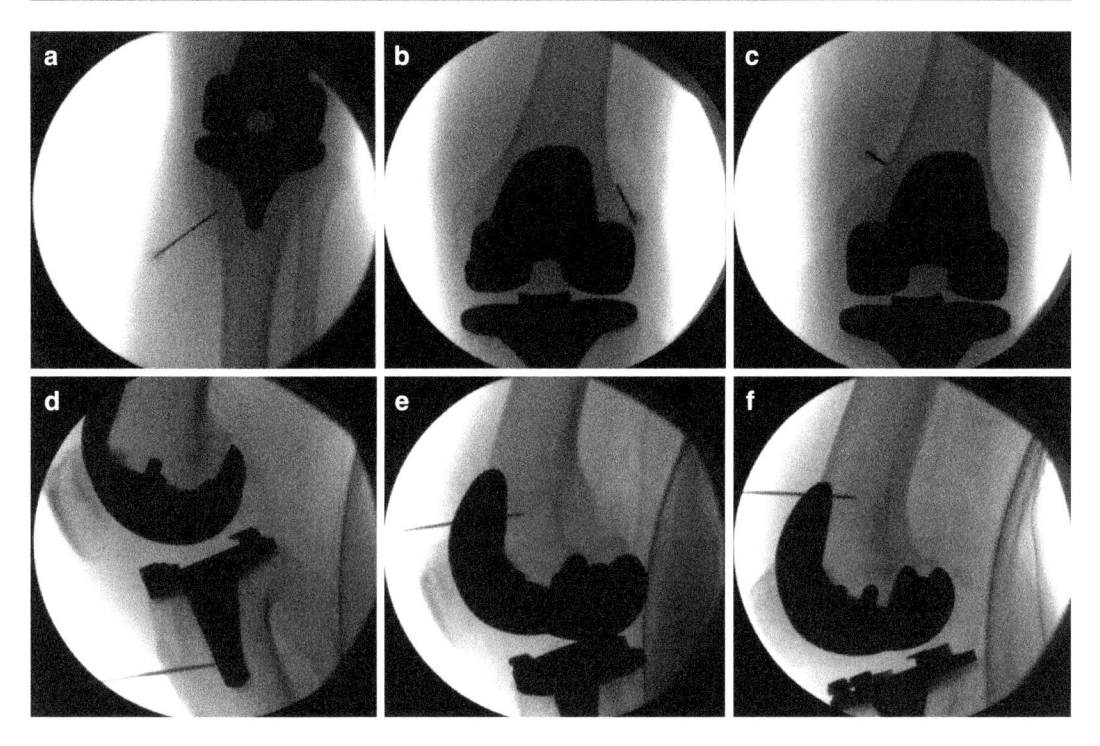

Fig. 11.16 The performance of genicular nerve cooled RFA. (**a**, **d**) Procedure on the IMGN. (**b**, **e**) Procedure on the SLGN. (**c**, **f**) Procedure on the SMGN

the depth from the skin to the target is shallower than this, a burn injury may occur on the skin. Although it is extremely rare, the operator should be especially careful when performing the procedure on a person of low weight. If the patient complains of severe pain, the procedure must be stopped immediately, and the patient should be checked for burn injuries.

11.3.3 Diagnostic Genicular Nerve Block

RF lesioning may not be effective, and the risk of complications cannot be completely dismissed. Therefore, selecting the patients for whom this procedure would be effective is more important than performing the procedure well.

McCormick et al. performed cooled RFA on the genicular nerve and observed the effects of the procedure for the subsequent 6 months. The results indicated that patients in whom an improvement effect of ≥80% was achieved with diagnostic genicular nerve block and the administration of local anesthetic, as well as those who had experienced pain for no more than 5 years, were associated with the highest likelihood of improvement.

We also reported favorable results after performing RFA on patients who had maintained a pain reduction of ≥50% for more than 24 h following diagnostic genicular nerve block and local anesthetic.

Cooled RFA has a higher probability of being effective than does conventional RFA. However, the procedure itself is very expensive. Considering these points, the procedure should only be performed on patients for whom a successful procedure is more likely: those who have experienced pain for no more than 5 years and who have demonstrated a reduction in pain of ≥50% for at least 12 h after a diagnostic block.

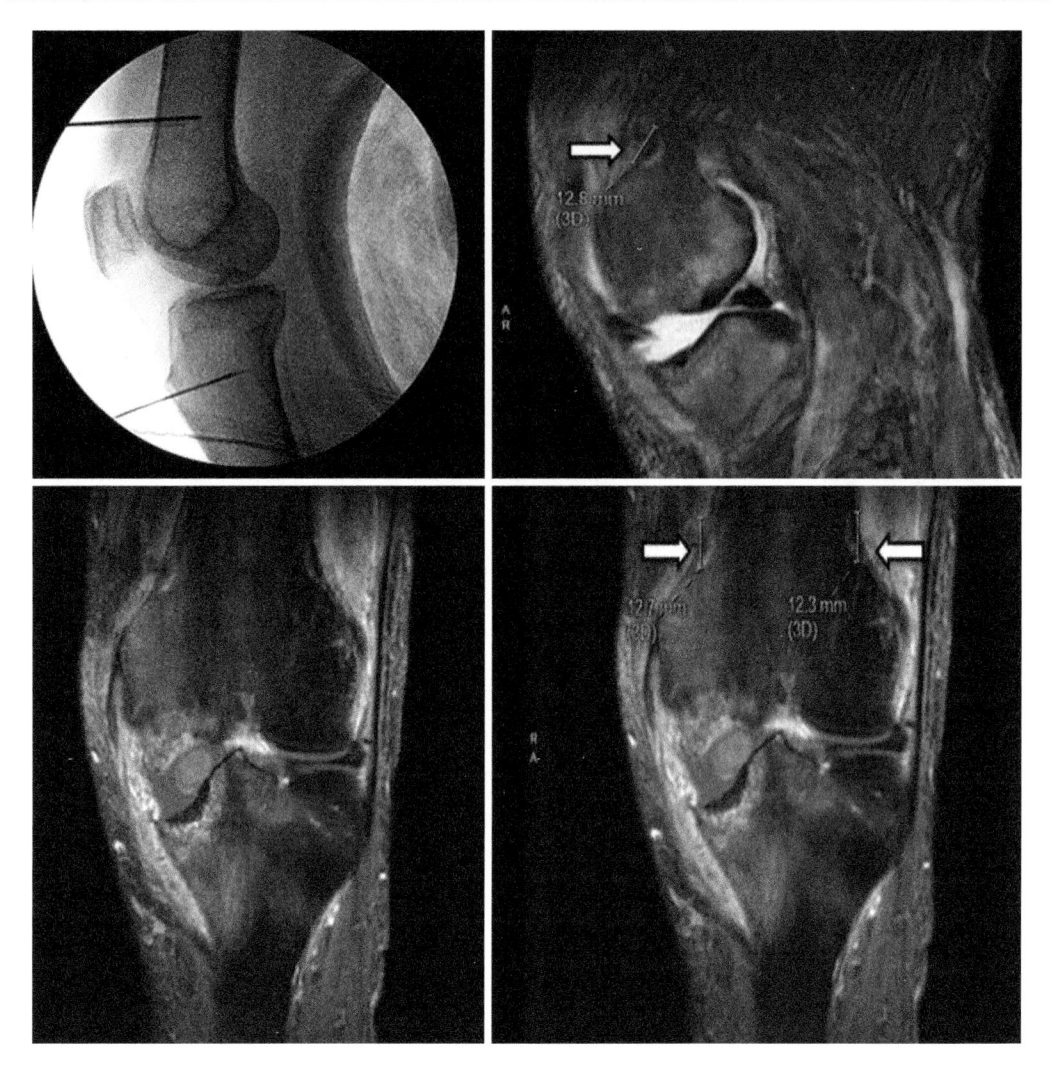

Fig. 11.17 MRI findings. Appearance and size of lesions generated by genicular nerve cooled RFA. Arrow: Appearance of the lesions

11.3.4 Ultrasound-Guided Genicular Nerve Block

Pain Physician 2018; 21:41-51 • ISSN 1533-3159

Randomized Trial

Ultrasound-Guided Genicular Nerve Block for Knee Osteoarthritis: A Double-Blind, Randomized Controlled Trial of Local Anesthetic Alone or in Combination with Corticosteroid

Doo-Hwan Kim, MD, Seong-Soo Choi, MD, PhD, Syn-Hae Yoon, MD, So-Hee Lee, MD, Dong-Kyun Seo, MD, In-Gyu Lee, MD, Woo-Jong Choi, MD, PhD, and Jin-Woo Shin, MD, PhD

11.4 Comparison of Outcomes According to Procedure

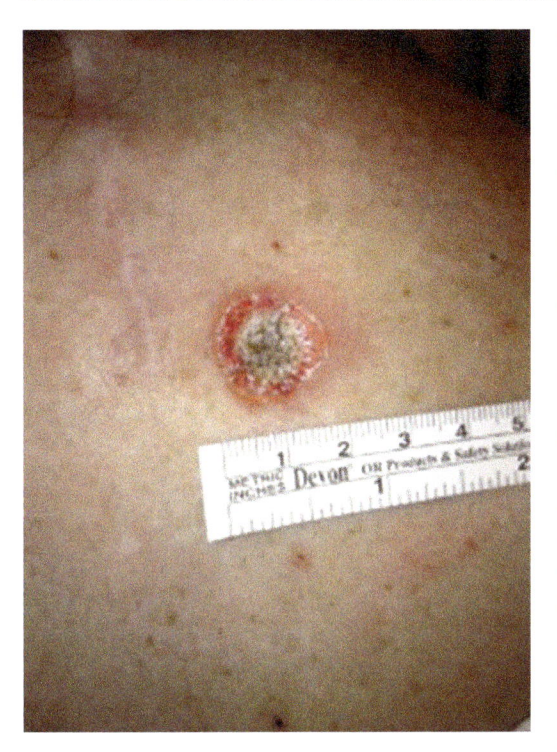

Fig. 11.18 A third-degree burn that occurred after cooled RFA was performed on the thoracic medial branch of a 61-year-old female patient who had a BMI of 21.8 kg/m² and a history of C3-T1 posterior instrumented fusion surgery

The following explanation is informed by a 2018 report on ultrasound-guided genicular nerve block.

Because the genicular nerve is situated at a comparatively shallow depth relative to the skin surface, an outpatient procedure on the nerve could be easily performed using ultrasound. While ultrasound-guided RFA could also be used, RFA requires more precision; hence, the use of a C-arm is recommended. For other diagnostic block procedures or simple genicular nerve block, the use of ultrasound is recommended over C-arm.

The operator performs the procedure while changing the patient's posture according to the requirements of the ultrasound. The area connecting the medial and lateral shaft and epicondyle, where the SMGN, SLGN, and IMGN pass through, is often palpable: as long as the patient is not overweight, feeling along the shaft toward the knee allows for the detection of a sudden change in slope. By placing a linear 10–15 MHz probe on that site and moving parallel along the shaft toward the knee at the same angle, a location when the slope changes on the ultrasound can be found. The probe must be moved while it is maintained at an orientation that is parallel with the shaft line to allow the change in slope to be detected easily.

By applying a color Doppler, the genicular artery can be easily located, and the operator can assume that the genicular nerve runs adjacent to this artery (Fig. 11.19).

Although the procedure can be performed in either in-plane or out-plane modes, inserting the needle in the latter facilitates the procedure since the target area is shallow relative to the skin. Despite the fact that the nerve cannot be clearly identified on ultrasound since it is small and is almost attached to the periosteum, the procedure is simplified when the genicular artery is used as a reference. With respect to the drug(s) used, a local anesthetic alone or a steroid/anesthetic, as in other nerve block procedures, can be used.

11.4 Comparison of Outcomes According to Procedure

In a randomized controlled trial of 38 patients with intractable degenerative arthritis, the RFA procedure group showed significant differences in all indicators during a 3-month follow-up period relative to a control group that only received an administration of a steroid/local anesthetic mixture. The report indicated no cases of adverse events, such as dysesthesia, exacerbation of pain, hypoesthesia, or decline in motor function (Figs. 11.20, 11.21 and 11.22).

Based on these study results, it is believed that improvement in pain and function achieved with genicular nerve RFA is sustained for approximately 3 months; i.e., the level and duration of improvement are increased relative to when only the drug injection is administered.

Concerning the performance of ultrasound-guided genicular nerve block in patients with

Fig. 11.19 Ultrasound findings of superolateral, superomedial, and inferomedial genicular arteries. The genicular nerve runs adjacent to this artery. Arrow: Genicular artery. Arrowhead: Genicular Nerve

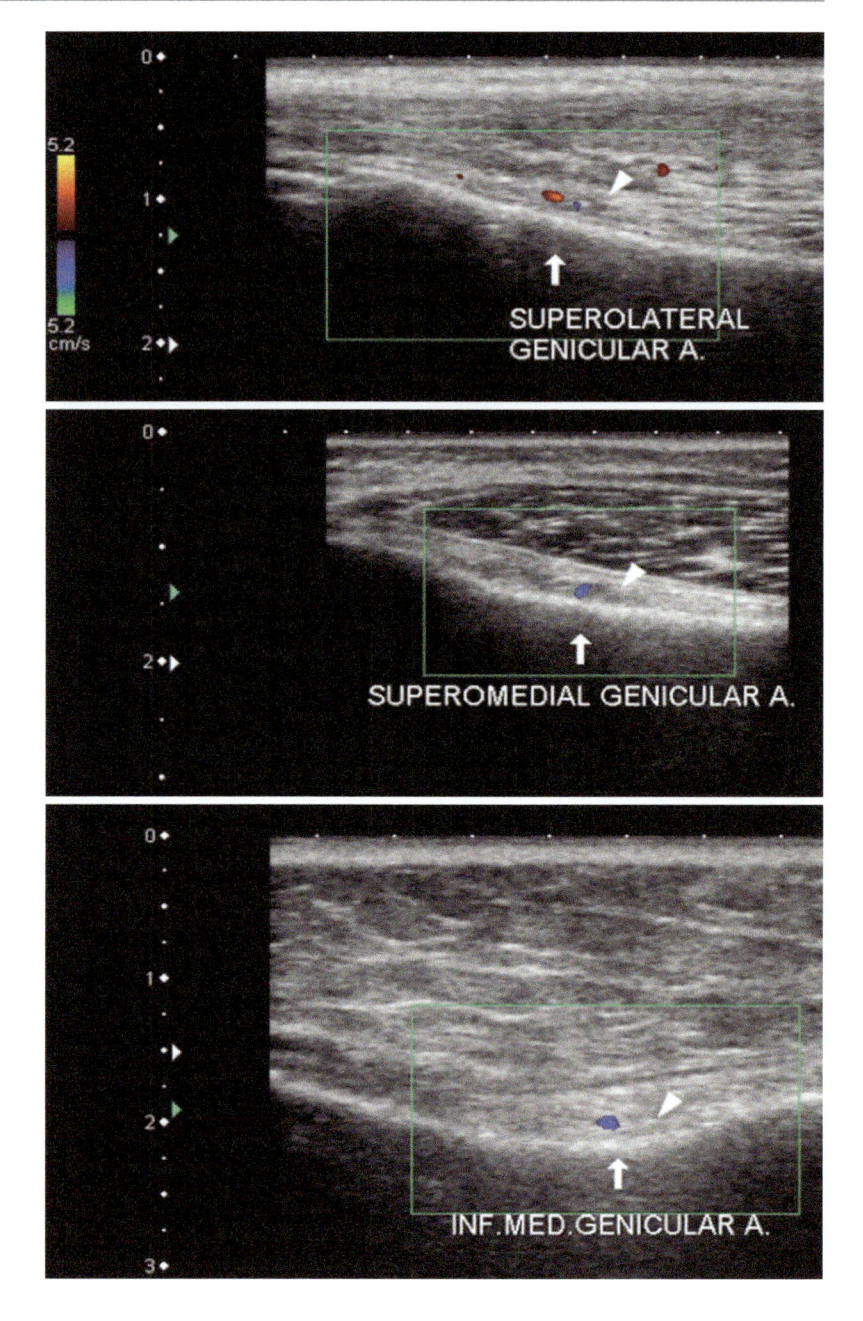

intractable chronic degenerative arthritis, the article also reported that the administration of Lidocaine alone yielded an improvement effect that lasted for approximately 2 weeks; by contrast, the combined use of Lidocaine and triamcinolone achieved an improvement effect that lasted for approximately 4 weeks. A significant difference between the two groups with respect to functional improvement and satisfaction was found only at 4 weeks following the procedure (Figs. 11.23, 11.24 and 11.25).

In summary, clinical trials have demonstrated that genicular nerve RFA, cooled RFA, and the administration of only local anesthetic as well as that of steroid and local anesthetic to patients with intractable chronic generative arthritis mitigated pain and improved motor functioning for

11.4 Comparison of Outcomes According to Procedure

3–4 months, 6–12 months, 2 weeks, and 4 weeks, respectively.

In clinical practice, procedures other than cooled or conventional RFA required repeated performance since the effect is after each procedure is of relatively short duration. In such cases, the repeated administration of steroids could cause adverse events. From the perspective of cost-effectiveness, this strategy is thus a poor option. The repeated administration of local anesthetic is associated with less adverse events, decreases in neuronal excitability, and the reduction of onset of neuropathic pain; hence, this option warrants consideration.

The development of genicular nerve block, conventional RFA, and cooled RFA has to varying degrees helped to attenuate pain in many patients with intractable knee pain. I am extremely pleased and thankful to find, with the establishment of their academic basis, that they are being accepted by physicians worldwide. I sincerely hope that these procedures can be actively applied by the readers of this book and be of significant help in the treatment of patients.

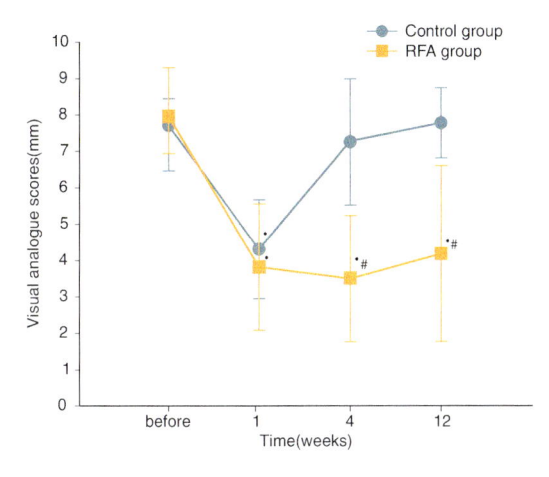

Fig. 11.20 Compared to the control group, the RFA group showed significant pain reduction across 3 months. The control group showed pain reduction for only 1 week

Clinical and Functional Outcomes after Radiofrequency (RF) Neurotomy and Changes from Baseline Values

Post-procedure time	Control (n-18)	RFA (n-17)	Changes from baseline Control	Changes from baseline RFA	p-value
OKS (12-60 points)					
1 week	26.8±4.5	23.6±7.5	12.4±4.3	16.2±9.5	0.296
4 weeks	36.9±3.5	25.8±8.0	2.3±4.8	14.1±9.7*	<0.001
12 weeks	38.9±4.9	27.4±10.2	0.3±1.3	12.4±10.7*	<0.001
Patient satisfaction with GPE**					
1 week	5.3±0.8	5.5±0.7			0.457
4 weeks	4.3±0.8	5.9±0.9***			<0.001
12 weeks	3.7±0.5	5.5±1.1***			<0.001

All data values are means ±SD. VAS: visual analogue scale; OKS: Oxford knee score
* $p < 0.05$ compared to the change from baseline in the control froup
** Global perceived effect (GPE) with 7-point scale (1 – worst ever, 2 – much worse, 3 – worse, 4 – not improved not worse, 5 – improved, 6 – much improved, 7 – best ever).
*** $p < 0.05$ compared to control group

Fig. 11.21 Compared to the control group, the RFA group showed significant differences in functional improvement (OKS) and satisfaction (GPE) after 4 and 12 weeks

Fig. 11.22 Compared to the control group, the RFA group featured a significantly higher percentage of patients who showed pain reduction of ≥50% for up to 12 weeks

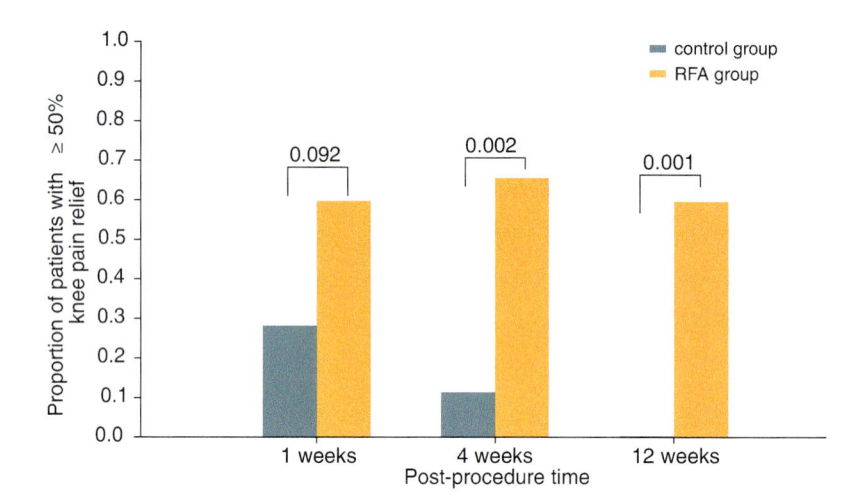

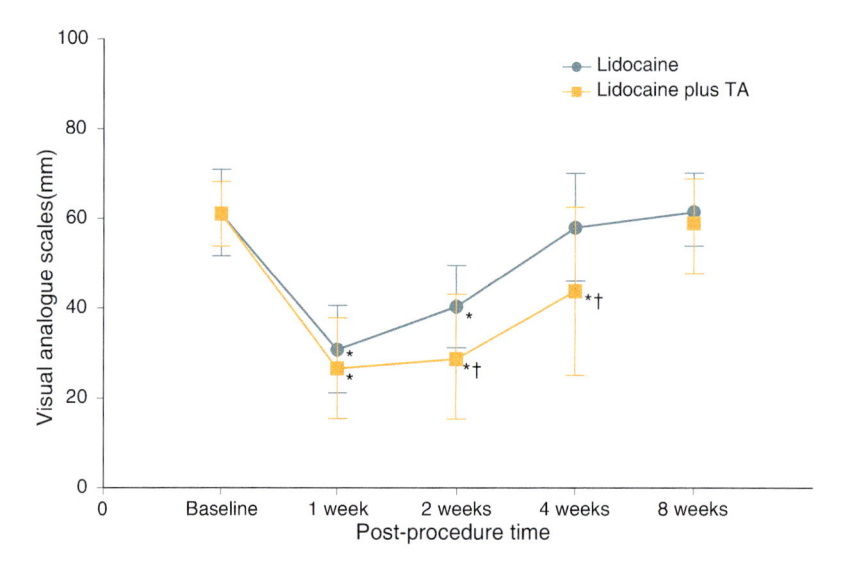

Fig. 11.23 Lidocaine administration produced an improvement effect that lasted for approximately 2 weeks. The administration of Lidocaine and triamcinolone together yielded an improvement effect that lasted for approximately 4 weeks. At 2–4 weeks, the administration of Lidocaine + triamcinolone achieved a significantly greater improvement effect relative to the use of Lidocaine alone. $^*P < 0.05$ vs. baseline. $^+P < 0.05$ vs. Lidocaine group

11.4 Comparison of Outcomes According to Procedure

Clinical and Functional Outcomes after genicular nerve block with lidocaine or lidocaine plus triamcinolone

Post-procedure time	Lidocaine(n=24)	Lidocaine plusTA(n=24)	Changes from baseline Lidocaine	Changes from baseline Lidocaine plus TA	P value
VAS(0-100mm)					
Baseline	60.8±7.2	62.1±9.8			
1 week	30.8±9.7*	28.4±11.2*	30.1±8.8	33.7±6.0	0.062
2 weeks	40.4±9.1*	31.1±14.9*	20.4±10.0	31.1±9.4	<0.001
4 weeks	57.9±12.2	45.3±19.8*	2.9±10.0	16.8±14.2	<0.001
8 weeks	61.3±7.4	59.5±11.8	-0.4±3.6	2.6±11.0	0.098
OKS(12-60 points)					
Baseline	37.1±2.8	37.6±3.8			
1 week	27.7±4.5*	28.3±5.8*	9.4±4.1	9.4±3.6	0.940
2 weeks	30.1±5.4*	28.7±6.6*	7.0±5.5	8.9±4.5	0.142
4 weeks	36.8±1.9	31.8±6.2*	0.3±1.6	5.8±4.2	<0.001
8 weeks	36.9±3.0	36.6±4.2	0.2±1.1	1.1±1.7	0.145
GPES(1-7)					
1 week	5.5±0.7	5.5±0.8			1.0
2 weeks	5.1±0.8	4.5±0.8			0.056
4 weeks	3.6±0.6	4.7±0.7			<0.001
8 weeks	3.3±0.5	3.3±0.8			0.820

All data values shown as means ± standard deviations. OKS = Oxford knee score; TA = triamcinolone; VAS = visual analogue; GPES = global perceived effect. * $P < 0.05$ compared with baseline values.

Fig. 11.24 Comparing the use of Lidocaine alone with the combined administration of Lidocaine and triamcinolone, significant differences in functional improvement (OKS) and satisfaction (GPES) were found only at 4 weeks

Fig. 11.25 The percentage of patients with a pain reduction of ≥50% was significantly higher in the Lidocaine + triamcinolone group than in Lidocaine group during the 2–4 weeks following the procedure

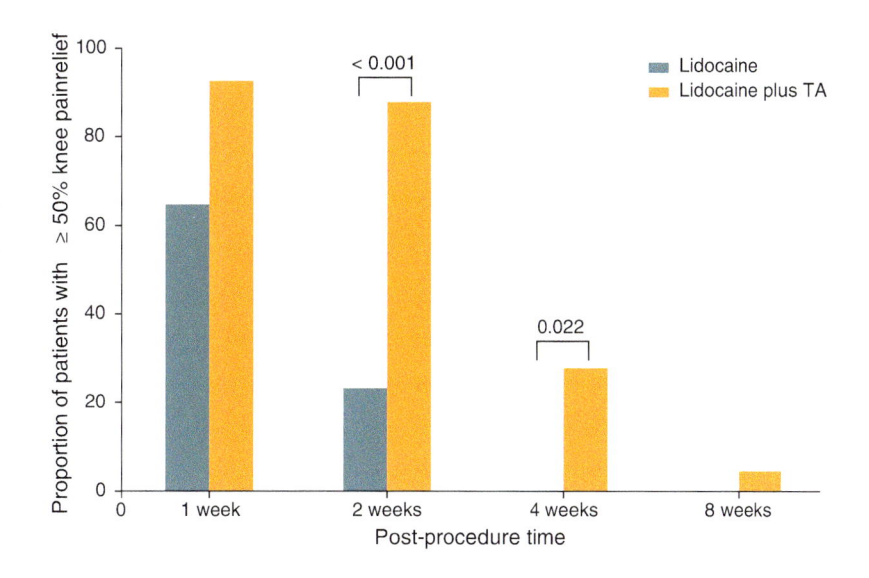

Bibliography

1. Bellini M, Barbieri M. Cooled radiofrequency system relieves chronic knee osteoarthritis pain: the first case-series. Anaesthesiol Intensive Ther. 2015;47(1):30–3.
2. Choi WJ, Hwang SJ, Song JG, Leem JG, Kang YU, Park PH, Shin JW. Radiofrequency treatment relieves chronic knee osteoarthritis pain: a double-blind randomized controlled trial. Pain. 2011;152:481–7.
3. Clemente CD. Anatomy of the human body by Henry Gray. Philadelphia: Lea & Febiger; 1985. p. 1239–41.
4. Cohen SP, Hurley RW, Buckenmaier CC 3rd, Kurihara C, Morlando B, Dragovich A. Randomized placebo-controlled study evaluating lateral branch radiofrequency denervation for sacroiliac joint pain. Anesthesiology. 2008;109(2):279–88.
5. Farrell ME, Gutierrez G, Desai MJ. Demonstration of lesions produced by cooled radiofrequency Neurotomy for chronic osteoarthritic knee pain: a case presentation. PM R. 2017;9(3):314–7.
6. Horner G, Dellon AL. Innervation of the human knee joint and implications for surgery. Clin Orthop Relat Res. 1994;301:221–6.
7. Kim DH, Choi SS, Yoon SH, Lee SH, Seo DK, Lee IG, Choi WJ, Shin JW. Ultrasound-guided genicular nerve block for knee osteoarthritis: a double-blind, randomized controlled trial of local Anesthetic alone or in combination with corticosteroid. Pain Physician. 2018;21(1):41–52.
8. McCormick ZL, Korn M, Reddy R, Marcolina A, Dayanim D, Mattie R, Cushman D, Bhave M, McCarthy RJ, Khan D, Nagpal G, Walega DR. Cooled radiofrequency ablation of the genicular nerves for chronic pain due to knee osteoarthritis: six-month outcomes. Pain Med. 2017;18(9):1631–41.
9. Walega D, Roussis C. Third-degree burn from cooled radiofrequency ablation of medial branch nerves for treatment of thoracic facet syndrome. Pain Pract. 2014;14(6):e154–8.
10. Keystone of pain intervention. Medianbooks Publication. p. 407–12.